GASTROESOPHAGEAL REFLUX DISEASE

Edited by **Mauro Bortolotti**

Gastroesophageal Reflux Disease
Edited by Mauro Bortolotti

Published by InTech
Janeza Trdine 9, 51000 Rijeka, Croatia

Publishing Process Manager Tajana Jevtic

Technical Editor Teodora Smiljanic

Cover Designer InTech Design Team

Additional hard copies can be obtained from orders@intechopen.com

Gastroesophageal Reflux Disease, Edited by Mauro Bortolotti
p. cm.
ISBN 978-953-51-0314-1

For EU product safety concerns:
IN TECH d.o.o., Prolaz Marije Krucifikse Kozulić 3, 51000 Rijeka, Croatia,
info@intechopen.com or visit our website at intechopen.com.

Meet the editor

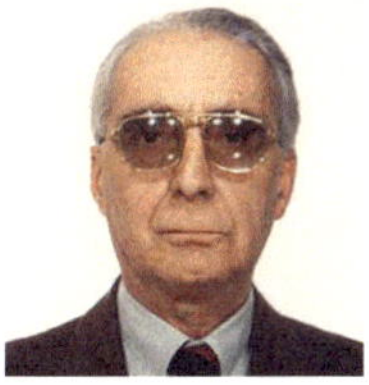

Prof Mauro Bortolotti, specialist in Gastroenterology and Internal Medicine, graduated cum laude in Medicine and Surgery at the Medical School of the University of Bologna. He is also First Level Director of the Internal Medicine Ward at the Department of Internal Medicine and Gastroenterology of the St. Orsola Polyclinic in Bologna. He is also Chief of the Gut Motility Laboratory and of the Section of Diagnosis and Therapy of Diseases of the Esophagus, and a professor at postgraduate Schools of Internal Medicine and Thoracic Surgery at the University of Bologna. His main fields of research are: pathophysiology, diagnosis, and treatment of functional gastrointestinal diseases from the esophagus to the anus. He discovered innovative pharmacological treatments for achalasia with nifedipine and sildenafil, and the treatment for functional dyspepsia and irritable bowel syndrome with capsaicin, contained in red pepper. He devised a novel magnetic valve to prevent gastroesophageal reflux and fecal incontinence. Prof. Bortolotti has organized several national and international congresses. His research has been accepted for presentation to many international and national congresses, some of which earned him awards. He was invited to illustrate his research as a visiting professor by the Department of Internal Medicine and Gastroenterology, the Department of Thoracic Surgery at the University of Toronto, Canada, and the Medical Clinic at the University of São Paulo, Brazil. He is the author of 95 publications in main medical journals, he has undertaken 12 book-related collaborations, and he authored an 800 page book titled Dispepsia. In 1982, he was a founding member of the European Society of Neurogastroenterology and Motility, a member of the editorial board of the journal Neurogastroenterology and Motility, and a member of the steering committee of GISMAD. In 1987, he became an international member of the American Gastroenterological Association. He is frequently asked to be a trusted reviewer for various manuscripts sent for publication to main medical journals.

Contents

Preface

Gastroesophageal reflux (GER) is a rather frequent occurrence that, when its factors overcome the resistance of the esophageal mucosa, may cause inflammatory lesions of various degrees. In some cases, metaplasia, dysplasia and neoplasia may start to develop. This non-physiological disorder may also affect extraesophageal organs, such as the pharynx, larynx, bronchopulmonary tree, ear, nose, and oral cavities, and may also influence the heart through nervous reflexes.

In this book, contributions from international experts in this field have been collected. Interesting aspects of this disease are highlighted, including pathophysiology, diagnostic problems, and medical or surgical treatment. These aspects are examined through reviews, original investigations, and clinical experiences, spreading from esophageal to extra-esophageal manifestations of the disease.

Prof. Mauro Bortolotti
MD, Department of Internal Medicine and Gastroenterology,
University of Bologna,
Bologna,
Italy

Part 1

Pathophysiology and Symptomatology

1

Neural Regulatory Mechanisms of Esophageal Motility and Its Implication for GERD

Takahiko Shiina and Yasutake Shimizu
Department of Basic Veterinary Science, Laboratory of Physiology, The United Graduate School of Veterinary Sciences, Gifu University, Gifu, Japan

1. Introduction

Gastroesophageal reflux disease (GERD) is one of the representative esophageal disorders and can severely influence the quality of life in humans (Jung, 2011; Moayyedi & Talley, 2006; Salvatore & Vandenplas, 2003). In GERD patients, abnormal reflux of gastric contents to the esophagus causes chest pain and heartburn (Moayyedi & Talley, 2006; Salvatore & Vandenplas, 2003). Esophageal mucosal erosions and/or ulcers are formed by acid exposure (Moayyedi & Talley, 2006; Salvatore & Vandenplas, 2003). On the other hand, patients with nonerosive reflux disease (NERD), one phenotype of GERD, have typical reflux symptoms induced by intraesophageal reflux of gastric contents but have no visible esophageal mucosal injury (Long & Orlando, 2008; Tack, 2005; Winter & Heading, 2008). GERD is caused mainly by acid reflux due to abnormal relaxation of the lower esophageal sphincter (LES) and/or low activity of clearance in the esophageal body (DeMeester et al., 1979; Grossi et al., 1998; Grossi et al., 2006; Moayyedi & Talley, 2006; Nagahama et al., 2003). Abnormal relaxation of the LES and low activity of clearance might be associated with dysmotility of the esophagus. The motility in the esophageal body and LES is regulated by both the central and peripheral nervous systems (Clouse & Diamant, 2006; Conklin & Christensen, 1994; Cunningham & Sawchenko, 1990; Jean, 2001; Neuhuber et al., 2006; Park & Conklin, 1999; Wörl & Neuhuber, 2005). Therefore, dysfunction of neural regulation seems to cause abnormal motility in the esophagus, resulting in excessive acid reflux and then GERD (Moayyedi & Talley, 2006; Orlando, 1997; Parkman & Fisher, 1997; Salvatore & Vandenplas, 2003; Vandenplas & Hassall, 2002).

In fact, there are many reports about the involvement of esophageal dysmotility in the pathogenic mechanism of GERD (Dogan & Mittal, 2006; Moayyedi & Talley, 2006; Orlando, 1997; Parkman & Fisher, 1997; Salvatore & Vandenplas, 2003; Shiina et al., 2010; Vandenplas & Hassall, 2002). On the other hand, since neural regulatory mechanisms of esophageal motiliy, especially roles of the intrinsic nervous system in the striated muscle portion, have remained to be clarified (Clouse & Diamant, 2006; Conklin & Christensen, 1994; Goyal & Chaudhury, 2008), little attention has been paid to the relationship between intrinsic neural regulatory mechanisms for esophageal motility and pathophysiology of GERD. Discussion of this relationship is important and might indicate novel therapeutic targets for GERD. In this chapter, we describe neural regulation of the esophageal motility on the basis of results of our studies, and we discuss the relationship between pathogenic mechanisms of GERD and esophageal dysmotility.

2. Neural regulation of esophageal motility

The tunica muscularis of the stomach, small intestine and large intestine is constituted entirely of smooth muscle (Makhlouf & Murthy, 2009). Gastrointestinal smooth muscle motility is regulated by the enteric nervous system (Furness, 2006; Hansen, 2003; Kunze & Furness, 1999; Olsson & Holmgren, 2001; 2011). The sequence of peristaltic events does not depend on extrinsic autonomic innervation but rather involves the activation of intrinsic sensory neurons, which are coupled via modulatory interneurons to excitatory and inhibitory motor neurons projecting into the smooth muscle layer (Furness, 2006; Hansen, 2003; Kunze & Furness, 1999; Olsson & Holmgren, 2001; 2011).

In contrast to other gastrointestinal tracts, the external muscle layer of the mammalian esophagus contains striated muscle fibers, which extend from the pharyngoesophageal junction to the thoracic or even abdominal portion, depending on the species (Izumi et al., 2002; Neuhuber et al., 2006; Shiina et al., 2005; Wooldridge et al., 2002; Wörl & Neuhuber, 2005) (Fig.1). In humans, horses, cats and pigs, the upper and lower portions of the esophagus are composed of striated and smooth muscles, respectively, with a mixed portion between them. In dogs, ruminants and rodents including mice, rats and hamsters, the muscle layer of the esophagus consists mostly of striated muscle fibers. On the other hand, the tunica muscularis of the LES consists of smooth muscles (Neuhuber et al., 2006; Wörl & Neuhuber, 2005). Esophageal motility is controlled centrally by an extrinsic neuronal mechanism and peripherally by an intrinsic neuronal mechanism (Clouse & Diamant, 2006; Conklin & Christensen, 1994; Cunningham & Sawchenko, 1990; Goyal & Chaudhury, 2008; Jean, 2001; Neuhuber et al., 2006; Park & Conklin, 1999; Wörl & Neuhuber, 2005). Below, we describe the neuronal controls of these two muscle types in the esophageal body and smooth muscles in the LES.

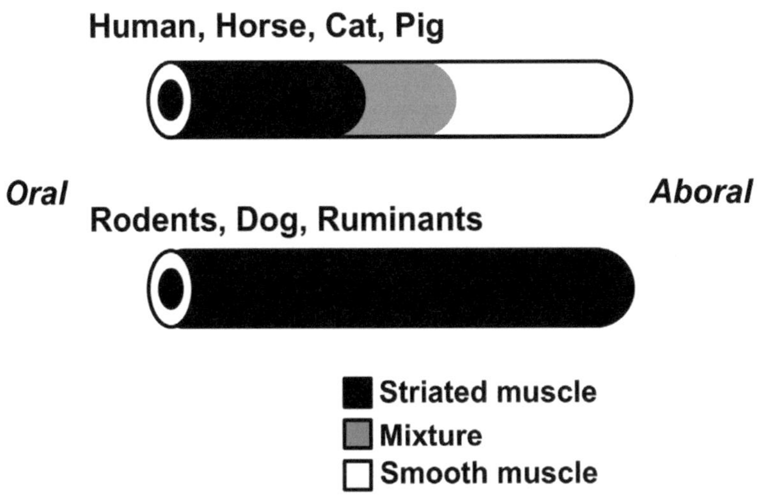

Fig. 1. Tunica muscularis of the esophageal body in mammals. Left is oral side and right is aboral side.

2.1 Esophageal body

The mechanisms of peristalsis control are different between striated muscle and smooth muscle in the esophageal body. However, in both portions, esophageal peristalsis is controlled by the swallowing pattern generator (SPG) located in the brainstem (Bieger, 1993; Bieger & Neuhuber, 2006; Conklin & Christensen, 1994; Jean, 2001; Jean & Dallaporta, 2006), depending on extrinsic neurons unlike other gastrointestinal tracts.

2.1.1 Neural control of peristalsis in the esophageal striated muscle portion

According to the conventional view, the SPG both initiates and organizes peristalsis in the striated esophageal muscle, i.e., both primary and secondary peristaltic contractions are centrally mediated in the striated muscle portion (Bieger, 1993; Bieger & Neuhuber, 2006; Conklin & Christensen, 1994; Goyal & Chaudhury, 2008; Jean & Dallaporta, 2006). Striated muscle fibers are innervated exclusively by excitatory vagal efferents that arise from motor neurons localized in the nucleus ambiguus and terminate on motor endplates (Bieger & Hopkins, 1987; Cunningham & Sawchenko, 1990; Neuhuber et al., 1998). We could confirm this view additionally by demonstrating that vagal nerve stimulation evokes twitch contractile responses of the striated muscle in an isolated segment of mammalian esophagus, which are abolished by d-tubocurarine, an antagonist of nicotinic acetylcholine receptors on the striated muscle, but not by atropine, an antagonist of muscarinic acetylcholine receptors on the smooth muscle, or hexamethonium, a blocker of ganglionic acetylcholine receptors (Boudaka et al., 2007a; Boudaka et al., 2007b; Izumi et al., 2003; Shiina et al., 2006). Peristalsis in the striated esophageal muscle is executed according to a sequence pre-programmed in the compact formation of the nucleus ambiguus (Andrew, 1956). The compact formation of the nucleus ambiguus receives projections from the central subnucleus of the nucleus of the solitary tract (Barrett et al., 1994; Cunningham & Sawchenko, 1989; Lu & Bieger, 1998), which in turn receives vagal afferents from the esophagus (Altschuler et al., 1989; Ross et al., 1985), thus closing a reflex loop for esophageal motor control (Bieger, 1993; Cunningham & Sawchenko, 1990; Lu & Bieger, 1998). Neural controls of motility in the striated muscle esophagus are illustrated in Fig. 2.

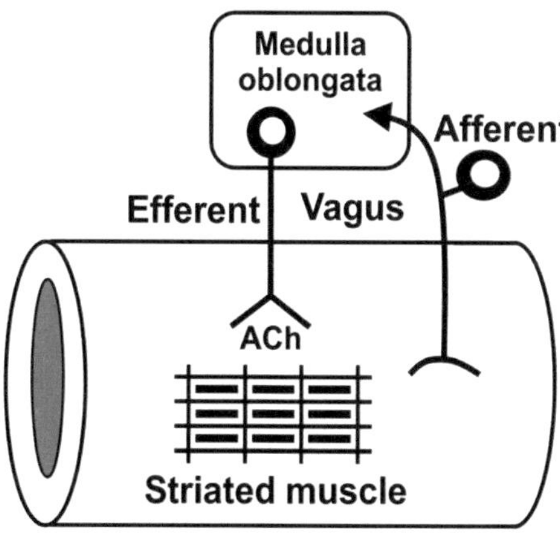

Fig. 2. Neural control of peristalsis in the striated muscle portion of the esophagus by vago-vagal reflex. ACh; acetylcholine.

2.1.2 Neural control of peristalsis in the esophageal smooth muscle portion

In contrast to striated muscle, motor innervation of the smooth muscle esophagus is more complex. Here, the SPG initiates peristalsis via preganglionic neurons in the dorsal motor nucleus of the vagus that project to the myenteric ganglia in the esophagus, i.e., the primary peristalsis involves both central and peripheral mechanisms (Conklin & Christensen, 1994). The smooth muscle is innervated by myenteric motor neurons that can release acetylcholine, tachykinins or nitric oxide (NO) (Conklin & Christensen, 1994; Furness, 2006). However, the progressing front of contraction is organized by virtue of their local reflex circuits that are composed of sensory neurons, interneurons and motor neurons as elsewhere in the gut, i.e., the secondary peristalsis is entirely due to peripheral mechanisms in the smooth muscle esophagus (Clouse & Diamant, 2006; Conklin & Christensen, 1994; Goyal & Chaudhury, 2008). In fact, the smooth muscle esophagus can exhibit propulsive peristaltic contractions in response to an intraluminal bolus of food even in a vagotomy model (Cannon, 1907; Tieffenbach & Roman, 1972). Moreover, peristaltic reflexes can be elicited by distention in an isolated segment of the smooth muscle esophagus from the opossum (Christensen & Lund, 1969). Neural controls of motility in the smooth muscle esophagus are illustrated in Fig. 3.

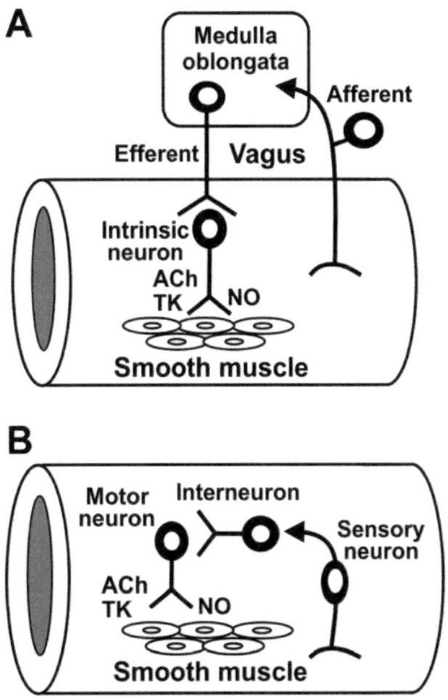

Fig. 3. Neural control of peristalsis in the smooth muscle portion of the esophagus. (A) Vagal innervation for primary peristalsis. (B) Local reflex circuit by enteric neurons for secondary peristalsis. ACh; acetylcholine. TK; tachykinin. NO; nitric oxide.

2.2 Involvement of intrinsic neurons in motility of the esophageal striated muscle

The striated muscle fibers in the esophagus were hitherto considered as 'classical' skeletal muscle fibers, innervated exclusively by excitatory vagal motor neurons, which terminate on motor endplates (Bieger & Hopkins, 1987; Cunningham & Sawchenko, 1990; Neuhuber et al., 1998). It is believed that peristalsis in the striated esophageal muscle is executed according to a sequence pre-programmed in a medullary swallowing network and modulated via vago-vagal reflexes as described above (Clouse & Diamant, 2006; Conklin & Christensen, 1994; Jean, 2001; Mukhopadhyay & Weisbrodt, 1975; Park & Conklin, 1999; Roman & Gonella, 1987). On the other hand, the presence of a distinct ganglionated myenteric plexus in the striated muscle portion of the mammalian esophagus, comparable to other gastrointestinal tracts, has been well known for a long time (Gruber, 1968; Stefanelli, 1938). However, functional roles of the intrinsic nervous system in peristalsis of the striated muscle in the esophagus have remained enigmatic and have been neglected in concepts of peristaltic control (Clouse & Diamant, 2006; Conklin & Christensen, 1994; Diamant, 1989; Wörl & Neuhuber, 2005). To clarify roles of the intrinsic nervous system in motility of the esophageal striated muscle, morphological and then functional studies have been performed.

2.2.1 Morphological investigation

Investigation of the regulatory role of intrinsic neurons in the esophagus was advanced by the discovery of 'enteric co-innervation' of esophageal motor endplates (Neuhuber et al., 1994; Wörl et al., 1994). The enteric co-innervation challenged the conventional view of peristalsis control in the striated esophageal muscle. Originally described in the rat, esophageal striated muscle receives dual innervation from both vagal motor fibers originating in the brainstem and varicose intrinsic nerve fibers originating in the myenteric plexus (Neuhuber et al., 1994; Wörl et al., 1994). This new paradigm of striated muscle innervation has meanwhile been confirmed in a variety of species including humans, underlining its significance (Kallmunzer et al., 2008; Wörl & Neuhuber, 2005). It has been demonstrated that neuronal nitric oxide synthase (nNOS) was highly colocalized with vasoactive intestinal peptide (VIP), neuropeptide Y (NPY), galanin and Met-enkephalin in enteric nerve terminals on esophageal motor endplates (Kuramoto & Endo, 1995; Neuhuber et al., 2001; Neuhuber et al., 1994; Wörl et al., 1998; Wörl et al., 1994; Wörl et al., 1997; Wu et al., 2003). These markers are suggestive of inhibitory modulation of vagally-induced striated muscle contraction (Wörl & Neuhuber, 2005). Since morphological studies revealed further that spinal afferent nerve fibers closely innervate myenteric neurons in the esophagus (Holzer, 1988; Kuramoto et al., 2004; Mazzia & Clerc, 1997; Wörl & Neuhuber, 2005), the presence of 'a peripheral mechanism' regulating the motility of esophageal striated muscle including afferent and enteric neurons in the esophagus was suggested (Neuhuber et al., 2001; Wörl & Neuhuber, 2005).

2.2.2 Functional aproaches

Efforts have been made to demonstrate 'a peripheral mechanism' regulating the motility of esophageal striated muscle by functional experiments, but it had been difficult to prove the hypothesis. For example, in an approach using a vagus nerve–esophagus preparation from the rat, Storr et al. tested effects of exogenous application of VIP, galanin, a NOS inhibitor, and an NO-donor on vagally induced contraction of the striated esophageal muscle, but no significant effect could be ascertained (Storr et al., 2001). They also demonstrated inhibitory effects of exogenous application of endomorphin-1 and -2 on striated and smooth muscle contraction in the rat esophagus but did not provide evidences that endogenously released intrinsic neural components can affect the esophageal motility (Storr et al., 2000).

However, our research group demonstrated roles of intrinsic neuorns in the esophageal striated muscle by functional studies using stimulants of sensory neurons such as capsaicin and piperine, which are main pungents from red pepper and black pepper, respectively (Boudaka et al., 2007a; Boudaka et al., 2007b; Boudaka et al., 2009; Izumi et al., 2003; Shiina et al., 2006). In brief, we isolated rodent esophagi and performed electrical stimulation of the vagal nerves, which evoked contractile responses of the striated esophageal muscle. Capsaicin or piperine inhibited the vagally-mediated contractions of the esophageal preparations via attenuating acetylcholine release from the vagus nerve. In addition, the inhibitory effects of capsaicin or piperine on the contractile responses were blocked by inhibitors to prevent funtions of several neurotransmitters in enteric or sensory neurons such as NO, tachykinins and galanin (Boudaka et al., 2007a; Boudaka et al., 2007b; Boudaka et al., 2009; Izumi et al., 2003; Shiina et al., 2006). The experiments demonstrated that capsaicin or piperine can induce release of endogenous neurotransmitters, which exert the inhibitiory effects on motility of the esophagus. These findings indicate that the mammalian esophagus has a putative local neural reflex that regulates the motility of striated muscle by inhibiting acetylcholine release from vagal motor neurons pre-synaptically (Figs. 4, 5 and 6), which solidify and extend the recently raised hypothesis on the basis of results of morphological studies (Wörl & Neuhuber, 2005). This reflex arc consists of capsaicin-sensitive, transient receptor potential vanilloid 1 (TRPV1)-positive, afferent neurons and inhbitory myenteric neurons. The local neural reflex might be involved in coordinating esophageal peristalsis in the striated muscle portion (Shiina et al., 2010).

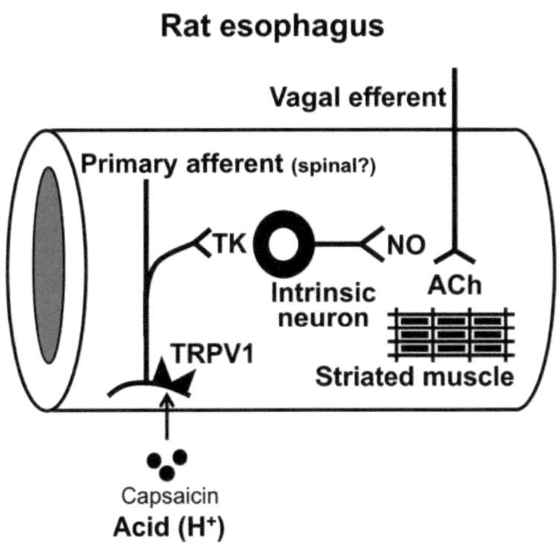

Fig. 4. Local neural reflex in the striated muscle portion of the rat esophagus. Acid as well as capsaicin can stimulate primary afferent neurons and then activate the local reflex arc. ACh; acetylcholine. TK; tachykinin. NO; nitric oxide. TRPV1; transient receptor potential vanilloid 1.

For these experiments, hamsters, rats and mice have been used. Interestingly, neuronal pathways for the inhibitory effects of capsaicin or piperine are slightly different depending on the species. In the rat esophagus, the inhibitory effect of capsaicin on contractile responses was blocked by a NOS inhibitor or a tachykinin NK_1 receptor antagonist, suggesting that the local neural reflex invloves tachykininergic afferent neurons and intrinsic nitrergic neurons (Shiina et al., 2006) (Fig. 4). Hamsters and mice also have a similar neural pathway (Figs. 5 and 6). In addition to trials using capsacin as a stimulator for afferents, piperine was used in experiments with mice and hamsters. In the hamster esophagus, the piperine-activated neural pathway seems to be similar to the capsaicin-activated one, which invloves caisain-sensitive afferent neurons and myenteric nitrergic neurons (Izumi et al., 2003) (Fig. 5).

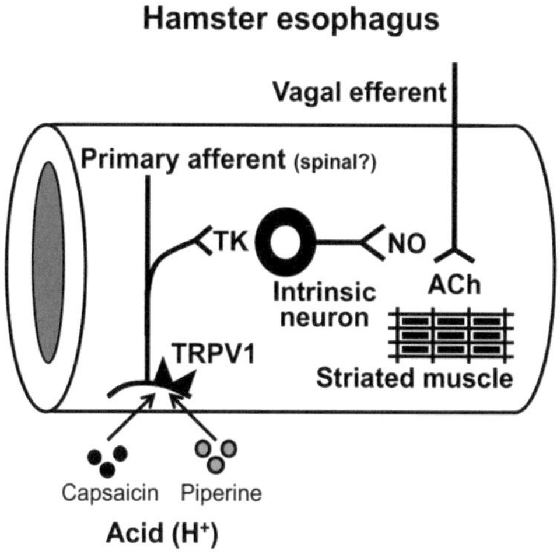

Fig. 5. Local neural reflex in the striated muscle portion of the hamster esophagus. Acid as well as capsaicin and piperine can stimulate primary afferent neurons and then activate the local reflex arc. ACh; acetylcholine. TK; tachykinin. NO; nitric oxide. TRPV1; transient receptor potential vanilloid 1.

However, in the mouse esophagus, these two pathways are independent because piperine can exert inhibitory action on esophageal contractions even after desentitization of capsaisin-sensitive neurons by pretreatment with capsaicin (Boudaka et al., 2007a) (Fig. 6). This is supported by evidence that the capsaicin-mediated inhibition was reversed by a NOS inhibitor or a tachykinin NK_1 receptor antagonist but that the piperine-sensitive pathway was not affected by the same treatments (Boudaka et al., 2007a). In addition, it has been demonstrated that mice have another neural reflex arc including myenteric galaninergic neurons in the esophagus (Boudaka et al., 2009) (Fig. 6).

Rodents including the rat, mouse, guinea pig and hamster have mainly been used as model animals for analysis of the intrinsic nervous system in the esophageal striated muscle because their esophagi are composed entirely of striated muscles (Wörl & Neuhuber, 2005). *Suncus murinus* (a house musk shrew; 'suncus' used as a laboratory name) is a small laboratory animal that belongs to a species of insectivore (Tsutsui et al., 2009; Ueno et al., 1987). Suncus has the ability to vomit in response to mild shaking or ingestion of chemicals (Andrews et al., 1996; Ueno et al., 1987). Since rodents including rats and mice do not show an emetic reflex, suncus has been extensively used to examine the mechanism of emetic responses and to develop antiemetic drugs (Andrews et al., 1996; Cheng et al., 2005; Sam et al., 2003; Uchino et al., 2002; Yamamoto et al., 2009). Hempfling et al. reported that the suncus esophagus has morphological features similar to those in rats and mice: intrinsic nitrergic nerves innervate motor endplates on striated muscle cells, which is called 'enteric co-innervation' (Hempfling et al., 2009). In addition, our examinations demonstrated functionally that the striated muscle portion in the suncus esophagus has a peripheral neuronal mechanism by nitrergic neurons as in rodent esophagi (unpublished data). This fact indicates that the presence of intrinsic nervous regulation on esophageal striated muscle is across species, which might imply pathological and physiological significance of the intrinsic nervous system in the regulation of esophageal motility.

It should be noted that the majority of findings described is related to the striated muscle of the animal esophagus and cannot be simply transferred to the human esophagus. Thus, more progress in basic research on the human esophagus may be required to elucidate the pathogenesis of GERD.

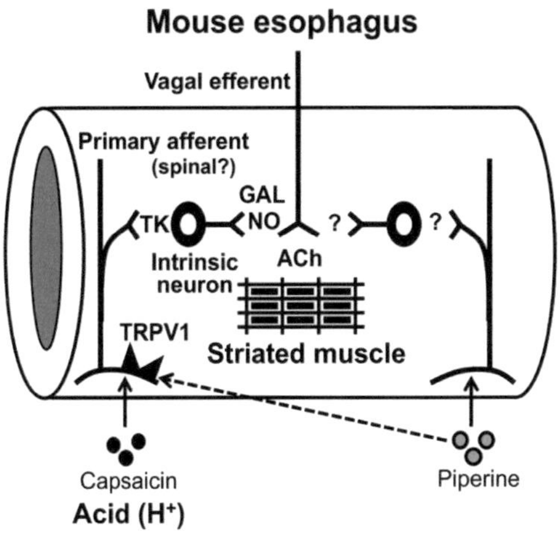

Fig. 6. Local neural reflex in the striated muscle portion of the mouse esophagus. Acid as well as capsaicin can stimulate primary afferent neurons and then activate the local reflex arc. ACh; acetylcholine. TK; tachykinin. NO; nitric oxide. GAL; galanin. TRPV1; transient receptor potential vanilloid 1.

2.3 LES

The LES is a specialized region of the esophageal circular smooth muscle that allows the passage of a swallowed bolus to the stomach and prevents reflux of gastric contents into the esophagus (Farre & Sifrim, 2008; Clouse & Diamant, 2006; Conklin & Christensen, 1994; Goyal & Chaudhury, 2008). Appropriate opening and closure of the LES is controlled by neuronal mechanisms that normally maintain tonic contration of the musculature to prevent reflux and cause relaxation during swallowing (Mittal et al., 1995; Yuan et al., 1998). The LES is innervated by both extatory and inhibitory motor neurons that are located in the myenteric plexus of the LES and the esophgeal body (Brookes et al., 1996). Acetylcholine and NO are the main excitatory and inhibitory neurotransmitters involved in LES contraction and relaxation, respectively (Farre & Sifrim, 2008). In addition, VIP, ATP, carbon monoxide (CO), and calcitonin gene-related peptide (CGRP) also have been proposed as putative neurotransmitters in the LES (Chang et al., 2003; Farre et al., 2006; Farre & Sifrim, 2008; Uc et al., 1999). A subclass of intrinsic neurons are innervated by vagal preganglionic fibers as postganglionic neurons (Diamant, 1989; Goyal & Chaudhury, 2008). Neural controls of motility in the LES are illustrated in Fig. 7.

3. Dysmotility of the esophagus and GERD

As described above, esophageal motility is regulated centrally by vagal motor neurons and peripherally by myenteric neurons, especially cholinergic and nitrergic neurons (Figs. 2 and 3). Here, we have discussed the hypothesis that dysmotility of the esophagus is involved in the pathogenic mechanisms of GERD.

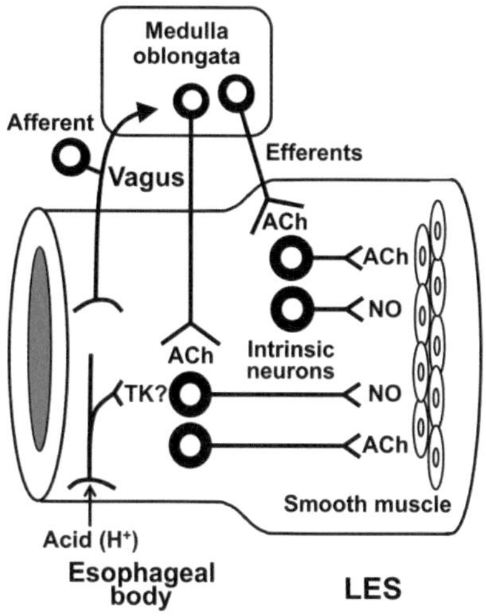

Fig. 7. Neural control of the the lower esophageal sphincter (LES). Acid can stimulate primary afferent neurons and then activate intrinsic motor neurons. ACh; acetylcholine. TK; tachykinin. NO; nitric oxide.

3.1 Gastroesophageal reflux and dysfunction of neural controls of esophageal motility

GERD is caused mainly by acid reflux due to abnormal relaxation of the LES and/or low activity of clearance in the esophageal body (DeMeester et al., 1979; Grossi et al., 2006; Grossi et al., 1998; Moayyedi & Talley, 2006; Nagahama *et al.*, 2003). Gastroesophageal reflux itself occurs in almost all individuals to some degree (Holloway, 2000; Vandenplas & Hassall, 2002). The esophageal body is a major component of the antireflux mechanism. Once reflux has occured, the reflux contents can be cleared by peristaltic sequences (Holloway, 2000). An intact peristaltic mechanism is essential for effective acid clearance. Thus, disruption of esophageal persistalsis affects clearance of the refluxate, resulting in exceccive acid reflux and then onset of GERD (Kahrilas et al., 1988; Moayyedi & Talley, 2006).

In fact, it has been suggested that the pathogenesis of some esophageal disorders icluding GERD is involved in dysfunction of neural regulation such as imbalance of excitatory and inhibitory components of neurons and disruption of neural components (Banerjee et al., 2007; Kim et al., 2008; Mittal & Bhalla, 2004; Shiina et al., 2010). In GERD patients, ineffective esophageal motility (IEM), a typical hypocontractile disorder, is the most common motor abnormality (Lemme et al., 2005). IEM patients have more than the normal number of nNOS-positive neurons in circular muscle in the esophagus, which might result in enhancement of inhibitory neural components (Leite et al., 1997; Lemme et al., 2005). On the other hand, esophageal dysfunctions and then GERD occur frequently in patients with diabetes mellitus (Phillips et al., 2006; Sellin & Chang, 2008). This is a typical symptom of diabetic neuropathy in which enteric neurons decrease (Chandrasekharan & Srinivasan, 2007). These facts indicate that imbalance of excitatory and inhibitory innervations, resulting in disfunction of esophageal persistalsis in the esophageal body, can be associated with onset of GERD possibly via attenuation of clearance activity and then excessive acid reflux.

3.2 Involvement of excessive activation of the local inhibitory neural reflex in onset of GERD

We have reported that application of capsaicin remarkably can attenuate the mechanical activity of the esophageal striated muscle via activation of the local neural reflex including primary afferents and intrinsic neuorns in our experimental conditions *in vitro* (Boudaka et al., 2007a; Boudaka et al., 2007b; Izumi et al., 2003; Shiina et al., 2006). Thus, the local neural reflex might be involved in not only coordinating esophageal peristalsis but also dysmotility of the esophagus and then the pathogenesis of GERD. Acid exposure not only induces inflammation in the esophageal mucosa (Rieder et al., 2010) but also might influence afferent neurons expressing TRPV1, which can be stimulated by protons (Tominaga & Tominaga, 2005). If acid excessively activates local neural reflex in the esophageal body, esophageal motility might be attenuated, resulting in decrease of clearance activity (Figs. 4, 5, 6). In accordance with this, low pH can attenuate contractile activity in isolated esophageal segments from rats and mice like as capsaicin and piperine (unpublished data). In addition, functional changes of TRPV1 by proinflammatory mediators such as prostaglandin E2 (Adcock, 2009; Lopshire & Nicol, 1998) might facilitate activation of the inhibitory local neural reflex, resulting in low clearance activity. Decrease of clearance activity might permit further acid reflux, which would cause severe symptoms of GERD. Therefore, it is presumed that excessive activation of the local inhibitory neural reflex might be involved in the pathophysiology of GERD.

Challenge of acid exposure enhances TRPV1 and substance P expression in TRPV1-positive neurons accompanying esophageal mucosa inflammation (Banerjee et al., 2007). In accordance with this, acid-induced esophagitis is not so severe in TRPV1-deficient mice (Fujino et al., 2006). Interestingly, it has been reported that TRPV1-positive neurons are local effectors of mucosal protection (Bass et al., 1991) and are associated with a protective effect of an H_2-receptor antagonist on reflux esophagitis (Nagahama et al., 2003). Enhancement of TRPV1 and tachykinins expression also might result in intensification of local neural regulation, which is an exacerbating factor of GERD.

Of course, dysmotility of the striated muscle portion of the esophagus described here might not directly be involved in gastroesophageal reflux in human because the external muscle layer in the distal portion of human esophagus is composed with smooth muscle fibers (Wörl & Neuhuber, 2005). The inhibitory neural pathway activated by acid reflex has not been demonstrated in smooth muscle of the human esophagus. In fact, spastic contractions are induced by acid reflux in the distal esophagus (diffuse esophageal spasm), which frequently are responsible of chest pain in GERD (Richter, 2007; Tutuian & Castell, 2006). This excessive contraction of smooth muscle is in contrast to the inhibition of striated muscle contraction via the local neural reflex activated by acid reflex.

3.3 Abnormal relaxation of the LES and GERD

Abnormal relaxation of the LES is one of causes for GERD. LES hypotension may be due to a number of potential disturbances, including abnormality of the muscle function itself, lack of normal cholinergic activation, decreased reflex excitation, decreased responsiveness to circulating substances such as gastrin, and activation of inhibitory system (Clouse & Diamant, 2006). The LES is innervated by inhbitory and excitatory intrinsic neurons that are located in the myenteric plexus not only of the LES but also of the esophgeal body (Fig. 7) (Brookes et al., 1996). Abnormal activation of vagal afferents and/or efferents might activate inhibitory intrinsic neurons and cause LES relaxation and then excessive acid reflux from the stomach to the esophagus (Mittal et al., 1995). Kuramto et al. reported that a subpopulation of myenteric nitrergic neurons is immunoreactive for a tachykinin receptor in the rat esophageal body (Kuramoto et al., 2004). Considering that myenteric neurons are closely innervated by spinal afferents in which TRPV1 and tachykinins might be expressed in the esophagus (Holzer, 1988; Kuramoto & Endo, 1995; Mazzia & Clerc, 1997; Wörl & Neuhuber, 2005) as well as vagal afferent neurons, it is possible that acid can induce release of tachykinins from afferent neurons and subsequently tachykinins would act on intrinsic nitrergic neurons innervated to the LES (Fig. 7). This suggests that excessive acid reflux to the esophageal body might evoke abnormal relaxation of the LES by NO, resulting in severe GERD.

3.4 A putative vicious circle in onset and exacerbation of GERD

Chronic esophagitis, a symptom of GERD, may damage not only the mucosa but also intrinsic neurons (Rieder et al., 2010). In fact, it has been reported that proinflammatory cytokines contribute to reducing esophageal contraction by inhibiting release of acetylcholine from myenteric neurons (Cao et al., 2004). Esophageal dysmotility might subject the mucosa to further acid exposure, which would cause more severe inflammation by directly influencing the mucosa or neurogenic mechanism via TRPV1-positive neurons and peptidergic neurotransmitters (Bozic et al., 1996; Richardson & Vasko, 2002). Considering that the severity of myenteric plexus damage is positively correlated with the duration of history of esophageal diseases (Gockel et al., 2008), there might be a vicious circle in GERD (Fig. 8).

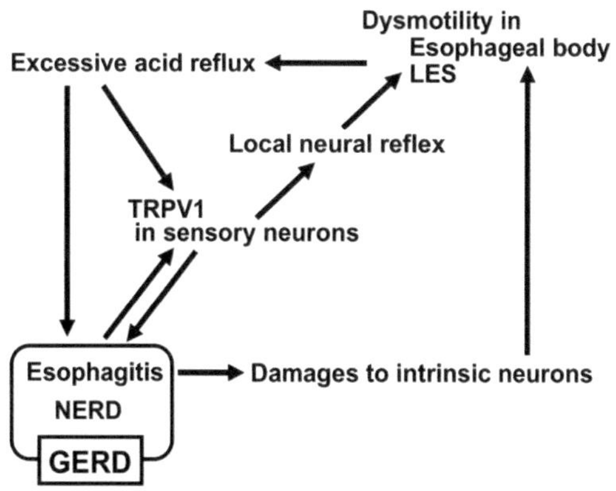

Fig. 8. A predicted vicious circle model of GERD. The circle might exacerbate GERD. GERD; gastroesophageal reflux disease. NERD; nonerosive reflux disease. LES; lower esophageal sphincter. TRPV1; transient receptor potential vanilloid 1.

4. Conclusion

Motor functions of the esophagus are controlled by both vagal neurons arising in the brainstem and locally intrinsic neurons in the striated and smooth muscles. The pathogenesis of GERD might be involved in dysfunction of neural networks in the esophagus. We propose new aspects of the involvement of pathophysiology of GERD in excessive activation of the local neural reflex by intrinsic neurons on the basis of results of our morphological and functional studies on esophageal motility.

5. Acknowledgments

We are grateful to Dr. Hirofumi Kuramoto, Kyoto Institute of Technology, Japan and Prof. Jürgen Wörl, University of Erlangen-Nuremberg, Germany for their valuable supports of morphological studies. The reviewed results obtained in our laboratory were supported in part by Grants-In-Aid for Scientific Research from the Ministry of Education, Culture, Sports, Science, and Technology of Japan.

6. References

Adcock, J.J. (2009). TRPV1 receptors in sensitisation of cough and pain reflexes. *Pulmonary pharmacology & therapeutics,* 22(2): 65-70, ISSN 1094-5539.

Altschuler, S.M., Bao, X.M., Bieger, D., Hopkins, D.A. & Miselis, R.R. (1989). Viscerotopic representation of the upper alimentary tract in the rat: sensory ganglia and nuclei of the solitary and spinal trigeminal tracts. *The Journal of Comparative Neurology,* 283(2): 248-268, ISSN 0021-9967.

Andrew, B.L. (1956). The nervous control of the cervical oesophagus of the rat during swallowing. *The Journal of Physiology,* 134(3): 729-740, ISSN 0022-3751.

Andrews, P., Torii, Y., Saito, H. & Matsuki, N. (1996). The pharmacology of the emetic response to upper gastrointestinal tract stimulation in Suncus murinus. *European Journal of Pharmacology,* 307(3): 305-313, ISSN 0014-2999.

Banerjee, B., Medda, B.K., Lazarova, Z., Bansal, N., Shaker, R. & Sengupta, J. N. (2007). Effect of reflux-induced inflammation on transient receptor potential vanilloid one (TRPV1) expression in primary sensory neurons innervating the oesophagus of rats. *Neurogastroenterology and Motility,* 19(8): 681-691, ISSN 1350-1925.

Barrett, R. T., Bao, X., Miselis, R.R. & Altschuler, S.M. (1994). Brain stem localization of rodent esophageal premotor neurons revealed by transneuronal passage of pseudorabies virus. *Gastroenterology,* 107(3): 728-737, ISSN 0016-5085.

Bass, B.L., Trad, K.S., Harmon, J.W. & Hakki, F. Z. (1991). Capsaicin-sensitive nerves mediate esophageal mucosal protection. *Surgery,* 110(2): 419-425; discussion 425-426, ISSN 0039-6060.

Bieger, D. (1993). The brainstem esophagomotor network pattern generator: a rodent model. *Dysphagia,* 8(3): 203-208, ISSN 0179-051X.

Bieger, D. & Hopkins, D.A. (1987). Viscerotopic representation of the upper alimentary tract in the medulla oblongata in the rat: the nucleus ambiguus. *The Journal of Comparative Neurology,* 262(4): 546-562, ISSN 0021-9967.

Bieger, D., & Neuhuber, W.L. (2006). Neural circuits and mediators regulating swallowing in the brainstem. *GI Motility online,* doi:10.1038/gimo1074.

Boudaka, A., Wörl, J., Shiina, T., Neuhuber, W.L., Kobayashi, H., Shimizu, Y. & Takewaki, T. (2007a). Involvement of TRPV1-dependent and -independent components in the regulation of vagally induced contractions in the mouse esophagus. *European Journal of Pharmacology*, 556(1-3): 157-165, ISSN 0014-2999.

Boudaka, A., Wörl, J., Shiina, T., Saito, S., Atoji, Y., Kobayashi, H., Shimizu, Y. & Takewaki, T. (2007b). Key role of mucosal primary afferents in mediating the inhibitory influence of capsaicin on vagally mediated contractions in the mouse esophagus. *The Journal of Veteterinary Medical Science*, 69(4): 365-372, ISSN 0916-7250.

Boudaka, A., Wörl, J., Shiina, T., Shimizu, Y., Takewaki, T., & Neuhuber, W. L. (2009). Galanin modulates vagally induced contractions in the mouse oesophagus. *Neurogastroenterology and Motility*, 21(2): 180-188, ISSN 1350-1925.

Bozic, C.R., Lu, B., Hopken, U.E., Gerard, C. & Gerard, N.P. (1996). Neurogenic amplification of immune complex inflammation. *Science*, 273(5282): 1722-1725, ISSN 0036-8075.

Brookes, S.J., Chen, B.N., Hodgson, W.M. & Costa, M. (1996). Characterization of excitatory and inhibitory motor neurons to the guinea pig lower esophageal sphincter. *Gastroenterology*, 111(1): 108-117, ISSN 0016-5085.

Cannon, W. (1907). Oesophageal peristalsis after bilateral vagotomy. *American Journal of Physiology*, 19: 436-444, ISSN 0193-1857.

Cao, W., Cheng, L., Behar, J., Fiocchi, C., Biancani, P. & Harnett, K.M. (2004). Proinflammatory cytokines alter/reduce esophageal circular muscle contraction in experimental cat esophagitis. *American Journal of Physiology. Gastrointestinal and Liver Physiology*, 287(6): G1131-1139, ISSN 0193-1857.

Chandrasekharan, B. & Srinivasan, S. (2007). Diabetes and the enteric nervous system. *Neurogastroenterology and Motility*, 19(12): 951-960, ISSN 1350-1925.

Chang, H.Y., Mashimo, H. & Goyal, R.K. (2003). Musings on the wanderer: what's new in our understanding of vago-vagal reflex? IV. Current concepts of vagal efferent projections to the gut. *American Journal of Physiology. Gastrointestinal and Liver Physiology*, 284(3): G357-366, ISSN 0193-1857.

Cheng, F.H., Andrews, P.L., Moreaux, B., Ngan, M.P., Rudd, J.A., Sam, T.S., Wai, M.K. & Wan, C. (2005). Evaluation of the anti-emetic potential of anti-migraine drugs to prevent resiniferatoxin-induced emesis in Suncus murinus (house musk shrew). *European Journal of Pharmacology*, 508(1-3): 231-238, ISSN 0014-2999.

Christensen, J. & Lund, G.F. (1969). Esophageal responses to distension and electrical stimulation. *The Journal of Clinical Investigation*, 48(2): 408-419, ISSN 0021-9738.

Clouse, R.E. & Diamant, N.E. (2006). Motor Function of the Esophagus. In: *Physiology of the Gastrointestinal Tract (4th ed.)*, L.R. Johnson (ed.), pp. 913-926, Elsevier Academic Press, ISBN 978-0-120883950 , Burlington.

Conklin, J. L. & Christensen, J. (1994). Motor Functions of the Pharynx and Esophagus. In: *Physiology of the Gastrointestinal Tract (3rd ed.)*, L.R. Johnson (ed.), pp. 903-928, Raven Press, ISBN 978-0781701327, New York.

Cunningham, E.T.Jr. & Sawchenko, P.E. (1989). A circumscribed projection from the nucleus of the solitary tract to the nucleus ambiguus in the rat: anatomical evidence for somatostatin-28-immunoreactive interneurons subserving reflex control of esophageal motility. *The Journal of Neuroscience*, 9(5): 1668-1682, ISSN 0270-6474.

Cunningham, E.T.Jr. & Sawchenko, P.E. (1990). Central neural control of esophageal motility: a review. *Dysphagia*, 5(1): 35-51, ISSN 0179-051X.

DeMeester, T.R., Wernly, J.A., Bryant, G.H., Little, A.G. & Skinner, D.B. (1979). Clinical and in vitro analysis of determinants of gastroesophageal competence. A study of the principles of antireflux surgery. *American Journal of Surgery*, 137(1): 39-46, ISSN 0002-9610.

Diamant, N.E. (1989). Physiology of esophageal motor function. *Gastroenterology Clinics of North America*, 18(2): 179-194, ISSN 0889-8553.

Dogan, I. & Mittal, R.K. (2006). Esophageal motor disorders: recent advances. *Current Opinion in Gastroenterology*, 22(4): 417-422, ISSN 0267-1379.

Farre, R., Auli, M., Lecea, B., Martinez, E. & Clave, P. (2006). Pharmacologic characterization of intrinsic mechanisms controlling tone and relaxation of porcine lower esophageal sphincter. *The Journal of Pharmacology and Experimental Therapeutics*, 316(3): 1238-1248, ISSN 0022-3565.

Farre, R. & Sifrim, D. (2008). Regulation of basal tone, relaxation and contraction of the lower oesophageal sphincter. Relevance to drug discovery for oesophageal disorders. *British Journal of Pharmacology*, 153(5): 858-869, ISSN 0007-1188.

Fujino, K., de la Fuente, S.G., Takami, Y., Takahashi, T. & Mantyh, C. R. 2006. Attenuation of acid induced oesophagitis in VR-1 deficient mice. *Gut*, 55(1): 34-40, ISSN 0017-5749.

Furness, J.B. (2006). *The Enteric Nervous System*, Blackwell Publishing, ISBN 978-1-4051-3376-0, Malden.

Gockel, I., Bohl, J.R., Eckardt, V.F. & Junginger, T. (2008). Reduction of interstitial cells of Cajal (ICC) associated with neuronal nitric oxide synthase (n-NOS) in patients with achalasia. *The American Journal of Gastroenterology*, 103(4): 856-864, ISSN 1572-0241.

Goyal, R.K. & Chaudhury, A. (2008). Physiology of normal esophageal motility. *Journal of Clinical Gastroenterology*, 42(5): 610-619, ISSN 0192-0790.

Grossi, L., Cappello, G. & Marzio, L. (2006). Effect of an acute intraluminal administration of capsaicin on oesophageal motor pattern in GORD patients with ineffective oesophageal motility. *Neurogastroenterol Motil*, 18(8): 632-636, ISSN 1350-1925.

Grossi, L., Ciccaglione, A. F., Travaglini, N., & Marzio, L. (1998). Swallows, oesophageal and gastric motility in normal subjects and in patients with gastro-oesophageal reflux disease: a 24-h pH-manometric study. *Neurogastroenterology and Motility*, 10(2): 115-121, ISSN 1350-1925.

Gruber, H. (1968). Structure and innervation of the striated muscle fibres of the esophagus of the rat. *Z Zellforsch Mikrosk Anat*, 91(2): 236-247, ISSN 0340-0336.

Hansen, M.B. (2003). Neurohumoral control of gastrointestinal motility. *Physiological Research*, 52(1): 1-30, ISSN 0862-8408.

Hempfling, C., Seibold, R., Shiina, T., Heimler, W., Neuhuber, W.L. & Wörl, J. (2009). Enteric co-innervation of esophageal striated muscle fibers: a phylogenetic study. *Autonomic Neuroscience : Basic & Clinical*, 151(2): 135-141, ISSN 1566-0702.

Holloway, R.H. (2000). Esophageal body motor response to reflux events: secondary peristalsis. *The American Journal of Medicine*, 108 Suppl 4a: 20S-26S, ISSN 0002-9343.

Holzer, P. (1988). Local effector functions of capsaicin-sensitive sensory nerve endings: involvement of tachykinins, calcitonin gene-related peptide and other neuropeptides. *Neuroscience*, 24(3): 739-768, ISSN 0306-4522.

Izumi, N., Matsuyama, H., Ko, M., Shimizu, Y. & Takewaki, T. (2003). Role of intrinsic nitrergic neurones on vagally mediated striated muscle contractions in the hamster oesophagus. *The Journal of Physiology*, 551(Pt 1): 287-294, ISSN 0022-3751.

Izumi, N., Matsuyama, H., Yamamoto, Y., Atoji, Y., Suzuki, Y., Unno, T. and Takewaki, T. (2002). Morphological and morphometrical characteristics of the esophageal intrinsic nervous system in the golden hamster. *European Journal of Morphology*, 40(3): 137-144, ISSN 0924-3860.

Jean, A. (2001). Brain stem control of swallowing: neuronal network and cellular mechanisms. *Physiological Reviews*, 81(2): 929-969, ISSN 0031-9333.

Jean, A. & Dallaporta, M. (2006). Electrophysiologic characterization of the swallowing pattern generator in the brainstem. *GI Motility online*, doi:10.1038/gimo1039.

Jung, H.K. (2011). Epidemiology of gastroesophageal reflux disease in Asia: a systematic review. *Journal of Neurogastroenterology and Motility*, 17(1): 14-27, ISSN 2093-0879.

Kahrilas, P.J., Dodds, W.J. & Hogan, W.J. (1988). Effect of peristaltic dysfunction on esophageal volume clearance. *Gastroenterology*, 94(1): 73-80, ISSN 0016-5085.

Kallmunzer, B., Sorensen, B., Neuhuber, W.L. & Wörl, J. (2008). Enteric co-innervation of striated muscle fibres in human oesophagus. *Neurogastroenterology and Motility*, 20(6): 597-610, ISSN 1365-2982.

Kim, H.S., Park, H., Lim, J.H., Choi, S.H., Park, C., Lee, S.I. & Conklin, J.L. (2008). Morphometric evaluation of oesophageal wall in patients with nutcracker oesophagus and ineffective oesophageal motility. *Neurogastroenterology and Motility*, 20(8): 869-876, ISSN 1365-2982.

Kunze, W.A. & Furness, J.B. (1999). The enteric nervous system and regulation of intestinal motility. *Annual Review of Physiology*, 61: 117-142, ISSN 0066-4278.

Kuramoto, H. & Endo, Y. (1995). Galanin-immunoreactive nerve terminals innervating the striated muscle fibers of the rat esophagus. *Neuroscience Letters*, 188(3): 171-174, ISSN 0304-3940.

Kuramoto, H., Oomori, Y., Murabayashi, H., Kadowaki, M., Karaki, S. & Kuwahara, A. (2004). Localization of neurokinin 1 receptor (NK1R) immunoreactivity in rat esophagus. *The Journal of Comparative Neurology*, 478(1): 11-21, ISSN 0021-9967.

Leite, L.P., Johnston, B.T., Barrett, J., Castell, J.A. & Castell, D.O. (1997). Ineffective esophageal motility (IEM): the primary finding in patients with nonspecific esophageal motility disorder. *Digestive Diseases and Sciences*, 42(9): 1859-1865, ISSN 0163-2116.

Lemme, E.M., Abrahao-Junior, L.J., Manhaes, Y., Shechter, R., Carvalho, B.B. & Alvariz, A. (2005). Ineffective esophageal motility in gastroesophageal erosive reflux disease and in nonerosive reflux disease: are they different? *Journal of Clinical Gastroenterology*, 39(3): 224-227, ISSN 0192-0790.

Long, J.D. & Orlando, R.C. (2008). Nonerosive reflux disease: a pathophysiologic perspective. *Current Gastroenterology Reports*, 10(3): 200-207, ISSN 1522-8037.

Lopshire, J.C. & Nicol, G.D. (1998). The cAMP transduction cascade mediates the prostaglandin E2 enhancement of the capsaicin-elicited current in rat sensory neurons: whole-cell and single-channel studies. *The Journal of Neuroscience*, 18(16): 6081-6092, ISSN 0270-6474.

Lu, W.Y. & Bieger, D. (1998). Vagovagal reflex motility patterns of the rat esophagus. *American Journal of Physiology*, 274(5 Pt 2): R1425-1435, ISSN 0002-9513.

Makhlouf, G.M. & Murthy, K.S. (2009). Smooth muscle and the gut. In: *Textbook of gasrtoenterology (fifth ed.)*, T. Yamada (ed.), pp. 103-132, Blackwell Publishing Ltd, ISBN 978-1-4051-6911-0, Oxford.

Mazzia, C. & Clerc, N. (1997). Ultrastructural relationships of spinal primary afferent fibres with neuronal and non-neuronal cells in the myenteric plexus of the cat oesophago-gastric junction. *Neuroscience*, 80(3): 925-937, ISSN 0306-4522.

Mittal, R. K. & Bhalla, V. (2004). Oesophageal motor functions and its disorders. *Gut*, 53(10): 1536-1542, ISSN 0017-5749.

Mittal, R.K., Holloway, R.H., Penagini,R., Blackshaw, L.A. & Dent, J. (1995). Transient lower esophageal sphincter relaxation. *Gastroenterology*, 109(2): 601-610, ISSN 0016-5085.

Moayyedi, P. & Talley, N.J. (2006). Gastro-oesophageal reflux disease. *Lancet*, 367(9528): 2086-2100, ISSN 1474-547X.

Mukhopadhyay, A.K. & Weisbrodt, N.W. (1975). Neural organization of esophageal peristalsis: role of vagus nerve. *Gastroenterology*, 68(3): 444-447, ISSN 0016-5085.

Nagahama, K., Yamato, M., Kato, S. & Takeuchi, K. (2003). Protective effect of lafutidine, a novel H2-receptor antagonist, on reflux esophagitis in rats through capsaicin-sensitive afferent neurons. *Journal of Pharmacological Sciences*, 93(1): 55-61, ISSN 1347-8613.

Neuhuber, W.L., Eichhorn, U. & Wörl, J. (2001). Enteric co-innervation of striated muscle fibers in the esophagus: just a "hangover"? *The Anatomical Record*, 262(1): 41-46, ISSN 0003-276X.

Neuhuber, W.L., Kressel, M., Stark, A. & Berthoud, H.R. (1998). Vagal efferent and afferent innervation of the rat esophagus as demonstrated by anterograde DiI and DiA tracing: focus on myenteric ganglia. *Journal of the Autonomic Nervous System*, 70(1-2): 92-102, ISSN 0165-1838.

Neuhuber, W.L., Raab, M., Berthoud, H.R. & Wörl, J. (2006). Innervation of the mammalian esophagus. *Advances in Anatomy,Embryology, and Cell Biology*, 185: 1-73, back cover, ISSN 0301-5556.

Neuhuber, W.L., Wörl, J., Berthoud, H.R. & Conte, B. (1994). NADPH-diaphorase-positive nerve fibers associated with motor endplates in the rat esophagus: new evidence for co-innervation of striated muscle by enteric neurons. *Cell and Tissue Research*, 276(1): 23-30, ISSN 0302-766X.

Olsson, C. & Holmgren, S. (2001). The control of gut motility. *Comparative Biochemistry and Physiology. Part A, Molecular & Integrative Physiology*, 128(3): 481-503, ISSN 1095-6433.

Olsson, C. & Holmgren, S. (2011). Autonomic control of gut motility: A comparative view. *Autonomic Neuroscience : Basic & Clinical*, doi:10.1016/j.autneu.2010.07.002, ISSN 1566-0702.

Orlando, R.C. (1997). The pathogenesis of gastroesophageal reflux disease: the relationship between epithelial defense, dysmotility, and acid exposure. *The American Journal of Gastroenterology*, 92(4 Suppl): 3S-5S; discussion 5S-7S, ISSN.

Park, H. & Conklin, J.L. (1999). Neuromuscular control of esophageal peristalsis. *Current Gastroenterology Reports*, 1(3): 186-197, ISSN 1522-8037.

Parkman, H.P. & Fisher, R.S. (1997). Contributing role of motility abnormalities in the pathogenesis of gastroesophageal reflux disease. *Digestive Diseases*, 15 Suppl 1: 40-52, ISSN 0257-2753.

Phillips, L.K., Rayner, C.K., Jones, K.L. & Horowitz, M. (2006). An update on autonomic neuropathy affecting the gastrointestinal tract. *Current Diabetes Reports*, 6(6): 417-423, ISSN 1534-4827.

Richardson, J.D. & Vasko, M.R. (2002). Cellular mechanisms of neurogenic inflammation. *The Journal of Pharmacology and Experimental Therapeutics*, 302(3): 839-845, ISSN 0022-3565.

Richter, J.E. (2007). Gastrooesophageal reflux disease. *Best Practice & Research Clinical Gastroenterology*, 21(4): 609-631.

Rieder, F., Biancani, P., Harnett, K., Yerian, L. & Falk, G.W. (2010). Inflammatory mediators in gastroesophageal reflux disease: impact on esophageal motility, fibrosis, and carcinogenesis. *American Journal of Physiology. Gastrointestinal and Liver Physiology*, 298(5): G571-581, ISSN 0193-1857.

Roman, C. & Gonella, J. (1987). Extrinsic control of digestive tract motility. In: *Physiology of the Gastrointestinal Tract (2nd ed.)*, L.R. Johnson (ed.), pp. 507-553, Raven Press, ISBN 978-0881671650, New York:

Ross, C.A., Ruggiero, D.A. & Reis, D.J. (1985). Projections from the nucleus tractus solitarii to the rostral ventrolateral medulla. *The Journal of Comparative Neurology*, 242(4): 511-534, ISSN 0021-9967.

Salvatore, S. & Vandenplas, Y. (2003). Gastro-oesophageal reflux disease and motility disorders. *Best Practice & Research. Clinical Gastroenterology*, 17(2): 163-179, ISSN 1521-6918.

Sam, T.S., Cheng, J.T., Johnston, K.D., Kan, K.K., Ngan, M.P., Rudd, J.A., Wai, M.K. & Yeung, J.H. (2003). Action of 5-HT3 receptor antagonists and dexamethasone to modify cisplatin-induced emesis in Suncus murinus (house musk shrew). *European Journal of Pharmacology*, 472(1-2): 135-145, ISSN 0014-2999.

Sellin, J.H. & Chang, E.B. (2008). Therapy Insight: gastrointestinal complications of diabetes--pathophysiology and management. *Nature Clinical Practice. Gastroenterology & Hepatology*, 5(3): 162-171, ISSN 1743-4378.

Shiina, T., Shima, T., Wörl, J., Neuhuber, W.L. & Shimizu, Y. (2010). The neural regulation of the mammalian esophageal motility and its implication for esophageal diseases. *Pathophysiology*, 17(2): 129-133, ISSN 0928-4680.

Shiina, T., Shimizu, Y., Boudaka, A., Wörl, J. & Takewaki, T. (2006). Tachykinins are involved in local reflex modulation of vagally mediated striated muscle contractions in the rat esophagus via tachykinin NK1 receptors. *Neuroscience*, 139(2): 495-503, ISSN 0306-4522.

Shiina, T., Shimizu, Y., Izumi, N., Suzuki, Y., Asano, M., Atoji, Y., Nikami, H. & Takewaki, T. (2005). A comparative histological study on the distribution of striated and smooth muscles and glands in the esophagus of wild birds and mammals. *The Journal of Veterinary Medical Science*, 67(1): 115-117, ISSN 0916-7250.

Stefanelli, A. (1938). Considerazioni ed osservazioni sulla struttura microscopica del tessuto nervoso autonomo alla periferia nei vertebrati superiori. *Z. Zellforsch.*, 28: 485-511, ISSN 0340-0336.

Storr, M., Geisler, F., Neuhuber, W.L., Schusdziarra, V. & Allescher, H.D. (2000). Endomorphin-1 and -2, endogenous ligands for the mu-opioid receptor, inhibit striated and smooth muscle contraction in the rat oesophagus. *Neurogastroenterology and Motility*, 12(5): 441-448, ISSN 1350-1925.

Storr, M., Geisler, F., Neuhuber, W.L., Schusdziarra, V. & Allescher, H.D. (2001). Characterization of vagal input to the rat esophageal muscle. *Autonomic Neuroscience : Basic & Clinical*, 91(1-2): 1-9, ISSN 1566-0702.

Tack, J. (2005). Recent developments in the pathophysiology and therapy of gastroesophageal reflux disease and nonerosive reflux disease. *Current Opinion in Gastroenterology*, 21(4): 454-460, ISSN 0267-1379.

Tieffenbach, L. & Roman, C. (1972). The role of extrinsic vagal innervation in the motility of the smooth-musculed portion of the esophagus: electromyographic study in the cat and the baboon. *Journal de Physiologie*, 64(3): 193-226, ISSN 0021-7948.

Tominaga, M. & Tominaga, T. (2005). Structure and function of TRPV1. *Pflügers Archiv*, 451(1): 143-150, ISSN 0031-6768.

Tsutsui, C., Kajihara, K., Yanaka, T., Sakata, I., Itoh, Z., Oda, S. & Sakai, T. (2009). House musk shrew (Suncus murinus, order: Insectivora) as a new model animal for motilin study. *Peptides*, 30(2): 318-329, ISSN 0196-9781.

Tutuian, R. & Castell, D.O. (2996). Review article: oesophageal spasm - diagnosis and management. *Alimentary Pharmacology & Therapeutics*, 23(10): 1393-1402.

Uc, A., Oh, S. T., Murray, J. A., Clark, E. & Conklin, J.L. (1999). Biphasic relaxation of the opossum lower esophageal sphincter: roles of NO., VIP, and CGRP. *American Journal of Physiology*, 277(3 Pt 1): G548-554, ISSN 0002-9513.

Uchino, M., Ishii, K., Kuwahara, M., Ebukuro, S. & Tsubone, H. (2002). Role of the autonomic nervous system in emetic and cardiovascular responses in Suncus murinus. *Autonomic Neuroscience : Basic & Clinical*, 100(1-2): 32-40, ISSN 1566-0702.

Ueno, S., Matsuki, N. & Saito, H. (1987). Suncus murinus: a new experimental model in emesis research. *Life Sciences*, 41(4): 513-518, ISSN 0024-3205.

Vandenplas, Y. & Hassall, E. (2002). Mechanisms of gastroesophageal reflux and gastroesophageal reflux disease. *Journal of Pediatric Gastroenterology and Nutrition*, 35(2): 119-136, ISSN 0277-2116.

Winter, J.W. & Heading, R.C. (2008). The nonerosive reflux disease-gastroesophageal reflux disease controversy. *Current Opinion in Gastroenterology*, 24(4): 509-515, ISSN 0267-1379.

Wooldridge, A.A., Eades, S.C., Hosgood, G.L. & Moore, R.M. (2002). In vitro effects of oxytocin, acepromazine, detomidine, xylazine, butorphanol, terbutaline, isoproterenol, and dantrolene on smooth and skeletal muscles of the equine esophagus. *American Journal of Veterinary Research*, 63(12): 1732-1737, ISSN 0002-9645.

Wörl, J., Fischer, J. & Neuhuber, W.L. (1998). Nonvagal origin of galanin-containing nerve terminals innervating striated muscle fibers of the rat esophagus. *Cell and Tissue Research*, 292(3): 453-461, ISSN 0302-766X.

Wörl, J., Mayer, B. & Neuhuber, W.L. (1994). Nitrergic innervation of the rat esophagus: focus on motor endplates. *Journal of Autonomic Nervous System*, 49(3): 227-233, ISSN 0165-1838.

Wörl, J., Mayer, B. & Neuhuber, W.L. (1997). Spatial relationships of enteric nerve fibers to vagal motor terminals and the sarcolemma in motor endplates of the rat esophagus: a confocal laser scanning and electron-microscopic study. *Cell and Tissue Research*, 287(1): 113-118, ISSN 0302-766X.

Wörl, J. & Neuhuber, W.L. (2005). Enteric co-innervation of motor endplates in the esophagus: state of the art ten years after. *Histochemistry and Cell Biology*, 123(2): 117-130, ISSN 0948-6143.

Wu, M., Majewski, M., Wojtkiewicz, J., Vanderwinden, J.M., Adriaensen, D. & Timmermans, J.P. (2003). Anatomical and neurochemical features of the extrinsic and intrinsic innervation of the striated muscle in the porcine esophagus: evidence for regional and species differences. *Cell and Tissue Research*, 311(3): 289-297, ISSN 0302-766X.

Yamamoto, K., Chan, S. W., Rudd, J.A., Lin, G., Asano, K. & Yamatodani, A. (2009). Involvement of hypothalamic glutamate in cisplatin-induced emesis in Suncus murinus (house musk shrew). *Journal of Pharmacological Sciences*, 109(4): 631-634, ISSN 1347-8613.

Yuan, S., Costa, M. & Brookes, S.J. (1998). Neuronal pathways and transmission to the lower esophageal sphincter of the guinea Pig. *Gastroenterology*, 115(3): 661-671, ISSN 0016-5085.

2

Gastroesophageal Reflux Disease: Molecular Predictors in Neoplastic Progression of Barrett's Esophagus

Fritz Francois, Abraham Khan,
Liying Yang, Sam M. Serouya and Zhiheng Pei
New York University Langone Medical Center
USA

1. Introduction

Barrett's esophagus (BE) represents a metaplastic change from squamous epithelium to intestinal epithelium as a result of chronic gastroesophagheal reflux. Since the development of esophageal adenocarcinoma (EAC) is not universal among patients with BE, it is important to understand and to gauge the factors that influence risk of progression to dysplasia and cancer. While heartburn symptoms have been reported to be associated with BE (Eisen et al., 1997; Lagergren et al., 1999a), the severity of gastroesophageal reflux symptoms is not a reliable indicator for the presence of BE (Eloubeidi and Provenzale, 2001). There is a vital need to explore factors other than symptoms that not only may elucidate the pathophysiology of BE development but also that may be predictive of progression to EAC. Significant advances have been made along key areas such as cell cycle abnormalities, growth factors, adiposity, and the gut microbiome. This chapter aims to review some of these elements as well as the prognostic value of biomarkers for progression from BE to EAC. The importance of fulfilling the promise that these biomarkers hold is underscored by the notable increase in the risk of progression to cancer from 0.5% per year in non-dysplastic BE, to 13% in the setting of low-grade dysplasia, and to 40% in high-grade dysplasia (Curvers et al., 2010; Wani et al., 2009).

2. Cell cycle abnormalities

The normal cell cycle by which cells proliferate is comprised of an intricate system of checkpoints and regulations designed to carefully modulate growth. Cell cycle regulation is dependent on the members of several protein classes, including cyclins and cyclin dependent kinase (CDK) complexes, tumor suppressors, and pro as well as anti-apoptotic proteins. Derangements in this system result in dysregulation of the cell cycle and provide opportunity for uncontrolled proliferation, as well as the potential for neoplastic progression (Evan and Vousden, 2001). The tissue invasion and metastatic progression phases of the neoplastic change are also dependent on cellular as well as extracellular proteins that are normally involved in cell cycle regulation. The pathophysiologic mechanisms through which these proteins function have been implicated in most cancers and are the focus of current research due to their possible prognostic value and implication for therapeutic targeting. The association of chronic GERD with the development of BE, dysplasia, and EAC (Gerdes, 1990; Herbst et al., 1978; Pellish et al., 1980; Preston-Martin et al., 1990; Reid et al., 1993; Ronkainen et al., 2005) provides an opportunity to explore the underlying cellular mechanisms that drive the transformation. This section will discuss the mechanisms by which cell cycle proteins may confer a survival advantage for transformation of BE to EAC.

As a class, tumor suppressor genes code for proteins that protect the cell by arresting the cellular growth cycle or by promoting apoptosis. Proteins such as p53, p16, and adenomatous polyposis coli (APC), normally recognize DNA damage and halt progression through the cell cycle, allowing for repair, senescence, or cell death. Therefore allelic mutations leading to loss of function of these proteins can be carcinogenic (Sherr, 2004). Mutations of the p53 protein have been implicated in nearly every cancer and may be one of the most common derangements in BE and EAC (Greenblatt et al., 1994; Vaninetti et al., 2008). Normally the detection of DNA damage results in p53 activation via signals that promote p21 transcription with subsequent binding and inhibition of cyclin dependent kinase-complexes that prevent progression into the next stage of the cell cycle (Levine, 1997). Additionally p53 triggers apoptosis through the intrinsic pathway mediated by Bax and Bak as well as the extrinsic pathway via Fas action. Through different downstream pathways these proteins lead to the release of cytochrome C and other intermitochrondrial proteins into the cytosol including caspace formation, leading to cellular degradation (Levine, 1997; Levine et al., 2006; Petros et al., 2004; Vousden, 2005). Mutated p53 has a prolonged half-life and its overexpression can be detected as deposits in the cell nucleus (Hinds et al., 1990). Without normal p53 regulation damaged cells are no longer inhibited from progressing through the cell cycle and are not marked for repair, senescence, or apoptosis. Furthermore the damaged DNA leads to additional genetic mutations that perpetuate cancerous gene formation as well as cells that are resistant to treatment. Several studies have found overexpression of p53 throughout the different stages of carcinogenesis to be a risk factor for progression from BE to EAC, however the exact mechanism has not been completely elucidated (Krishnadath et al., 1995; Murray et al., 2006; Ramel et al., 1992). As a clinical prognostic indicator alterations in p53 expression have been found to be predictive of response to chemotherapy and overall survival (Heeren et al., 2004; Madani et al., 2010).

P16, the protein product of the INK4A/CDKN2A gene, is a cyclin dependent kinase inhibitor that has been demonstrated to be mutated in a variety of cancers including EAC. P16 tumor suppression is initiated by cellular stress leading to the binding of p16 to CDK4 and CDK6. CDK4/p16 and CDK6/p16 complexes inhibit formation CDK-cyclin D complexes, leading to the destruction of cyclin D (Diehl and Sherr, 1997; Rocco and Sidransky, 2001). Without cyclin D, $p27^{KIPI}$ accumulation occurs, which in turn prevents CDK2/cyclin E and CDK2/cyclin A complexes from phosphorylating the retinoblastoma protein (Rb). The Rb protein is required for activation of the transcriptional complex E2F-DB and subsequent gene transcription. Additionally the Rb-E2F complexes that form serve as inhibitors of transcription. Given this series of steps, proper p16 regulation responds to cell stress by inhibiting transcription, which is required for the cell to continue through the G_1/S cell cycle checkpoint (Rocco and Sidransky, 2001). Mutation in p16 genes, occur through point mutations, loss of heterozygosity, and/or silencing of the gene through promoter hypermethylation (Maley et al., 2004; Rocco and Sidransky, 2001). Therefore, loss of p16 activity in the context of DNA damage and cellular stressors, permit the cell to undergo unregulated transcription and proliferation. There exists an increasing amount of evidence showing that p16 inactivation is a critical step in the development of EAC. In fact the most prevalent genetic alteration in BE is the result of INK4A/CDKN2A hypermethylation, which is an early epigenetic change that occurs in the progression from BE to EAC (Bian et al., 2002; Hardie et al., 2005; Powell et al., 2005; Souza et al., 2001; Vieth et al., 2004).

As a tumor suppressor, the adenomatous polyposis coli (APC) protein has been implicated in the development of EAC (Clement et al., 2006a, b). APC is part of the Wnt signaling pathway which modulates the levels of β-catenin, a key protein for cell-cell adhesion and transcription. This pathway is activated by Wnt proteins binding to receptors of the Frizzled transmembrane protein family and LDL-receptor-related protein, which in turn trigger the phosphorylation of Dishevelled protein. The Dishevelled protein blocks the phosphorylating activity of GSK3β, which is a complex composed of APC, Axin and casein kinase 1 (CK1). When activated, GSK3β phosphorylates β-catenin initiating its destruction. When β-catenin is in its unphosphorylated state it translocates to the cell nucleus, binds to DNA-binding proteins TCF/LEF, and activates gene transcription of growth promoting genes myc, COX-2, matrilysin/matrix metalloproteinase 7, and cyclin D (Clement et al., 2006a; Giles et al., 2003; Logan and Nusse, 2004; Rocco and Sidransky, 2001). Therefore loss of APC, as implicated in a number of cancers, may result in increased β-catenin in the nucleus and uncontrolled cellular proliferation and tumorigensis (Bian et al., 2000; Clement et al., 2006a; Logan and Nusse, 2004; Trigg, 1998). Furthermore, it has been demonstrated that APC is involved with microtubule function. Without functional APC there is an increase in abnormal mitotic spindles and subsequently chromosomal defects. Several studies have demonstrated that APC inactivation leads to β-catenin accumulation in EAC, but is not necessary or sufficient for activation of the Wnt pathway since β-catenin accumulates without APC inactivation (Clement et al., 2006a). Despite this patients with APC gene hypermethylation in BE samples were more likely to progress to EAC and several studies have shown that all EACs have APC promoter methylation (Wang et al., 2009b). Therefore while the exact mechanism by which loss of APC leads to EAC has not been completely elucidated, its detection might provide prognostic value in assessing the progression from BE to EAC.

Cyclins and cyclin dependent kinases (CDKs) are integral parts of the cell cycle regulation control system. Cyclins bind to CDKs and lead to phosphorylation of proteins necessary for progression through the cell cycle (Stamatakos et al., 2010). In addition to these regulators, p21 acts as a cyclin dependent kinase inhibitor in tumor suppression as well as a possible oncogene, inhibiting apoptosis and promoting proliferation (Abbas and Dutta, 2009; Gartel, 2006). Derangements in the function of these proteins have been implicated in nearly all tumors and their involvement in the progression to BE and EAC is an area of active investigation. Cyclin D1 regulates cell cycle activity by forming a complex with CDK4/6 and controlling activity through G1. Once bound, cyclin D1/CDK 4/6 complexes phosphorylate the retinoblastoma protein (Rb), deactivating it and activating E2F transcription complex. E2F leads to the transcription of genes required for transition through G_1 (Shapiro and Harper, 1999; Traganos, 2004). One of the genes transcribed when E2F is activated, cyclin E binds CDK2 leading to phosphorylation of downstream targets that are necessary for replication initiation, histone synthesis, and replication of centrosomes. This allows transition through G_1 checkpoint to the S phase (Ma et al., 2000). Additionally, cyclin E/CDK2 complexes further phosphorylate Rb leading to additional transcriptional activity (Fu et al., 2004). P21 has been described initially in the tumor suppression cascade of p53 as described above, however new research suggests that it may also have the opposite action as an oncogene promoting tumorinogensis (Gartel, 2006).

Cyclin D1 has been implicated in a number of cancers and is overexpressed due to derangements that include chromosomal translocations, gene amplification and anomalies in proper intercellular trafficking and proteolysis (Kim and Diehl, 2009; Stamatakos et al., 2010). When overexpressed cyclin D1 leads to tumor formation through several mechanisms. First, high levels of cyclin D1 lead to increased activation of CDK4/6 leading to increased proliferation. Second, cyclin D1/CDK complexes inhibit p21 and p27 activity, two CDK inhibitors, and therefore with abnormal levels of p21/p27 inhibition there is decreased inhibitory control over the cell cycle (Cheng et al., 1998). Third cyclin D1 also has non-CDK dependent actions including increasing estrogen receptor transcription (Neuman et al., 1997) as well as abnormalities in the repression of PPARγ, a transcriptional protein modulated by abnormal binding of HDAC by cyclin D1 (Fu et al., 2005). In addition cyclin D1 has been reported to lead to increased expression of fibroblast growth factor 1 (Tashiro et al., 2007) as well as increased production of reactive oxygen species (ROS) leading to metastasis of tumors (Stamatakos et al., 2010). Although the exact mechanism of action in EAC has not been completely elucidated, studies have demonstrated cyclin D1 overexpression in BE and early stages of tumorigensis (Arber et al., 1996; Bani-Hani et al., 2000).

Aberration in cyclin E activity, from gene amplification (Marone et al., 1998; Stamatakos et al., 2010) or defective degradation (Buckley et al., 1993), leads to constitutive expression and increased activity of the protein, which results in increased cellular proliferation (Stamatakos et al., 2010). Increased levels of cyclin E lead to increased activity of CDK2, subsequent activation of transcription proteins, as well as increased phosphorylation of Rb. Given the pathway described above, these anomalies may all lead to deregulated progression into the S phase and consequently amplified proliferation. This has been noted as a shortened G_1 phase, decreased cell size due to decreased time for growth, and decreased requirement for proper environmental factors necessary for replication (Sala et al., 1997; Stamatakos et al., 2010). The relevance of cyclin E and its deregulation in the development of EAC is currently unclear.

Although P21, a cyclin dependent kinase inhibitor, was thought to solely act in the tumor suppression cascade of p53 as described above, recent evidence suggests that it also has the opposite role as an oncogene, inhibiting apoptosis and promoting cellular proliferation (Abbas and Dutta, 2009; Gartel, 2006; Roninson, 2002). In the tumor suppression cascade of p53, loss of p21 inhibition of cyclin-CDK complexes, especially CDK2, in cells with DNA damage may lead to uncontrolled progression through the cell cycle and carcinogenesis (Abbas and Dutta, 2009). Additionally, it is hypothesized that p21 contains antiapoptotic activity and therefore, when overexpressed, damaged cells avoid degradation and proliferate to form tumors (Roninson, 2002). P21 might also promote cyclin D1 accumulation in the nucleus, therefore avoiding destruction, and facilitating binding with CDK4/6, leading to increased transcription (LaBaer et al., 1997; Liu et al., 2007). P21 has not been extensively studied in BE and EAC, but some evidence suggests that similar to p53 changes in the expression pattern of p21 may lead to a better response to treatment in these patients (Heeren et al., 2004).

In addition to the main regulatory proteins described above, several other proteins have been implicated in carcinogenesis and may have a role in BE and EAC. Apoptosis is a key component of normal cellular functioning that serves to limit cells with DNA damage by triggering them to self destruct. Two proteins have been implicated in cells evading proper apoptotic pathways, cyclooxygenase 2 (COX-2) and B cell lymphoma 2 protein.

While COX-2 is not constitutively expressed in all tissues, it is found in response to inflammation or mitogenic stimuli ultimately leading to increased production of prostaglandins (PGs) (Konturek et al., 2005). Recent evidence has demonstrated that COX-2 expression increases with worsening grades of dysplasia in esophageal carcinogenesis (Cheong et al., 2003; Konturek et al., 2004) and that the increased COX-2 expression in the esophageal epithelium might be secondary to gastric acid and bile exposure (Shirvani et al., 2000). The mechanisms by which COX-2 overexpression leads to the development of EAC is related to COX-2 derived PGs' actions. These prostaglandins are involved in evasion of apoptosis by inhibiting release of cytochrome c, decreasing activation of caspase-9 and -3, increasing activity of bcl-2 (Wang et al., 2005) and blocking Fas mediated cell death (Nzeako et al., 2002). BE cells with overexpression of COX-2 have lower rates of apoptosis (Wilson et al., 1998). Additionally, COX-2 produced PGs have been implicated in invasion and metastasis, theorized to be due to increased metalloproteinase-2 activity (Nzeako et al., 2002). Furthermore, COX-2 derived PGs have been demonstrated to lead to cell proliferation through stimulation of epidermal growth factor receptors (Baatar et al., 2002), angiogenesis by increasing VEGF levels (Wang and DuBois, 2004); (Shiff et al., 2003) and inhibition of immune anti-tumor responses by hampering the activity of natural killer cells, macrophages, and dendritic cells, and decreasing production of Th1 cytokines. Given these mechanisms, it is not surprising that multiple studies have demonstrated a decreased risk of progression to cancer (Buttar et al., 2002), and decreased cell proliferation in BE epithelium when treated with COX inhibitors (Kaur et al., 2002).

B cell lymphoma 2 protein (Bcl-2) is an integral part in regulation of cell survival by inhibiting apoptosis. Overexpression of Bcl-2 has been documented in a number of cancers as well as all phases of reflux-associated esophageal carcinogenesis including esophagitis, nondysplastic BE, dysplatic BE, and EAC (Metzger et al., 2004). Overexpression of Bcl-2 leads to inhibition of apoptosis early in carcinogenesis leading to decreased cell death and elongated cell lifespan (Metzger et al., 2004) (Lehrbach et al., 2009) (Thomadaki and Scorilas, 2006). The extended cell survival is hypothesized to allow for accumulation of oncogenic mutations leading to carcinogenesis (Zhivotovsky and Orrenius, 2006). Bcl-2 overexpression leads to apoptotic evasion by inhibiting mitochondrial release of cytochrome c and eventual caspase formation (Thomadaki and Scorilas, 2006). In fact, cells with elevated Bcl-2 production are more resistant to chemotherapy and radiation treatment (Thomadaki and Scorilas, 2006). However, its exact role in EAC development has not been extensively studied.

In order for tumors to survive, invade, and metastasize there are a number of proteins involved including Tissue inhibitors of metalloproteinase (TIMPs). These classes of proteins have distinct roles in this aspect of tumorigenesis and have been associated with BE and EAC.

TIMPs are enzymes that regulate the production and actions of metalloproteinases (MMPs), which are responsible for turnover and remodeling of the extracellular matrix and cell signaling, in addition to non-MMP dependent actions. TIMPs have been evaluated in a number of cancers and have demonstrated multi-factorial and contradictory roles in cancer, with both overexpression and silencing observed. Furthermore, it is theorized that TIMPs exhibit different actions depending on the level of expression. Mechanisms by which TIMPs are involved in carcinogenesis include apoptosis and cell proliferation, angiogenesis, and metastasis and cell adhesion (Bourboulia and Stetler-Stevenson, 2010; Cruz-Munoz and Khokha, 2008; Jiang et al., 2002; Sun, 2010). In cancer cell lines, TIMP-1 enhanced cell survival and growth by increasing expression of IL-10 and anti-apoptotic protein bcl-xl (Chirco et al., 2006). TIMPs promote cell proliferation by increasing p65 phosphorylation, which increases NF-Kβ, a protein that binds gene promoters and leads to cell proliferation. This, however, was observed at late stages of tumor growth while upregulation of NF-Kβ has also demonstrated slowing tumor growth in its early stages. The exact role in proliferation seems to depend on the stage of tumorigenesis (Sun, 2010). TIMPs are thought to enhance angiogenesis by increasing vascular endothelial growth factor (VEGF) production and inhibiting MMPs, which, produce angiogenesis inhibitors, endostatin and angiostatin (Jiang et al., 2002). As well, TIMP-2, which normally blocks microvascular endothelial cell growth in response to pro-angiogenic factors like FGF-2 or VEGF A is silenced through promoter hypermethylation in a number of cancers (Sun, 2010). Lastly, TIMPs normally inhibit cell adhesion and metastasis by blocking the breakdown of the extracellular matrix through inhibition of MMPs. However, in cancers there is a disruption of the balance between MMPs and TIMPs, with possible elevated levels of MMPs and increased disruption of the ECM and cell-cell adhesion leading to increased cell motility (Bourboulia and Stetler-Stevenson, 2010; Cruz-Munoz and Khokha, 2008). Given these mechanisms in a number of cancer, the exact role of TIMPs in esophageal adenocarcinoma development from BE has not been elucidated.

Lastly the plasmingonen acitvating system, which includes urokinase-type plasminogen activator (uPA), has been investigated for its prognostic value in BE. In normal physiologic states, this system regulates the fibrinoylitic system, however it has been implicated in a variety of pathologic states including tumor cell proliferation, apoptosis, cell migration and invasion, and angiogenesis (Laufs et al., 2006; McMahon and Kwaan, 2008). uPA, a serine protease has been demonstrated to be expressed in tumor cells, and is considered the most active component of this system. uPA is involved in cell proliferation, apoptosis, and angiogenesis through interaction with its cellular receptor uPAR and the epidermal growth factor receptor (EGFR), which stimulates cell growth through a cascade of intracellular mechanisms (McMahon and Kwaan, 2008). uPA is believed to assist in tumor cell migration and invasion by converting plasminogen to plasmin, which activates MMPs, which degrade ECM elements such as vitronectin, laminin, and type IV collagen, leading to altered cell adhesion, shape, and migration (Laufs et al., 2006; McMahon and Kwaan, 2008). Angiogenesis is altered by uPA by affecting endothelial cell proliferation leading to angiogenesis and by activating kringle structures, which inhibit microvascular endothelial cell proliferation through changes in angiostatin levels therefore inhibiting angiogenesis.

Several proteins have been implicated in tumorogenesis and may have prognostic implications in EAC including cadherins and Ki-67. The mechanism by which these proteins promote oncogenesis, provide opportunity for further investigation.

3. Growth factors

The mechanisms that promote evolution of BE to EAC are largely unknown. As derangements in the cell cycle are believed to be involved in carcinogenesis and the development of uncontrolled cellular replication, growth factors have been the focus of investigations in the neoplastic progression of BE. Three such factors that have been recognized as promoting growth in BE are: epidermal growth factor (EGF), vascular endothelial growth factor (VEGF), and transforming growth factor beta (TGF-β).

The epidermal growth factor receptor (EGFR) family of receptors has been studied as a potential biomarker in the progression of BE to EAC. This family of tyrosine kinase receptors initiates a signal transduction cascade that modulates cell proliferation, differentiation, adhesion, and migration (Yarden, 2001). EGFR is a transmembrane receptor that enables signals to be transmitted across the plasma membrane, affecting gene expression and a multitude of cellular responses. Overexpression of this receptor has been shown to occur in several malignancies, including EAC (Wang et al., 2007).

The correlation of EGFR expression with early neoplastic progression of BE has not been completely elucidated. Using PCR to evaluate gene expression, amplification of the EGFR locus was demonstrated in EAC without concomitant elevated expression in high-grade dysplasia with BE (Miller et al., 2003). However, another study did show gene locus amplification of EGFR in both BE associated high-grade dysplasia and EAC (Rygiel et al., 2008). There is also the possibility of a certain EGF polymorphism leading to an increased risk of EAC, as the specific EGFA61G G/G genotype has been shown to confer such a risk (Lanuti et al., 2008).

While there is evidence linking EGFR gene expression with EAC, until recently there was only limited evidence of this expression in regards to protein abundance (Li et al., 2006; Wilkinson et al., 2004). Importantly, for EGFR to be considered a useful biomarker of histological progression of BE, it would increase in progression during neoplastic transformation. In addition, it would also be expressed on the luminal epithelial surface so as to be readily visualized during endoscopy, and be available for biopsy targeting. One recent study evaluated this potential dual role for EGFR using tissue microarray technology, exploring the possibility of EGFR as a relevant biomarker to monitor histological progression, and ultimately to allow for biopsy targeting of abnormal tissue (Cronin et al., 2011). The study showed a stepwise increase in EGFR abundance in BE, high-grade dysplasia, and EAC. As EGFR is a transmembrane protein expressed on the luminal esophageal surface, it also has potential for sampling during endoscopy.

VEGF is another growth marker that performs an important role in tumor formation. Increased vascularity is associated with a poor prognosis in several human malignancies, and VEGF is important for angiogenesis in neoplastic progression. By using immunohistochemistry to examine VEGF expression, one study specifically studied vascularization in both BE and associated EAC (Couvelard et al., 2000). An increase in angiogenesis was found in precancerous lesions, and VEGF expression correlated with the increase in vascularization. However VEGF in the study had no prognostic significance.

As it is accepted that BE develops from esophageal mucosal injury incurred after acid and bile reflux, a study looked at VEGF expression in a bile acid environment. By quantitative

PCR, VEGF expression to increased after exposure to certain bile acids (Burnat et al., 2007). Another study looked at the possibility of an "angiogenic switch" in the transition from metaplasia to dysplasia to carcinoma in BE (Mobius et al., 2003). This study showed that VEGF expression increased during the sequence of metaplasia to advanced carcinoma. More specifically, the data suggested that the related impact on neovascularization occurred early on in the course of this transformation, as the only true significant difference in VEGF expression occurred between Barrett's metaplasia and high-grade dysplasia. This entailed that the importance of VEGF and related angiogenesis in the progression to EAC may occur before actual tumor growth.

TGF-β is a growth factor predominantly involved in cellular proliferation and differentiation, and several studies suggest that loss of TGF-β signaling is an important factor in BE-related EAC. Smad4, a protein that is part of a TGF-β mediated complex important in downstream gene activation, has been shown to potentially have a dual importance in the neoplastic progression of BE. In response to TGF-β, a majority of EAC cell lines in one study failed to growth arrest, and specific modulation of Smad4 was inhibited. However, the cell lines also upgraded the expression of certain proteases that led to a more invasive cell phenotype, suggesting a dual role for TGF-β (Onwuegbusi et al., 2007). By PCR, FISH, and sequencing, Smad4 expression has also been shown to be progressively reduced in the metaplasia to dysplasia to adenocarcinoma sequence (Onwuegbusi et al., 2006).

Other evidence propose additional roles for the downstream TGF-β pathway and its importance in the neoplastic progression of BE. One study showed that hypermethylation and inactivation of RUNX3, a target gene of TGF-β, is associated with the progression of BE to dysplasia and ultimately adenocarcinoma (Schulmann et al., 2005). TGF-β also has known significance in the epithelial to mesenchymal transition, which promotes cellular motility, invasion, and cytoskeletal rearrangement in a range of tumor cells. One study looked specifically at the ability of TGF-β to induce esophageal to mesenchymal transition in esophageal cell lines in vitro. The data from this study suggested a role for this transition in EAC, as TGF-β induced alterations in aggregation and invasion, and thus a more invasive phenotype (Rees et al., 2006).

There has been clear value in the investigation of EGF, VEGF, and TGF-β as performing critical roles in the progression of BE to EAC. More examination is needed to clarify the independent function of these growth factors and their downstream proteins in the progression of this disease.

4. Adiposity and adipokines

Obesity, as defined by a body mass index (BMI) >30, has been increasing steadily over the past twenty years and has become an epidemic in the US. In 1989 the prevalence of obesity among adults did not surpass 15% in any state. By contrast in 2009, the prevalence of obesity among adults is greater than 15% in every state [Ref: http://www.cdc.gov/obesity/data/trends.html#State]. It is estimated that 68% of adults twenty years of age or older in the US are either overweight or obese and nearly 34% of these are obese (Flegal et al., 2010). Obesity is associated not only with metabolic disorders such as diabetes (Bray, 1992; Pontiroli and Galli, 1998; Scott et al., 1997) but also with neoplastic conditions such as EAC (Chow et al., 1998; Dvoyrin et al., 2011; Lagergren et al., 1999b). Elucidating the biomolecular mechanisms that link adiposity with the development of GERD, BE, and EAC is an active area of investigation. Such information could provide novel targets for the treatment of conditions along the GERD spectrum.

Increased adiposity, defined by BMI or waist circumference, has been shown to be an independent risk factor for GERD epidemiologically, while being consistently linked to reflux symptoms as well as mucosal injury (Hampel et al., 2005). Increasing BMI and waist circumference separately lead to an increased frequency of GERD symptoms, esophageal acid exposure, (El-Serag et al., 2007; El-Serag et al., 2005; Locke et al., 1999; Murray et al., 2003) and reflux related hospitalizations (Ruhl and Everhart, 1999). In fact, those with a BMI greater than 30 kg/m^2 have been shown to be approximately three times more likely to develop GERD symptoms at least once per week (Locke et al., 1999; Murray et al., 2003). Even among those who are morbidly obese, those with a higher BMI have a higher percentage of time during which the esophageal pH is less than four (Fisher et al., 1999).

Obesity has also been linked to complications of GERD including the development of BE and EAC. These develop due to an imbalance between injurious elements and esophageal protective mechanisms (Vaezi and Richter, 1996). It is estimated that obesity leads to a two and a half fold increased risk of BE. Furthermore Stein and colleagues concluded that for every 10-pound increase in weight the risk of BE increases by 10%, and for each five point increase in BMI the risk increases by 35% (Stein et al., 2005). Recent evidence also suggests that abdominal obesity, specifically visceral fat, is a stronger risk factor for BE than BMI (Corley et al., 2007; Edelstein et al., 2007). In terms of EAC, a linear relationship with obesity seems to exists as higher BMI levels are associated with an increased risk of the malignancy (Brown et al., 1995; Chow et al., 1998; Lagergren et al., 1999b; Wu et al., 2001).

Several mechanisms have been proposed to explain the association between the level of adiposity and the development of GERD. The "transmitted pressure" hypothesis suggests that direct mechanical pressure from the large abdominal panus can lead to an increased intragastric pressure, which when relayed to the lower esophageal sphincter, can result in reflux by way of non-swallow induced transient relaxation (El-Serag, 2008; El-Serag et al., 2006; Lambert et al., 2005; Mercer et al., 1985; Pandolfino et al., 2006). Pandolfino et al. demonstrated a multi-faceted mechanism by which fat, especially visceral adiposity, leads to reflux. Utilizing high-resolution manometry, this study demonstrated that for every inch of increased waist circumference, there is a significant increase in intragastric and intraesophageal pressures, 0.4 mm Hg and 0.1 mm Hg, respectively. Additionally both the mean gastroesophageal pressure gradient (GEPG) as well as the disruption of the esophagogastric junction (EGJ), measured as separation of the lower esophageal sphincter and extrinsic crural diagphram, were higher among obese patients. Furthermore, EGJ disruption allows for the development of a hiatal hernia. Finally, patients with GERD symptoms when compared to non-GERD patients had increased GEPG and EGJ disruption. Given these pressure morphologies among overweight and obese patients, it appears that increasing panus size creates a pathophysiologic mechanism allowing for the flow of gastric contents into the esophagus (Pandolfino et al., 2006).

As an active endocrine organ, adipose tissue is also important metabolically, and produces adipocytokines such as leptin, and adiponectin. In addition while the gastric epithelium produces acid, it is also the primary source for the adipokine ghrelin. Evidence suggests that these hormones are associated mechanistically in the development of BE and esophageal adenocarcinoma.

Leptin, a proteohormone produced mostly in proportion to the amount of white adipose tissue, is a diverse hormone involved in energy homeostasis and satiety management (Housa et al., 2006). Leptin is also produced by the gastric epithelium and we have found that fundic levels to be significantly associated with risk of BE (Francois et al., 2008). In esophageal cell lines, leptin has been shown to have actions as a growth factor leading to increased proliferation (Beales and Ogunwobi, 2007; Lipetz, 1984; Somasundar et al., 2003) and inhibition of apoptosis, which may predispose to an increased risk of BE and esophageal adenocarcinoma (Beales and Ogunwobi, 2007). These effects have been demonstrated to be synergistic when leptin is combined with acid pulses (Beales and Ogunwobi, 2007). The most current research has demonstrated a complex signaling pathway by which leptin causes these aberrations, however the exact mechanism has not been completely elucidated. It is postulated that leptin stimulates a transmembrane leptin receptor, which activates both P38 MAP kinase and janus kinase JAK2 pathways. JAK2 also activates P38 MAP kinase, as well as, extracellular signal related kinase (ERK) and Akt, which all increase COX-2 mRNA levels. Upregulation of COX-2 leads to increased PGE-2 production, which subsequently activates an EP-4 receptor. The EP-4 receptor then causes activation of PKC, src, and MMPs, which increase cleavage and extracellular shedding of EGFR ligands, HB-EGF and TGFα. These transactivate an epidermal growth factor receptor (EGFR) (Beales and Ogunwobi, 2007; Ogunwobi et al., 2006; Ogunwobi and Beales, 2008b). Ultimately, C-jun NH_2 terminal kinase (JNK) is then activated which leads to the inhibition of apoptosis and increased proliferation. It is by this pathway which leptin may predispose obese patients to an increased risk of EAC (Beales and Ogunwobi, 2007; Ogunwobi et al., 2006).

Adiponectin is produced solely by white adipose tissue and has been shown to have anti-atherogenic, anti-inflammatory, and anti-diabetic actions (Housa et al., 2006; Nishida et al., 2007). It is a protein found in multiple isoforms, high molecular weight (HMW), medium molecular weight (MMW), and low molecular weight (LMW) (Suzuki et al., 2007). Unlike leptin, adiponectin levels are decreased in obesity, and low levels of adiponectin have been associated with an increased risk of BE and EAC (Rubenstein et al., 2008; Yildirim et al., 2009). Its role in the development of cancer is believed to be protective through anti-proliferative (Ogunwobi and Beales, 2008a) and pro-apoptotic effects (Konturek et al., 2008). Adiponectin leads to a dose-dependent increase in the rate of apoptosis in esophageal cancer cell lines, which can be explained by a dose dependent increase and decrease in mRNA and protein expression of pro-apoptotic BAX and anti-apoptotic Bcl-2, respectively (Konturek et al., 2008). Its anti-proliferative effects may be mediated through its actions on adiponectin receptor-1 as well as activation of adenosine monophosphate activated protein kinase and serine/threonine phosphatases, which ultimately lead to modulation of p53 and p21(Ogunwobi and Beales, 2008a);(Rubenstein et al., 2009). More recent evidence suggests unique roles of each adiponectin multimer in the development of BE High levels of LMW adiponectin have been shown to be associated with a decreased risk of BE, and conversely, high levels of HMW adiponectin are associated with an increased risk (Rubenstein et al., 2009). LMW adiponectin may prevent the inflammatory reaction of esophageal mucosa by suppressing the release of pro-inflammatory interleukin-6 and increasing release of anti-inflammatory interleukin-10. Therefore, low levels of LMW adiponectin might permit an aberrant response to reflux thus leading to metaplastic changes (Schober et al., 2007). Other possible mechanisms of adiponectin that have been postulated include suppression of extracellular signal related kinases 1 and 2, which when exuberantly activated lead to increased proliferation and decreased apoptosis, and possibly an exacerbated pathologic response to reflux (Rubenstein et al., 2008).

Lastly, ghrelin is a hormone that is produced primarily in the fundus of the stomach, (Kojima and Kangawa, 2005) and has a variety of roles which include stimulation of appetite as well as gastric acid secretion (Masuda et al., 2000; Wren et al., 2001). Ghrelin levels have been shown to be inversely related to adiposity and EAC risk (de Martel et al., 2007), but the biomolecular mechanism underlying this association has not been completely elucidated. There may be an anti-inflammatory component to the mechanism, as evidence suggests that ghrelin inhibits the increased production of COX-2 and interleukin-1β (IL-1β) by tumor necrosis factor alpha (TNFα) (Konturek et al., 2008). In addition, ghrelin stimulates gastric motility by stimulating the vagus nerve and myenteric neurons. By shortening gastric emptying time, this decreases the acid exposure of the lower esophageal and potentially decreases the risk of EAC (de Martel et al., 2007).

By further elucidating the mechanisms behind adipocytokines and their relationships to BE and EAC, there may be opportunities for both diagnostic as well as therapeutic approaches to these sequelae of GERD.

5. Microbiome and cancer

The human body is inhabited by ten times more bacteria than the number of human cells in the body (Savage, 1977). The bacteria form ecological communities on every external (skin) and internal (mucosal) surfaces of our body. Bacteria in the communities collectively are termed by Joshua Lederberg as "microbiome" (Lederberg and McCray, 2001). The host relationship with the microbiome can be commensal, symbiotic, and pathogenic. The general concept is that the host provides a nutrient-rich habitat, while the bacteria play important roles in the development of the mucosal immune system, the maintenance of a physiological environment, the provision of essential nutrients, and the prevention of colonization by pathogenic bacteria (Cunningham-Rundles et al., 2002; Eckburg et al., 2005). On the other hand, certain members of the human microbiome play a pathogenic role, as illustrated by traditional medical microbiology built upon concepts of infectious diseases in which a pathogen can often be identified and pathogenesis explained by toxins or virulent factors produced by the pathogen. These concepts have clearly demonstrated their usefulness in the identification of etiologic agents of a number of infectious diseases.

More recently, the concept that the microbiome is essential for the development of inflammation-induced carcinoma has emerged from studies of well-known colonic microbiome (Yang and Pei, 2006). In the TCRβ/p53, IL-10 and Gpx1/Gpx2 knockout mouse colitis models that mimic the development of adenocarcinoma in ulcerative colitis, carcinoma develops in conventional mice but not in mice raised under germ-free housing conditions (Balish and Warner, 2002; Chu et al., 2004; Kado et al., 2001). In IL-10, HLA-B27/β2m, and TCRα knockout mice, the colonic microbiome is also a prerequisite for the development of inflammation in the colon (Kawaguchi-Miyashita et al., 2001; Rath et al., 1996; Sellon et al., 1998; Song et al., 1999). Although intestinal bacteria are an important factor in the inflammation and tumorigenesis, their precise role remains elusive. One theory is that both "protective" species and "harmful" species exist within the normal enteric microbiome. A healthy balance between these two populations in a normal host might be detrimental for an inflammation-prone host. Alternatively, a breakdown in the balance between the two populations, termed "dysbiosis", could by itself promote inflammation in a normal host. Chronic inflammation could be carcinogenic. Although resident enteric bacteria are necessary for the development of spontaneous colitis in many rodent models, not all bacteria have an equivalent capability to induce inflammation. Germ-free IL-10-deficient mice populated with bacterial strains, including *Bacteroides vulgatus, Clostridium sordellii, Streptococcus viridans, Escherichia coli, Lactobacillus casei, Lactobacillus reuteri, Lactobacillus acidophilus*, and *Lactobacillus lactis* do not exhibit significant colitis (Balish and Warner, 2002; Sellon et al., 1998; Sydora et al., 2005). In contrast, *Citrobacter rodentium, Helicobacter hepaticus, Enterococcus faecalis* are examples of conditional cancer-causing bacteria that alone do not cause cancer, but are carcinogenic in certain genetically-engineered immunodeficient mice (Balish and Warner, 2002; Barthold and Jonas, 1977; Engle et al., 2002; Erdman et al., 2003; Newman et al., 2001; Sellon et al., 1998; Sydora et al., 2005; Ward et al., 1994).

The observations in rodent models which depict the role of the microbiome in tumorigenesis raise some interesting possibilities in relation to human cancers. Although there is no established bacterial pathogen for human colorectal cancer, unusual infections might precede the clinical diagnosis of cancer. A significant proportion (13%) of patients with *Streptococcus bovis* bacteremia have colon cancer (Panwalker, 1988). In some cases, the bacteremia occur months or years before the cancer is diagnosed. *Clostridium septicum* infections are rare, but are often (81%) associated with malignancy including colon cancer (34%) (Beebe and Koneman, 1995; Kornbluth et al., 1989).

The lessons learned from investigations of the colonic microbiome could serve as a general guide to studies of the etiology and pathogenesis of chronic inflammatory diseases and related cancers in other sites of the gastrointestinal tract. These include conditions such as reflux esophagitis and esophageal adenocarcinoma, *Helicobacter* gastritis and gastric adenocarcinoma and lymphoma, as well as inflammatory bowel diseases (IBD) and colorectal cancer.

5.1 *Helicobacter pylori* as a protective marker for esophageal adenocarcinoma

Helicobacter pylori is the most established bacterial cause of human cancer. In particular, *H. pylori* causes gastric adenocarcinoma, the fourth most common cancer and second leading cause of cancer-related death in the world (Ferlay et al., 2010; Parkin et al., 2005; Peek and Blaser, 2002). It is a Gram-negative, microaerophilic bacterium that colonizes the stomach of at least half the world's population (Pounder and Ng, 1995). *H. pylori* causes chronic active gastritis and the colonization and inflammation may persist in the stomach for life if not treated (Marshall and Warren, 1984). Although most individuals infected by *H. pylori* are asymptomatic, despite having chronic gastritis, approximately 10-20% of the patients will develop gastric and duodenal ulcers (Kusters et al., 2006). *H. pylori* infection is also associated with a 1-2% lifetime risk of stomach cancer and a less than 1% risk of gastric MALT lymphoma (Kusters et al., 2006). The risk of non-cardia gastric cancer was nearly six times higher for *H. pylori*-infected people than for uninfected people (Webb et al., 2001). In 1994, the International Agency for Research on Cancer (IARC) classified *H. pylori* as a group 1 carcinogen (IARC, 1994). *H. pylori* infection causes gastric cancer through interaction between bacterial virulent factors and human genes/pathways. *H. pylori* may directly damage the gastric mucosa by bacterial products such as ammonia, phospholipases, and toxins and causes mutations by promoting persistent tissue repair and cellular proliferation. Secondary response from the host, such as releasing free radicals, reactive oxygen metabolites, and cytokines can further damage the gastric mucosa (Bechi et al., 1996). *H. pylori* strains exhibit extensive genetic diversity and strain-specific proteins augment the risk for malignancy (Polk and Peek, 2010). Based on the presence or absence of cytotoxin-associated gene A (cagA), *H. pylori* can be divided into cagA-positive and cagA-negative strains (Covacci et al., 1993; Tummuru et al., 1993). Infection with cagA-positive *H. pylori* strains has been associated with more severe mucosal inflammation, atrophic gastritis and increased risk for the development of gastric carcinoma (Blaser et al., 1995; Kuipers et al., 1995; Parsonnet et al., 1997). There is a twofold increase in the risk of gastric carcinoma associated with cagA-positive strains compared to cagA-negative strains (Huang et al., 2003). *H. pylori* also augment its carcinogenicity by expression of active vacuolating cytotoxin (VacA) as well as blood-group antigen-binding adhesin (BabA1) (Figueiredo et al., 2002; Louw et al., 2001; Miehlke et al., 2001; Rhead et al., 2007). Eradication of *H. pylori* leads to a modest reduction in gastric cancer risk (Fuccio et al., 2009). On the host side, polymorphisms that are associated with increased expression of IL-1β and TNFα also increases the risk of gastric cancer (El-Omar et al., 2003).

Paradoxically, *H. pylori* infection might prevent against the development of EAC. In the majority of studies comparing the rates of *H. pylori* infection in patients with reflux disorders, *H. pylori* infection is associated with a reduced risk of BE and EAC (Islami and Kamangar, 2008; Rokkas et al., 2007; Ronkainen et al., 2005; Sorberg et al., 2003; Wang et al., 2009a). In particular, *H. pylori* infection is inversely associated with risk for EAC with an odds ratio (95% CI) of 0.56 (0.46-0.68), as shown in a meta analysis of 19 case control studies (Islami and Kamangar, 2008). The risk reduction is due to infection with CagA-positive strains (OR, 0.41; 95% CI, 0.28-0.62) as CagA-negative strains are not protective (OR, 1.08; 95% CI, 0.76-1.53). *H. pylori* infection and CagA-positive strains are also associated with a reduced risk for EAC in another meta analysis (Rokkas et al., 2007). Similarly, BE is inversely correlated with both the *H. pylori* prevalence (OR, 0.64; 95% CI, 0.43-0.94; P = .025) and the prevalence of *H. pylori* cagA-positive strain (OR, 0.39; 95% CI, 0.21-0.76; P = .005) (Rokkas et al., 2007). More recent meta analysis found that the prevalence of *H. pylori* infection is significantly lower in BE than in endoscopically normal healthy controls (23.1% vs. 42.7%, OR=0.50, 95% CI 0.27–0.93, P=0.03) but significantly higher in BE patients in studies using healthy blood donors as "normal controls" (71.2% vs. 48.1%, OR=2.21, 95% CI 1.07–4.55). The discrepancy appears to be due to difference in study designs (Wang et al., 2009a). The healthy blood donors are not appropriate controls because: i). the prevalence of *H. pylori* infection in the blood donors is different from that in the general population (Sorberg et al., 2003); ii). Some of the "healthy" blood donors may actually have unrecognized BE since they are not examined by endoscopy. BE is present in 1.6% of the general Swedish population (Ronkainen et al., 2005).

Although no simple theory can explain why *H. pylori infection* reduces the risk of BE and EAC, there are several plausible hypotheses. First, *H. pylori* infection may decrease the tissue damage caused by gastroesophageal reflux by lessening the acidity in the refluxate (Ye et al., 2004). The decrease in gastric acidity could be a result of chronic inflammation and atrophic gastritis associated with *H. pylori* infection as well as the action of bacterial urease that produces ammonia and neutralize gastric acid, independent of gastric atrophy (Richter et al., 1998). This hypothesis is consistent with the observed inverse relationship between indices of *H. pylori* infection and occurrence of gastroesophageal reflux symptoms (Raghunath et al., 2003). However, simple achlorhydria in patients with pernicious anemia does not appears be sufficient for reduction of the risk for EAC, contradicting this hypothesis (Ye and Nyren, 2003). Second, *H. pylori* infection suppresses levels of ghrelin, a potent appetite stimulant and potential contributor to obesity (Azuma et al., 2002; Jang et al., 2008; Nwokolo et al., 2003; Roper et al., 2008; Tatsuguchi et al., 2004; Thrift et al., 2011). Because obesity increases the risk for GERD, BE and EAC (Cook et al., 2008; Hampel et al., 2005; Kubo and Corley, 2006; Whiteman et al., 2008), it is possible that *H pylori* infection may decrease the risks for reflux disorders by reducing body weight. Paradoxically, high ghrelin levels (rather than low) reduce the risk for EAC (de Martel et al., 2007). Third, *H. pylori* is capable of inducing esophageal cancer cells to die through apoptosis *in vitro* experiments, which depends on the presence of CagA (Jones et al., 2003). Thus, *H. pylori* might reduce the EAC risk by killing the cancer cells. However, this finding may not be clinically relevant because *H. pylori* does not colonize Barrett's mucosa (Buttar and Wang, 2004). Ultimately the perceived mechanism behind which *H. pylori* infection may protect against BE and EAC remains unclear.

5.2 Microbiome alteration as a marker for Barrett's esophagus

The esophagus, as with other luminal organs of the digestive system, represents a suitable environment for bacteria to inhabit. Besides residential bacteria, extraneous bacteria could be introduced into the esophagus by swallowing or by reflux from the stomach. However, compared with the well-studied colonic and oral microbiomes, characterization of the esophageal microbiome has received less attention. Attempts to define the esophageal microbiome have been described in 9 reports (Table 1). Previous culture-based studies suggested that the esophagus is either sterile or contains only few transient bacteria (Gagliardi et al., 1998) but studies (Narikiyo et al., 2004; Pei et al., 2004; Pei et al., 2005; Yang et al., 2009) using cultivation-independent PCR have consistently identified indigenous bacteria associated with mucosal surfaces in tissue biopsies. Furthermore, the bacteria are visible on the mucosal surfaces of the distal esophagus (Figure 1) (Pei et al., 2004). Much of the interest to further study of the microbiome comes from its possible link to esophageal disease.

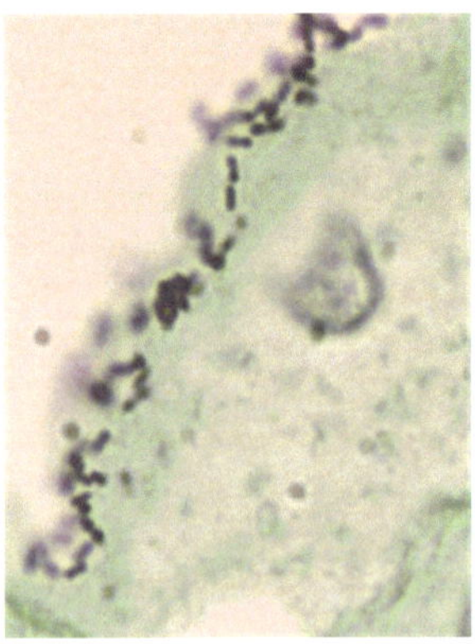

Fig. 1. Visualization of bacteria in the distal esophagus by gram stains in normal.

Category	Culture-based (1981-2007)					Non-culture-based (2004-2009) By Sanger sequencing			
	Lau 1981	Finlay 1982	Mannell 1983	Gagliardi 1998	Macfarlane 2007	Narikiyo 2004	Pei 2004	Pei 2005	Yang 2009
Disease	Cancer	Cancer	Cancer	Normal	BE	Cancer	Normal	RE, BE	RE, BE, Normal
Specimen	Aspirate	Resection	Aspirate	Aspirate	Biopsy Aspirate	Biopsy	Biopsy	Biopsy	Biopsy
No. cases	79	12	101	30	14	20	4	24	34
No. isolates or clones	61	85	377	30	ND	100	900	147	6,800
No. species	14	15	32	11	46	7	95	39	166
Mean species per case	1	6	4	1	ND	≤6	43	ND	24.7
% cases positive for bacteria	64	100	100	67	71	ND	100	100	100
% cases positive for *Streptococcus*	10	92	ND	ND	50	87	100	ND	100

Table 1. Summary of culture-based and non-culture-based studies on bacterial biota of the esophagus

A recent study of human distal esophagus microbiome (Yang et al., 2009) linked inflammation and BE to the change in the microbiome. The study used 16S rRNA gene survey to characterize the bacterial communities in biopsy samples taken from the distal esophagus of 34 individuals with either normal mucosa (n=12), esophagitis (n=12), or BE (intestinal metaplasia) (n=10). Two hundred 16S rRNA genes were cloned and sequenced from each sample. Overall, the 6800 sequences represented 9 phyla, 70 genera, or 166 species. Firmicutes is the only phylum consistently detected in all 34 samples, whereas the other 8 phyla, Bacteroidetes, Proteobacteria, Actinobacteria, Fusobacteria, TM7, Spirochaetes, Cyanobacteria and unclassified bacteria were less common. The samples from healthy subjects were dominated by *streptococci*. On average, 76% of the sequences from healthy esophageal mucosa were categorized to belong to *streptococcal* species and the numbers of some other species were low, but significantly increased in reflux esophagitis and BE.

With an unsupervised approach, samples of the microbiome form two distinct clusters or two microbiome types, type I and II (Figure 2), based on combined genetic distance between samples. Although neither of the two types of microbiome exclusively correlated with the 3 phenotypes, the type I microbiome is more closely associated with normal esophagus (11/12, 91.7%), whereas the type II microbiome is mainly associated with abnormal esophagus (13/22, 59.1%) (p=0.0173 among group comparison), including both esophagitis (7/12, 58.3%, OR=15.4) and BE (6/10, 60.0%, OR=16.5) (Table 2). The alteration of microbiome from type I to type II in distal esophagus, thus, is associated with host phenotypes and its disease progression.

Streptococcus is the most dominant genus in the esophageal microbiome and its relative abundance differs between the two types of microbiome and decreases in disease states. Overall, the 20 type I samples had a mean of 78.8% *Streptococcus* (range, 60.5%-97.0%), whereas the 14 type II samples had a mean of 30.0% (range, 8.0%- 46.5%) ($P < 1x10^{-10}$). The mean of relative abundance of *Streptococcus* in the normal esophagus group (75.9%) was significantly higher than that in the esophagitis (50.5%) and BE (54.1%) groups (Table 3) (Figure 3).

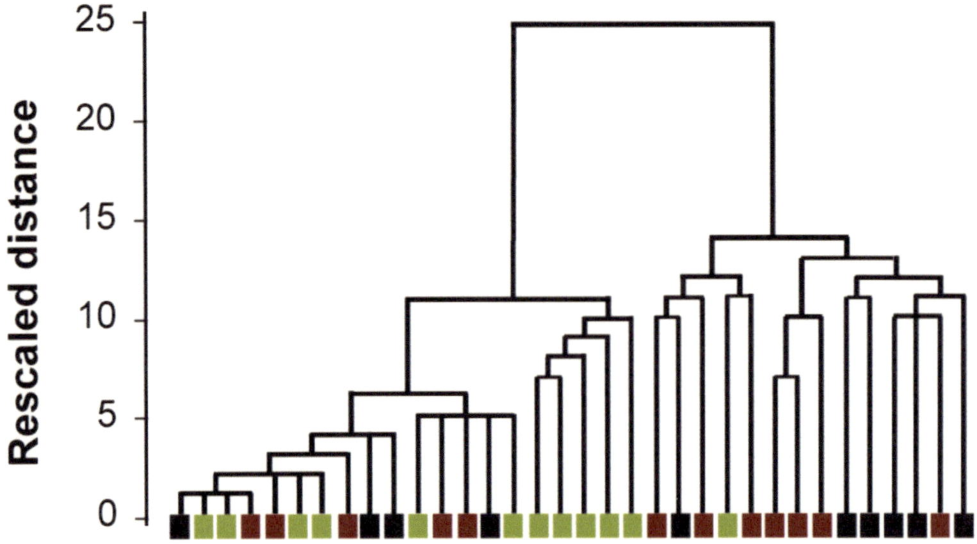

Fig. 2. Typing of esophageal microbiome. Detection of natural microbiome groups by unsupervised cluster analysis. The dendrogram was constructed using the average linkage algorithm and cosine measure of the genetic distance calculated from samples of the microbiome. Samples are represented by colored rectangles (green for normal, red for esophagitis, and black for Barrett's esophagus).

Omnibus test[A]							
Groups compared		Phenotype					
		Normal		Esophagitis		BE[B]	
Microbiome type	I	11		5		4	
	II	1		7		6	
P value		0.0173					
Follow-up tests[C]							
Groups compared		Phenotype					
		Normal	Esophagitis	Normal	BE	Esophagitis	BE
Microbiome type	I	11	5	11	4	5	4
	II	1	7	1	6	7	6
P value		0.027*		0.020*		1.000	
Odds ratio (95% C.I.)		15.4 (1.5-161.0)		16.5 (1.5-183.1)		1.1 (0.2-5.9)	

[A] The Omnibus test was performed using the two-tailed Fisher-Freeman-Halton 3 x 2 probability test.

[B] BE, Barrett's esophagus.

[C] The follow-up tests were performed with the two-tailed Fisher exact 2 x 2 probability test.
Tests that are statistically different at the false discovery rate < 5% [21] are marked by *.

Table 2. Association between host phenotypes and microbiome types in the distal esophagus

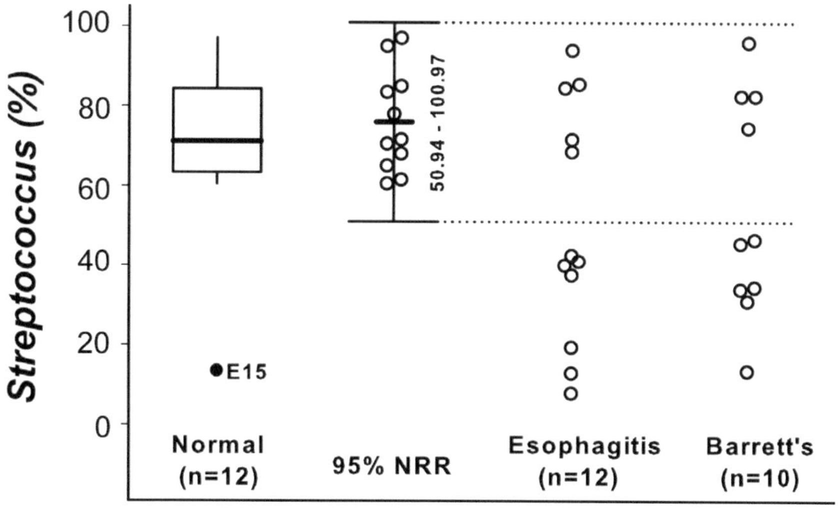

Fig. 3. Taxonomic definition of microbiome types. Classification of microbiome by the relative abundance of *Streptococcus*. An outlier (solid circle) was excluded using a box plot in which the upper whisker length is 1.5*IQR. The 95% normal reference range (NRR) (mean ± 1.96 S.D.) was calculated by the relative abundance of *Streptococcus* after excluding the outlier. The dotted line (50.3%) is the upper limit of the 95% normal reference range (NRR), which separates the 34 samples into normal (inside the NRR) and abnormal taxonomic types (outside the NRR).

Omnibus test[a]			
Groups compared	Phenotype		
	Normal[b] (n=11)	Esophagitis (n=12)	BE (n=10)
Relative abundance (%)	75.9	50.5	54.1
P value	0.043		

Follow-up tests[c]						
Groups compared	Phenotype					
	Normal	Esophagitis	Normal	BE	Esophagitis	BE
Relative abundance (%)	75.9	50.5	75.9		50.5	54.1
P value	0.016*		0.029*		0.773	

[a] The Omnibus test was performed using one-way ANOVA.
[b] An outlier (E15) in the normal group was not included in comparisons between esophageal phenotypic groups.
[c] The follow-up tests were performed with two-tailed independent *t*-test. Tests that are statistically different at the false discovery rate < 5% are marked by *.

Table 3. Comparisons of histological phenotypes in relative abundance of *Streptococcus*

In the disease-associated type II microbiome, the decrease in the relative abundance of *Streptococcus* is compensated by an increase in the relative abundance of 24 other genera. Specifically, the most prominent increase involves *Veillonella, Prevotella, Haemophilus, Neisseria, Rothia, Granulicatella, Campylobacter, Porphyromonas, Fusobacterium,* and *Actinomyces,* many of which are Gram-negative anaerobes or microaerophiles and are putative pathogens for periodontal disease. Anaerobic (type I: 11.0% vs. type II: 38.2%, P = 1.2 x 10^{-5}) and microaerophilic bacteria (5.4% vs. 23.0%, p= 1.1 x 10^{-4}) are more abundant in the type II microbiome than in the type I microbiome (Figure 4A). Gram-negative bacteria comprise 53.4% of type II microbiome but only 14.9% of type I microbiome (p= 8.0 x 10^{-10}) (Figure 4B). Overall, the type II microbiome is significantly more diverse (Shannon-Wiener diversity index mean of 2.69 vs. 1.51, P = 1.3 x 10 -7) and more even (Shannon-Wiener evenness index mean 0.78 vs. 0.51, P = 4.2 x 10-8) than the type I microbiome (Figure 5).

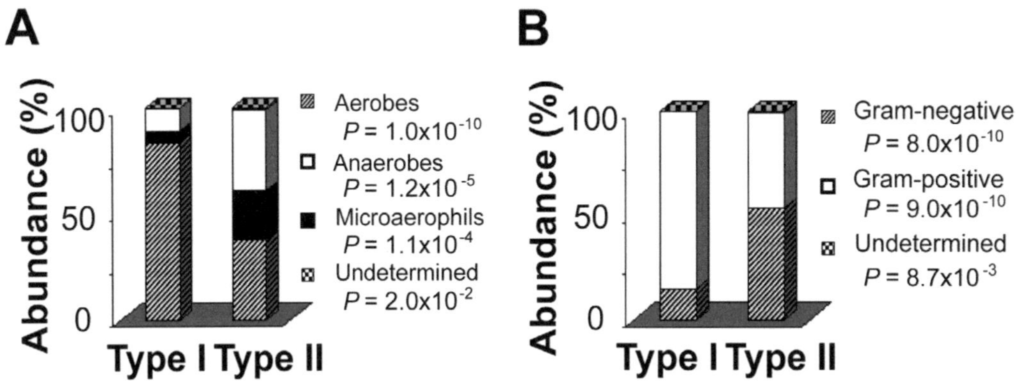

Fig. 4. Taxonomic characterization of microbiome by population of main bacterial groups. Comparisons of microbiome types according to culture conditions (Panel A) and staining properties (Panel B).

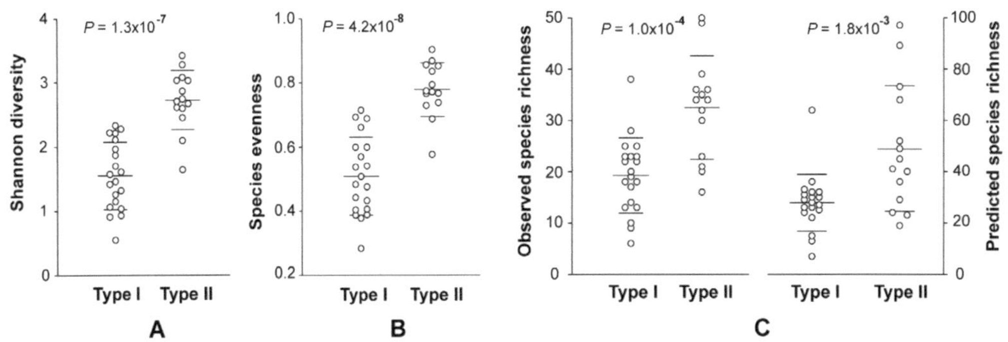

Fig. 5. Difference between the 2 types of microbiome in biologic diversity. (A) Shannon-Wiener diversity index. (B) Shannon-Wiener evenness index. (C) Richness by observed and estimated SLOTUs (Chao, 1984). Mean ± 1.96 SD is indicated by *horizontal lines.*

The type II microbiome appears to be the strongest (*OR* >15) amongst all known environmental factors that are associated with the pathological changes related to gastroesophageal reflux (Table 4). This finding has opened a new approach to

Category	Subcategory	Predictive factor	Predicted outcome (defining method)	Sample size	Odds ratio	95% C.I.	Reference
Host	Genetic	Immediate relatives	Heartburn (questionnaire)	1,524	2.6	1.8-3.7	Locke, 1999
		Parental family history		3,920	1.5	1.2-1.7	Mohammed, 2005
	Aging	Increasing age	GERD (ICD-9 code)	163,085	1.1	1.0-1.1	Kotzan, 2001
	Structural	Hiatus hernia			4.2	2.8-6.3	
			BE (histology)	457	3.9	2.5-6.0	Conio, 2001
			Esophagitis (endoscopy)	451	2.4	1.5-4.0	
		Papillae elongation	Heartburn (medical record)	1,128	2.2	1.5-3.2	Voutilainen, 2000
	Symptomatic	Heartburn/regurgitation	Esophagitis (endoscopy)	451	9.4	6.1-14.4	Ruigomez, 2004
			BE (histology)	457	5.8	4.0-8.4	
	Comorbid	Gallbladder disease	GERD (ICD-8 codes)	7,451	3.7	2.1-6.7	Ruigomez, 2004
		Asthma	GERD (ICD-9 code)	163,085	3.2	2.6-4.0	Kotzan, 2001
		Angina	GERD (ICD-8 codes)	7,451	3.2	2.1-4.9	Ruigomez, 2004
		Obesity	GERD (ICD-9 code)	163,085	2.8	2.1-3.6	Kotzan, 2001
		Peptic ulcer disease	GERD (ICD-8 codes)	7,451	2.5	1.7-3.6	Ruigomez, 2004
		Chest pain			2.3	1.8-2.8	
		Cough			1.7	1.4-2.1	
		Irritable bowel syndrome			1.6	1.2-2.1	
Environment	Behavioral	Tobacco	GERD (ICD-9 code)	163,085	2.6	1.9-3.5	Kotzan, 2001
		Alcohol			1.8	1.4-2.4	
	Medical	NSAID			1.8	1.6-2.1	
		Anticholinergic drug	Heartburn (questionnaire)	3,920	1.5	1.1-2.1	Mohammed, 2005
		Nitrates	GERD (ICD-8 codes)	7,451	1.5	1.1-2.0	Ruigomez, 2004
		Oral steroids			1.3	1.1-1.6	
	Bacterial	Type II microbiome	Esophagitis (histology)	24	15.4	1.5-161.0	Yang, 2009
			BE (histology)	22	16.5	1.5-183.1	

NSAID: Nonsteroidal anti-inflammatory drug.
GERD: gastroesophageal reflux disease.
BE: Barrett's esophagus.
ICD: international classification of diseases.
ICD-8 codes for GERD: gastroesophageal reflux, esophagitis, esophageal inflammation, or heartburn.
ICD-9 code for GERD: not specified in detail.

Table 4. Comparison of the type II microbiome with known risk factors in gastroesophageal reflux disorders

understanding the recent surge in the incidence/prevalence of GERD, BE and EAC, and suggest the possible role of dysbiosis in their pathogenesis. The diverse type II community with its larger content of Gram-negative bacteria might engage innate immune functions of the epithelial cells in a different way than the type I microbiome, owing to the release of a larger spectrum of microbial components, such as lipopolysaccharide (LPS) of Gram-negative bacteria stimulating pattern receptors (eg, Toll-like receptors). Furthermore, the type II microbiome that contains significant numbers of potential pathogens, such as *Campylobacter, Veillonella, Prevotella, Haemophilus, Neisseria, Porphyromonas, Fusobacterium, and Actinomyces* and a significantly higher percentage of Gram-negative bacteria, might play a role with relevance in the maintenance of inflammation. On the other hand, the type II microbiome might be secondary to changes caused by gastric reflux. The type I microbiome could represent a direct extension of the normal oral microbiome via saliva while the type II microbiome could represent regurgitated bacteria in gastric juice or a microbiome modified gastric acid by selecting against acid-sensitive bacteria in the esophagus. However, at this stage, it is unclear whether the presence of type II microbiome (or the absence of type I bacteria) plays a causal role in the pathogenesis of esophageal inflammation or BE. These hypotheses will have to be addressed by future studies, which should be conducted with a prospective design and involve a finer characterization of the microbiomes (Suerbaum, 2009). The microbiome alteration from type I to type II might prove to be an important step in the pathogenesis of esophageal tumorigenesis, and represent a biologically more plausible microbial component in GERD-BE-EAC progression. Consequently, it is essential to assess the type II microbiome and/or numbers of its potential pathogens as either a sole or a panel of biomarkers in order to decipher its relevance in GERD-BE-EAC progression.

6. Prognostic value of biomarkers

As discussed, biomarkers have an important role during the transition of BE to EAC. However, the diagnosis of dysplasia is still the principal marker that is monitored by endoscopic surveillance biopsies, with the aim of intervening prior to invasive adenocarcinoma. The shortcomings of this algorithm include undiagnosed disease, an unproven reduction in population mortality, and unnecessary surveillance. In addition, the current staging of EAC is based exclusively on the anatomical extent of the disease, and the tumor depth (T), lymph nodes involved (N), and the presence or absence of metastases (M); the TNM system. Despite the great number of relevant biomarkers that have been described, none are yet incorporated in a clear prognostic model in EAC. Much investigation is currently underway to identify prognostic biomarkers that may determine the best therapeutic course in this disease.

The development of cancer is generally accepted as being categorized by essential alterations in cell physiology that, when combined, dictate neoplasia: self-sufficiency in growth signals, insensitivity to antigrowth signals, evasion of apoptosis, limitless replicative potential, sustained angiogenesis, and tissue invasion and metastasis (Hanahan and Weinberg, 2000). For EAC, each of these physiologic changes is associated with relevant biomarkers that have been examined for prognostic potential. Two recent reviews detail the prognostic evidence of biomarkers by using these categories of mechanisms (Lagarde et al., 2007; Ong et al., 2010).

Several biomarkers are known to enable self-sufficiency in growth signals, and could have a vital impact on the different phenotypes of EAC. In a study of 124 EAC specimens, two of three specific genotypes of cyclin D1 were found to be predictive of overall survival time (Izzo et al., 2007). In addition, several studies have looked at the prognostic relevance of EGF and TGF-α, two growth factors that bind to the EGFR. TGF-α protein expression has been shown to be significantly associated with tumor progression and lymph node metastasis (D'Errico et al., 2000). Alternatively, in patients with node-negative esophageal cancer, low-level expression of TGF-α is associated with a worse prognosis (Aloia et al., 2001). These apparently conflicting findings are further complicated by studies of EGFR expression in EAC specimens, as one study showed a trend in its multivariate analysis towards expression and decreased survival, (Wang et al., 2007) and another showed significantly poorer survival in association with decreased expression in a univariate analysis (Langer et al., 2006). The mechanisms behind these seemingly discordant findings of the expression of EGFR and its related growth factors are yet to be elucidated. Furthermore, an oncogene HER-2/neu related to EGFR has been shown to significantly correlate with poorer survival in EAC, and may have independent prognostic significance (Brien et al., 2000).

Other biomarkers are thought to act in progression of EAC by insensitivity to growth-inhibitory signals, including TGF-β and APC. For TGF-β, there is some correlation on univariate analysis that overexpression of the gene is associated with depth of tumor infiltration, nodal involvement, and lymphatic vessel invasion, in addition to having a significant negative impact on survival (von Rahden et al., 2006). This evidence was reinforced in a intraoperative study of the mean levels of TGF-β1 from the azygos vein in patients with esophageal cancer, as higher levels significantly correlated with poorer survival. However, the majority of these cancers were esophageal squamous cell carcinoma, as opposed to adenocarcinoma (Fukuchi et al., 2004). The APC gene, a biomarker well known for its relationship with colon adenocarcinoma, has also been studied in esophageal carcinomas. One study found a dramatic and significant increase in the methylation of APC DNA in the plasma of patients with EAC, and this was associated with reduced patient survival (Kawakami et al., 2000).

Other potential predictive biomarkers in EAC are those that affect cell cycle arrest and the evasion of apoptosis. Immunohistochemical expression of both P21 and P53 have been studied in patients with EAC before and after treatment with chemotherapy. Some data suggests that loss of P53, surprisingly, and gain in expression of P21 have both correlated with better response to chemotherapy and survival (Heeren et al., 2004). The Bcl-2 family of genes have been well studied as apoptotic regulators of programmed cell death in several malignancies. In EAC, data show that expression of Bcl-2 is ultimately associated with improved survival, but does not predict response before neoadjuvant chemotherapy, suggesting a reliance on other factors in guiding response to this therapy (Raouf et al., 2003). Furthermore, NF-κβ, presumably by involvement in apoptosis, has been shown in a study of esophageal carcinoma specimens, with the vast majority being adenocarcinoma, to be activated and then significantly associated with overall and disease free survival after chemotherapy (Izzo et al., 2006).

The expression of COX-2, a marker of induction of apoptosis as well as increased angiogenesis, has shown promise in predicting prognosis in EAC. An original study of the intensity of immunohistochemical staining for COX-2 in EAC specimens revealed a significant association of higher COX-2 expression and amount of distant metastases, local recurrences, and decreased survival (Buskens et al., 2002). Poorer survival with increased COX-2 expression was substantiated in a smaller study of specimens from patients who underwent esophagectomy and either died within one year, or survived three years (France et al., 2004). Finally, a later study of 100 surgically resected specimens of EAC showed significant correlation of COX-2 expression and higher T stage, N stage, risk of tumor recurrence, and overall decreased survival (Bhandari et al., 2006).

Another mechanism thought necessary for neoplastic transformation is the acquisition of limitless replicative potential, as tumors stabilize their telomeres and halt the limited number of pre-defined cell divisions before growth arrest. In a study of 46 patients with resection of Barrett's related esophageal adenocarcinoma, telomere length was studied by Southern blot analysis. The telomere-length ratio of neoplastic to normal tissue was correlated with overall survival, as patients with higher ratios had significantly poorer survival (Gertler et al., 2008).

Angiogenesis is another necessary capability of malignant tumors, and its development has also been studied in regards to prognosis of EAC. CD105, or endoglin, as well as VEGF are both known factors that perform a major role in angiogenesis. In a study of 75 patients and specimens from esophagectomies to treat adenocarcinoma, endoglin or VEGF staining of microvessels was used to account for angiogenesis. Both endoglin and VEGF showed a prognostic significance and positive correlation with angiolymphatic invasion, lymph node metastases, and poorer survival (Saad et al., 2005).

The last classic mechanism thought to be vital for neoplastic transformation is tissue invasion and metastasis. Potential prognostic biomarkers involved in this invasion in EAC include the cell adhesion molecule E-cadherin, as well as uPA and TIMP-3, proteins involved in breaking down or preserving the extracellular matrix, respectively. Reduced levels of E-cadherin, by immunohistochemical staining of 59 Barrett's related esophageal adenocarcinoma specimens, was associated with significantly poorer prognosis (Falkenback et al., 2008). By also contributing to invasiveness of tumor cells, higher uPA expression was shown to be correlated with poorer survival, and correspondingly, in another study loss of TIMP-3 correlated with poorer survival and higher disease stage (Darnton et al., 2005; Nekarda et al., 1998).

Several of the aforementioned biomarkers are promising in deciphering prognosis in EAC, and show an association with tumor invasiveness or patient survival. However, the evidence for each individual marker has typically not been well replicated, and molecularly it is unlikely that any of these markers can correctly predict survival on their own, as many of the alterations are related. More recently, microarray technology has allowed for molecular signatures that examine several targets simultaneously. This is a rapidly evolving area of research, and several studies have already examined molecular signatures in EAC in order to attempt to accurately prognosticate.

The studies using microarray technology to generate molecular prognostic signatures for EAC have also attempted to externally validate their findings. One study on 75 resected esophageal specimens generated a set of four genes found to be prognostic at the protein level, which allows for more clinical applicability. This molecular signature was found to be significantly predictive of survival based on the amount of genes dysregulated, and was externally validated in a cohort of 371 cases (Peters et al., 2010). Other studies have not shown such promising results, as a study attempting to generate a prognostic gene expression profile for lymphatic dissemination in EAC was unsuccessful, but did identify an importance of argininosuccinate synthetase (ASS) in the development of this lymphatic dissemination (Lagarde et al., 2008). Microarray technology has also shown its potential for unexpected, though potentially important, results. In looking at response to neoadjuvant chemotherapy in EAC with microarray technology, one study showed a total of 86 genes that were differentially regulated , with the strongest difference in gene expression found with the gene encoding the ephrin B3 receptor, a tyrosine kinase receptor primarily described in the nervous system (Schauer et al., 2010).

In addition to the above methods of microarray technology, other approaches have been used to develop molecular signatures important in the prognosis of EAC. One study used protein expression profiling on 34 patients who underwent surgical resection for locally advanced EAC, and found a significant association between decreased expression of a particular protein, heat shock protein 27 (HSP27), and nonresponse to neoadjuvant chemotherapy. As overexpression of HSP27 has been shown to be associated with resistance to chemotherapy in several other cancers, including esophageal squamous cell carcinoma, this is a novel finding that needs to be further studied (Langer et al., 2008). Another study looked at a panel of genetic polymorphisms on survival outcomes in 210 esophageal carcinoma patients treated with fluorouracil, with 83% having adenocarcinoma. The study found five polymorphisms in three genes significantly associated with decreased recurrences and related disease free survival (Wu et al., 2006). Yet another study analyzed microRNA expression in 100 EAC patients, and found that reduced levels of microRNA-375 was associated with worse survival, suggesting a need for further study of microRNAs in the prognosis of this disease (Mathe et al., 2009). Finally, in a novel study looking at the total number of chromosomal aberrations in specimens of EAC using a multiplex ligation-dependent probe amplification technique, a significant negative correlation between patient survival and total number of aberrations was found. This finding may provide a more general, but still important, indicator of disease outcome (Pasello et al., 2009).

7. Conclusion

Overall, a lot of interest has been given to the study of biomarkers in EAC development, and to both identify prognostic indicators as well as guide therapy. Despite the large number of researched biomarkers showing a correlation with survival in EAC, it is unlikely that a single biomarker will adequately predict prognosis and survival in this disease. The wealth of data using traditional methods, in conjunction with new technologies geared towards molecular signatures, have identified both individual and panels of biomarkers important in predicting neoplastic transformation. However large-scale prospective cohorts are still needed to validate these biomarkers or molecular/microbiome signatures in development. Ultimately, these prognostic biomarkers will hopefully be incorporated into a model that can help with clinical management of patients with EAC.

8. Acknowledgements

Supported by grants from the National Cancer Institute and the National Institute for Allergy and Infectious Diseases K23CA107123, UH3CA140233, R01CA159036, R01AI063477, U19DE018385, as well as the RWJ Amos Medical Faculty Development Program.

9. References

Abbas, T., and Dutta, A. (2009). p21 in cancer: intricate networks and multiple activities. Nat Rev Cancer *9*, 400-414.

Aloia, T.A., Harpole, D.H., Jr., Reed, C.E., Allegra, C., Moore, M.B., Herndon, J.E., 2nd, and D'Amico, T.A. (2001). Tumor marker expression is predictive of survival in patients with esophageal cancer. Ann Thorac Surg *72*, 859-866.

Arber, N., Lightdale, C., Rotterdam, H., Han, K.H., Sgambato, A., Yap, E., Ahsan, H., Finegold, J., Stevens, P.D., Green, P.H., *et al.* (1996). Increased expression of the cyclin D1 gene in Barrett's esophagus. Cancer Epidemiol Biomarkers Prev *5*, 457-459.

Azuma, T., Suto, H., Ito, Y., Muramatsu, A., Ohtani, M., Dojo, M., Yamazaki, Y., Kuriyama, M., and Kato, T. (2002). Eradication of Helicobacter pylori infection induces an increase in body mass index. Aliment Pharmacol Ther *16 Suppl 2*, 240-244.

Baatar, D., Jones, M.K., Pai, R., Kawanaka, H., Szabo, I.L., Moon, W.S., Kitano, S., and Tarnawski, A.S. (2002). Selective cyclooxygenase-2 blocker delays healing of esophageal ulcers in rats and inhibits ulceration-triggered c-Met/hepatocyte growth factor receptor induction and extracellular signal-regulated kinase 2 activation. Am J Pathol *160*, 963-972.

Balish, E., and Warner, T. (2002). Enterococcus faecalis induces inflammatory bowel disease in interleukin-10 knockout mice. Am J Pathol *160*, 2253-2257.

Bani-Hani, K., Martin, I.G., Hardie, L.J., Mapstone, N., Briggs, J.A., Forman, D., and Wild, C.P. (2000). Prospective study of cyclin D1 overexpression in Barrett's esophagus: association with increased risk of adenocarcinoma. J Natl Cancer Inst *92*, 1316-1321.

Barthold, S.W., and Jonas, A.M. (1977). Morphogenesis of early 1, 2-dimethylhydrazine-induced lesions and latent period reduction of colon carcinogenesis in mice by a variant of Citrobacter freundii. Cancer Res *37*, 4352-4360.

Beales, I.L., and Ogunwobi, O.O. (2007). Leptin synergistically enhances the anti-apoptotic and growth-promoting effects of acid in OE33 oesophageal adenocarcinoma cells in culture. Mol Cell Endocrinol *274*, 60-68.

Bechi, P., Balzi, M., Becciolini, A., Maugeri, A., Raggi, C.C., Amorosi, A., and Dei, R. (1996). Helicobacter pylori and cell proliferation of the gastric mucosa: possible implications for gastric carcinogenesis. Am J Gastroenterol *91*, 271-276.

Beebe, J.L., and Koneman, E.W. (1995). Recovery of uncommon bacteria from blood: association with neoplastic disease. Clin Microbiol Rev *8*, 336-356.

Bhandari, P., Bateman, A.C., Mehta, R.L., Stacey, B.S., Johnson, P., Cree, I.A., Di Nicolantonio, F., and Patel, P. (2006). Prognostic significance of cyclooxygenase-2 (COX-2) expression in patients with surgically resectable adenocarcinoma of the oesophagus. BMC Cancer *6*, 134.

Bian, Y.S., Osterheld, M.C., Bosman, F.T., Fontolliet, C., and Benhattar, J. (2000). Nuclear accumulation of beta-catenin is a common and early event during neoplastic progression of Barrett esophagus. Am J Clin Pathol *114*, 583-590.

Bian, Y.S., Osterheld, M.C., Fontolliet, C., Bosman, F.T., and Benhattar, J. (2002). p16 inactivation by methylation of the CDKN2A promoter occurs early during neoplastic progression in Barrett's esophagus. Gastroenterology *122*, 1113-1121.

Blaser, M.J., Perez-Perez, G.I., Kleanthous, H., Cover, T.L., Peek, R.M., Chyou, P.H., Stemmermann, G.N., and Nomura, A. (1995). Infection with Helicobacter pylori strains possessing cagA is associated with an increased risk of developing adenocarcinoma of the stomach. Cancer Res *55*, 2111-2115.

Bourboulia, D., and Stetler-Stevenson, W.G. (2010). Matrix metalloproteinases (MMPs) and tissue inhibitors of metalloproteinases (TIMPs): Positive and negative regulators in tumor cell adhesion. Semin Cancer Biol *20*, 161-168.

Bray, G.A. (1992). Obesity increases risk for diabetes. Int J Obes Relat Metab Disord *16 Suppl 4*, S13-17.

Brien, T.P., Odze, R.D., Sheehan, C.E., McKenna, B.J., and Ross, J.S. (2000). HER-2/neu gene amplification by FISH predicts poor survival in Barrett's esophagus-associated adenocarcinoma. Hum Pathol *31*, 35-39.

Brown, L.M., Swanson, C.A., Gridley, G., Swanson, G.M., Schoenberg, J.B., Greenberg, R.S., Silverman, D.T., Pottern, L.M., Hayes, R.B., Schwartz, A.G., *et al.* (1995). Adenocarcinoma of the esophagus: role of obesity and diet. J Natl Cancer Inst *87*, 104-109.

Buckley, M.F., Sweeney, K.J., Hamilton, J.A., Sini, R.L., Manning, D.L., Nicholson, R.I., deFazio, A., Watts, C.K., Musgrove, E.A., and Sutherland, R.L. (1993). Expression and amplification of cyclin genes in human breast cancer. Oncogene *8*, 2127-2133.

Burnat, G., Rau, T., Elshimi, E., Hahn, E.G., and Konturek, P.C. (2007). Bile acids induce overexpression of homeobox gene CDX-2 and vascular endothelial growth factor (VEGF) in human Barrett's esophageal mucosa and adenocarcinoma cell line. Scand J Gastroenterol *42*, 1460-1465.

Buskens, C.J., Van Rees, B.P., Sivula, A., Reitsma, J.B., Haglund, C., Bosma, P.J., Offerhaus, G.J., Van Lanschot, J.J., and Ristimaki, A. (2002). Prognostic significance of elevated cyclooxygenase 2 expression in patients with adenocarcinoma of the esophagus. Gastroenterology *122*, 1800-1807.

Buttar, N.S., and Wang, K.K. (2004). Mechanisms of disease: Carcinogenesis in Barrett's esophagus. Nat Clin Pract Gastroenterol Hepatol *1*, 106-112.

Buttar, N.S., Wang, K.K., Leontovich, O., Westcott, J.Y., Pacifico, R.J., Anderson, M.A., Krishnadath, K.K., Lutzke, L.S., and Burgart, L.J. (2002). Chemoprevention of esophageal adenocarcinoma by COX-2 inhibitors in an animal model of Barrett's esophagus. Gastroenterology *122*, 1101-1112.

Chao, A. (1984). Nonparametric-Estimation of the Number of Classes in a Population. Scand J Stat *11*, 265-270.

Cheng, M., Sexl, V., Sherr, C.J., and Roussel, M.F. (1998). Assembly of cyclin D-dependent kinase and titration of p27Kip1 regulated by mitogen-activated protein kinase kinase (MEK1). Proc Natl Acad Sci U S A *95*, 1091-1096.

Cheong, E., Igali, L., Harvey, I., Mole, M., Lund, E., Johnson, I.T., and Rhodes, M. (2003). Cyclo-oxygenase-2 expression in Barrett's oesophageal carcinogenesis: an immunohistochemical study. Aliment Pharmacol Ther *17*, 379-386.

Chirco, R., Liu, X.W., Jung, K.K., and Kim, H.R. (2006). Novel functions of TIMPs in cell signaling. Cancer Metastasis Rev *25*, 99-113.

Chow, W.H., Blot, W.J., Vaughan, T.L., Risch, H.A., Gammon, M.D., Stanford, J.L., Dubrow, R., Schoenberg, J.B., Mayne, S.T., Farrow, D.C., *et al.* (1998). Body mass index and risk of adenocarcinomas of the esophagus and gastric cardia. J Natl Cancer Inst *90,* 150-155.

Chu, F.F., Esworthy, R.S., Chu, P.G., Longmate, J.A., Huycke, M.M., Wilczynski, S., and Doroshow, J.H. (2004). Bacteria-induced intestinal cancer in mice with disrupted Gpx1 and Gpx2 genes. Cancer Res *64,* 962-968.

Clement, G., Braunschweig, R., Pasquier, N., Bosman, F.T., and Benhattar, J. (2006a). Alterations of the Wnt signaling pathway during the neoplastic progression of Barrett's esophagus. Oncogene *25,* 3084-3092.

Clement, G., Braunschweig, R., Pasquier, N., Bosman, F.T., and Benhattar, J. (2006b). Methylation of APC, TIMP3, and TERT: a new predictive marker to distinguish Barrett's oesophagus patients at risk for malignant transformation. J Pathol *208,* 100-107.

Conio, M., Filiberti, R., Blanchi, S., Ferraris, R., Marchi, S., Ravelli, P., Lapertosa, G., Iaquinto, G., Sablich, R., and Giacosa, A., et al. (2001). Risk factors for Barrett's esophagus: a case-control study. Int J Cancer 97, 225-229.

Cook, M.B., Greenwood, D.C., Hardie, L.J., Wild, C.P., and Forman, D. (2008). A systematic review and meta-analysis of the risk of increasing adiposity on Barrett's esophagus. Am J Gastroenterol *103,* 292-300.

Corley, D.A., Kubo, A., Levin, T.R., Block, G., Habel, L., Zhao, W., Leighton, P., Quesenberry, C., Rumore, G.J., and Buffler, P.A. (2007). Abdominal obesity and body mass index as risk factors for Barrett's esophagus. Gastroenterology *133,* 34-41; quiz 311.

Couvelard, A., Paraf, F., Gratio, V., Scoazec, J.Y., Henin, D., Degott, C., and Flejou, J.F. (2000). Angiogenesis in the neoplastic sequence of Barrett's oesophagus. Correlation with VEGF expression. J Pathol *192,* 14-18.

Covacci, A., Censini, S., Bugnoli, M., Petracca, R., Burroni, D., Macchia, G., Massone, A., Papini, E., Xiang, Z., Figura, N., *et al.* (1993). Molecular characterization of the 128-kDa immunodominant antigen of Helicobacter pylori associated with cytotoxicity and duodenal ulcer. Proc Natl Acad Sci U S A *90,* 5791-5795.

Cronin, J., McAdam, E., Danikas, A., Tselepis, C., Griffiths, P., Baxter, J., Thomas, L., Manson, J., and Jenkins, G. (2011). Epidermal growth factor receptor (EGFR) is overexpressed in high-grade dysplasia and adenocarcinoma of the esophagus and may represent a biomarker of histological progression in Barrett's esophagus (BE). Am J Gastroenterol *106,* 46-56.

Cruz-Munoz, W., and Khokha, R. (2008). The role of tissue inhibitors of metalloproteinases in tumorigenesis and metastasis. Crit Rev Clin Lab Sci *45,* 291-338.

Cunningham-Rundles, S., Ahrn, S., Abuav-Nussbaum, R., and Dnistrian, A. (2002). Development of immunocompetence: role of micronutrients and microorganisms. Nutr Rev *60,* S68-72.

Curvers, W.L., ten Kate, F.J., Krishnadath, K.K., Visser, M., Elzer, B., Baak, L.C., Bohmer, C., Mallant-Hent, R.C., van Oijen, A., Naber, A.H., *et al.* (2010). Low-grade dysplasia in Barrett's esophagus: overdiagnosed and underestimated. Am J Gastroenterol *105,* 1523-1530.

D'Errico, A., Barozzi, C., Fiorentino, M., Carella, R., Di Simone, M., Ferruzzi, L., Mattioli, S., and Grigioni, W.F. (2000). Role and new perspectives of transforming growth factor-alpha (TGF-alpha) in adenocarcinoma of the gastro-oesophageal junction. Br J Cancer *82*, 865-870.

Darnton, S.J., Hardie, L.J., Muc, R.S., Wild, C.P., and Casson, A.G. (2005). Tissue inhibitor of metalloproteinase-3 (TIMP-3) gene is methylated in the development of esophageal adenocarcinoma: loss of expression correlates with poor prognosis. Int J Cancer *115*, 351-358.

de Martel, C., Haggerty, T.D., Corley, D.A., Vogelman, J.H., Orentreich, N., and Parsonnet, J. (2007). Serum ghrelin levels and risk of subsequent adenocarcinoma of the esophagus. Am J Gastroenterol *102*, 1166-1172.

Diehl, J.A., and Sherr, C.J. (1997). A dominant-negative cyclin D1 mutant prevents nuclear import of cyclin-dependent kinase 4 (CDK4) and its phosphorylation by CDK-activating kinase. Mol Cell Biol *17*, 7362-7374.

Dvoyrin, V.V., Sorokina, I.T., Mashinsky, V.M., Ischakova, L.D., Dianov, E.M., Kalashnikov, V.L., Yashkov, M.V., Khopin, V.F., and Guryanov, A.N. (2011). Tm3+-doped CW fiber laser based on a highly GeO2-doped dispersion-shifted fiber. Opt Express *19*, 7992-7999.

Eckburg, P.B., Bik, E.M., Bernstein, C.N., Purdom, E., Dethlefsen, L., Sargent, M., Gill, S.R., Nelson, K.E., and Relman, D.A. (2005). Diversity of the human intestinal microbial flora. Science *308*, 1635-1638.

Edelstein, Z.R., Farrow, D.C., Bronner, M.P., Rosen, S.N., and Vaughan, T.L. (2007). Central adiposity and risk of Barrett's esophagus. Gastroenterology *133*, 403-411.

Eisen, G.M., Sandler, R.S., Murray, S., and Gottfried, M. (1997). The relationship between gastroesophageal reflux disease and its complications with Barrett's esophagus. Am J Gastroenterol *92*, 27-31.

El-Omar, E.M., Rabkin, C.S., Gammon, M.D., Vaughan, T.L., Risch, H.A., Schoenberg, J.B., Stanford, J.L., Mayne, S.T., Goedert, J., Blot, W.J., *et al.* (2003). Increased risk of noncardia gastric cancer associated with proinflammatory cytokine gene polymorphisms. Gastroenterology *124*, 1193-1201.

El-Serag, H. (2008). Role of obesity in GORD-related disorders. Gut *57*, 281-284.

El-Serag, H.B., Ergun, G.A., Pandolfino, J., Fitzgerald, S., Tran, T., and Kramer, J.R. (2007). Obesity increases oesophageal acid exposure. Gut *56*, 749-755.

El-Serag, H.B., Graham, D.Y., Satia, J.A., and Rabeneck, L. (2005). Obesity is an independent risk factor for GERD symptoms and erosive esophagitis. Am J Gastroenterol *100*, 1243-1250.

El-Serag, H.B., Tran, T., Richardson, P., and Ergun, G. (2006). Anthropometric correlates of intragastric pressure. Scand J Gastroenterol *41*, 887-891.

Eloubeidi, M.A., and Provenzale, D. (2001). Clinical and demographic predictors of Barrett's esophagus among patients with gastroesophageal reflux disease: a multivariable analysis in veterans. J Clin Gastroenterol *33*, 306-309.

Engle, S.J., Ormsby, I., Pawlowski, S., Boivin, G.P., Croft, J., Balish, E., and Doetschman, T. (2002). Elimination of colon cancer in germ-free transforming growth factor beta 1-deficient mice. Cancer Res *62*, 6362-6366.

Erdman, S.E., Poutahidis, T., Tomczak, M., Rogers, A.B., Cormier, K., Plank, B., Horwitz, B.H., and Fox, J.G. (2003). CD4+ CD25+ regulatory T lymphocytes inhibit microbially induced colon cancer in Rag2-deficient mice. Am J Pathol *162*, 691-702.

Evan, G.I., and Vousden, K.H. (2001). Proliferation, cell cycle and apoptosis in cancer. Nature *411*, 342-348.

Falkenback, D., Nilbert, M., Oberg, S., and Johansson, J. (2008). Prognostic value of cell adhesion in esophageal adenocarcinomas. Dis Esophagus *21*, 97-102.

Ferlay, J., Shin, H.R., Bray, F., Forman, D., Mathers, C., and Parkin, D.M. (2010). Estimates of worldwide burden of cancer in 2008: GLOBOCAN 2008. Int J Cancer *127*, 2893-2917.

Figueiredo, C., Machado, J.C., Pharoah, P., Seruca, R., Sousa, S., Carvalho, R., Capelinha, A.F., Quint, W., Caldas, C., van Doorn, L.J., *et al.* (2002). Helicobacter pylori and interleukin 1 genotyping: an opportunity to identify high-risk individuals for gastric carcinoma. J Natl Cancer Inst *94*, 1680-1687.

Fisher, B.L., Pennathur, A., Mutnick, J.L., and Little, A.G. (1999). Obesity correlates with gastroesophageal reflux. Dig Dis Sci *44*, 2290-2294.

Flegal, K.M., Carroll, M.D., Ogden, C.L., and Curtin, L.R. (2010). Prevalence and trends in obesity among US adults, 1999-2008. JAMA *303*, 235-241.

France, M., Drew, P.A., Dodd, T., and Watson, D.I. (2004). Cyclo-oxygenase-2 expression in esophageal adenocarcinoma as a determinant of clinical outcome following esophagectomy. Dis Esophagus *17*, 136-140.

Francois, F., Roper, J., Goodman, A.J., Pei, Z., Ghumman, M., Mourad, M., de Perez, A.Z., Perez-Perez, G.I., Tseng, C.H., and Blaser, M.J. (2008). The association of gastric leptin with oesophageal inflammation and metaplasia. Gut *57*, 16-24.

Fu, M., Rao, M., Bouras, T., Wang, C., Wu, K., Zhang, X., Li, Z., Yao, T.P., and Pestell, R.G. (2005). Cyclin D1 inhibits peroxisome proliferator-activated receptor gamma-mediated adipogenesis through histone deacetylase recruitment. J Biol Chem *280*, 16934-16941.

Fu, M., Wang, C., Li, Z., Sakamaki, T., and Pestell, R.G. (2004). Minireview: Cyclin D1: normal and abnormal functions. Endocrinology *145*, 5439-5447.

Fuccio, L., Eusebi, L.H., Zagari, R.M., and Bazzoli, F. (2009). Helicobacter pylori eradication treatment reduces but does not abolish the risk of gastric cancer. Am J Gastroenterol *104*, 3100; author reply 3101-3102.

Fukuchi, M., Miyazaki, T., Fukai, Y., Nakajima, M., Sohda, M., Masuda, N., Manda, R., Tsukada, K., Kato, H., and Kuwano, H. (2004). Plasma level of transforming growth factor beta1 measured from the azygos vein predicts prognosis in patients with esophageal cancer. Clin Cancer Res *10*, 2738-2741.

Gagliardi, D., Makihara, S., Corsi, P.R., Viana Ade, T., Wiczer, M.V., Nakakubo, S., and Mimica, L.M. (1998). Microbial flora of the normal esophagus. Dis Esophagus *11*, 248-250.

Gartel, A.L. (2006). Is p21 an oncogene? Mol Cancer Ther *5*, 1385-1386.

Gerdes, J. (1990). Ki-67 and other proliferation markers useful for immunohistological diagnostic and prognostic evaluations in human malignancies. Semin Cancer Biol *1*, 199-206.

Gertler, R., Doll, D., Maak, M., Feith, M., and Rosenberg, R. (2008). Telomere length and telomerase subunits as diagnostic and prognostic biomarkers in Barrett carcinoma. Cancer *112*, 2173-2180.

Giles, R.H., van Es, J.H., and Clevers, H. (2003). Caught up in a Wnt storm: Wnt signaling in cancer. Biochim Biophys Acta *1653*, 1-24.

Greenblatt, M.S., Bennett, W.P., Hollstein, M., and Harris, C.C. (1994). Mutations in the p53 tumor suppressor gene: clues to cancer etiology and molecular pathogenesis. Cancer Res *54*, 4855-4878.

Hampel, H., Abraham, N.S., and El-Serag, H.B. (2005). Meta-analysis: obesity and the risk for gastroesophageal reflux disease and its complications. Ann Intern Med *143*, 199-211.

Hanahan, D., and Weinberg, R.A. (2000). The hallmarks of cancer. Cell *100*, 57-70.

Hardie, L.J., Darnton, S.J., Wallis, Y.L., Chauhan, A., Hainaut, P., Wild, C.P., and Casson, A.G. (2005). p16 expression in Barrett's esophagus and esophageal adenocarcinoma: association with genetic and epigenetic alterations. Cancer Lett *217*, 221-230.

Heeren, P.A., Kloppenberg, F.W., Hollema, H., Mulder, N.H., Nap, R.E., and Plukker, J.T. (2004). Predictive effect of p53 and p21 alteration on chemotherapy response and survival in locally advanced adenocarcinoma of the esophagus. Anticancer Res *24*, 2579-2583.

Herbst, J.J., Berenson, M.M., McCloskey, D.W., and Wiser, W.C. (1978). Cell proliferation in esophageal columnar epithelium (Barrett's esophagus). Gastroenterology *75*, 683-687.

Hinds, P.W., Finlay, C.A., Quartin, R.S., Baker, S.J., Fearon, E.R., Vogelstein, B., and Levine, A.J. (1990). Mutant p53 DNA clones from human colon carcinomas cooperate with ras in transforming primary rat cells: a comparison of the "hot spot" mutant phenotypes. Cell Growth Differ *1*, 571-580.

Housa, D., Housova, J., Vernerova, Z., and Haluzik, M. (2006). Adipocytokines and cancer. Physiol Res *55*, 233-244.

Huang, J.Q., Zheng, G.F., Sumanac, K., Irvine, E.J., and Hunt, R.H. (2003). Meta-analysis of the relationship between cagA seropositivity and gastric cancer. Gastroenterology *125*, 1636-1644.

IARC (1994). Schistosomes, liver flukes and Helicobacter pylori. IARC Working Group on the Evaluation of Carcinogenic Risks to Humans. Lyon, 7-14 June 1994. IARC Monogr Eval Carcinog Risks Hum *61*, 1-241.

Islami, F., and Kamangar, F. (2008). Helicobacter pylori and esophageal cancer risk: a meta-analysis. Cancer Prev Res (Phila) *1*, 329-338.

Izzo, J.G., Malhotra, U., Wu, T.T., Ensor, J., Luthra, R., Lee, J.H., Swisher, S.G., Liao, Z., Chao, K.S., Hittelman, W.N., *et al.* (2006). Association of activated transcription factor nuclear factor kappab with chemoradiation resistance and poor outcome in esophageal carcinoma. J Clin Oncol *24*, 748-754.

Izzo, J.G., Wu, T.T., Wu, X., Ensor, J., Luthra, R., Pan, J., Correa, A., Swisher, S.G., Chao, C.K., Hittelman, W.N., *et al.* (2007). Cyclin D1 guanine/adenine 870 polymorphism with altered protein expression is associated with genomic instability and aggressive clinical biology of esophageal adenocarcinoma. J Clin Oncol *25*, 698-707.

Jang, E.J., Park, S.W., Park, J.S., Park, S.J., Hahm, K.B., Paik, S.Y., Sin, M.K., Lee, E.S., Oh, S.W., Park, C.Y., *et al.* (2008). The influence of the eradication of Helicobacter pylori on gastric ghrelin, appetite, and body mass index in patients with peptic ulcer disease. J Gastroenterol Hepatol *23 Suppl 2*, S278-285.

Jiang, Y., Goldberg, I.D., and Shi, Y.E. (2002). Complex roles of tissue inhibitors of metalloproteinases in cancer. Oncogene *21*, 2245-2252.

Jones, A.D., Bacon, K.D., Jobe, B.A., Sheppard, B.C., Deveney, C.W., and Rutten, M.J. (2003). Helicobacter pylori induces apoptosis in Barrett's-derived esophageal adenocarcinoma cells. J Gastrointest Surg *7*, 68-76.

Kado, S., Uchida, K., Funabashi, H., Iwata, S., Nagata, Y., Ando, M., Onoue, M., Matsuoka, Y., Ohwaki, M., and Morotomi, M. (2001). Intestinal microflora are necessary for development of spontaneous adenocarcinoma of the large intestine in T-cell receptor beta chain and p53 double-knockout mice. Cancer Res *61*, 2395-2398.

Kaur, B.S., Khamnehei, N., Iravani, M., Namburu, S.S., Lin, O., and Triadafilopoulos, G. (2002). Rofecoxib inhibits cyclooxygenase 2 expression and activity and reduces cell proliferation in Barrett's esophagus. Gastroenterology *123*, 60-67.

Kawaguchi-Miyashita, M., Shimada, S., Kurosu, H., Kato-Nagaoka, N., Matsuoka, Y., Ohwaki, M., Ishikawa, H., and Nanno, M. (2001). An accessory role of TCRgammadelta (+) cells in the exacerbation of inflammatory bowel disease in TCRalpha mutant mice. Eur J Immunol *31*, 980-988.

Kawakami, K., Brabender, J., Lord, R.V., Groshen, S., Greenwald, B.D., Krasna, M.J., Yin, J., Fleisher, A.S., Abraham, J.M., Beer, D.G., *et al.* (2000). Hypermethylated APC DNA in plasma and prognosis of patients with esophageal adenocarcinoma. J Natl Cancer Inst *92*, 1805-1811.

Kim, J.K., and Diehl, J.A. (2009). Nuclear cyclin D1: an oncogenic driver in human cancer. J Cell Physiol *220*, 292-296.

Kojima, M., and Kangawa, K. (2005). Ghrelin: structure and function. Physiol Rev *85*, 495-522.

Konturek, P.C., Burnat, G., Rau, T., Hahn, E.G., and Konturek, S. (2008). Effect of adiponectin and ghrelin on apoptosis of Barrett adenocarcinoma cell line. Dig Dis Sci *53*, 597-605.

Konturek, P.C., Kania, J., Burnat, G., Hahn, E.G., and Konturek, S.J. (2005). Prostaglandins as mediators of COX-2 derived carcinogenesis in gastrointestinal tract. J Physiol Pharmacol *56 Suppl 5*, 57-73.

Konturek, P.C., Nikiforuk, A., Kania, J., Raithel, M., Hahn, E.G., and Muhldorfer, S. (2004). Activation of NFkappaB represents the central event in the neoplastic progression associated with Barrett's esophagus: a possible link to the inflammation and overexpression of COX-2, PPARgamma and growth factors. Dig Dis Sci *49*, 1075-1083.

Kornbluth, A.A., Danzig, J.B., and Bernstein, L.H. (1989). Clostridium septicum infection and associated malignancy. Report of 2 cases and review of the literature. Medicine (Baltimore) *68*, 30-37.

Kotzan, J., Wade, W., and Yu, H.H. (2001). Assessing NSAID Prescription Use as a Predisposing Factor for Gastroesophageal Reflux Disease in a Medicaid Population. Pharm Res 18,1367-1372.

Krishnadath, K.K., Tilanus, H.W., van Blankenstein, M., Bosman, F.T., and Mulder, A.H. (1995). Accumulation of p53 protein in normal, dysplastic, and neoplastic Barrett's oesophagus. J Pathol *175*, 175-180.

Kubo, A., and Corley, D.A. (2006). Body mass index and adenocarcinomas of the esophagus or gastric cardia: a systematic review and meta-analysis. Cancer Epidemiol Biomarkers Prev *15*, 872-878.

Kuipers, E.J., Perez-Perez, G.I., Meuwissen, S.G., and Blaser, M.J. (1995). Helicobacter pylori and atrophic gastritis: importance of the cagA status. J Natl Cancer Inst *87*, 1777-1780.

Kusters, J.G., van Vliet, A.H., and Kuipers, E.J. (2006). Pathogenesis of Helicobacter pylori infection. Clin Microbiol Rev *19*, 449-490.

LaBaer, J., Garrett, M.D., Stevenson, L.F., Slingerland, J.M., Sandhu, C., Chou, H.S., Fattaey, A., and Harlow, E. (1997). New functional activities for the p21 family of CDK inhibitors. Genes Dev *11*, 847-862.

Lagarde, S.M., ten Kate, F.J., Richel, D.J., Offerhaus, G.J., and van Lanschot, J.J. (2007). Molecular prognostic factors in adenocarcinoma of the esophagus and gastroesophageal junction. Ann Surg Oncol *14*, 977-991.

Lagarde, S.M., Ver Loren van Themaat, P.E., Moerland, P.D., Gilhuijs-Pederson, L.A., Ten Kate, F.J., Reitsma, P.H., van Kampen, A.H., Zwinderman, A.H., Baas, F., and van Lanschot, J.J. (2008). Analysis of gene expression identifies differentially expressed genes and pathways associated with lymphatic dissemination in patients with adenocarcinoma of the esophagus. Ann Surg Oncol *15*, 3459-3470.

Lagergren, J., Bergstrom, R., Lindgren, A., and Nyren, O. (1999a). Symptomatic gastroesophageal reflux as a risk factor for esophageal adenocarcinoma. N Engl J Med *340*, 825-831.

Lagergren, J., Bergstrom, R., and Nyren, O. (1999b). Association between body mass and adenocarcinoma of the esophagus and gastric cardia. Ann Intern Med *130*, 883-890.

Lambert, D.M., Marceau, S., and Forse, R.A. (2005). Intra-abdominal pressure in the morbidly obese. Obes Surg *15*, 1225-1232.

Langer, R., Ott, K., Specht, K., Becker, K., Lordick, F., Burian, M., Herrmann, K., Schrattenholz, A., Cahill, M.A., Schwaiger, M., *et al.* (2008). Protein expression profiling in esophageal adenocarcinoma patients indicates association of heat-shock protein 27 expression and chemotherapy response. Clin Cancer Res *14*, 8279-8287.

Langer, R., Von Rahden, B.H., Nahrig, J., Von Weyhern, C., Reiter, R., Feith, M., Stein, H.J., Siewert, J.R., Hofler, H., and Sarbia, M. (2006). Prognostic significance of expression patterns of c-erbB-2, p53, p16INK4A, p27KIP1, cyclin D1 and epidermal growth factor receptor in oesophageal adenocarcinoma: a tissue microarray study. J Clin Pathol *59*, 631-634.

Lanuti, M., Liu, G., Goodwin, J.M., Zhai, R., Fuchs, B.C., Asomaning, K., Su, L., Nishioka, N.S., Tanabe, K.K., and Christiani, D.C. (2008). A functional epidermal growth factor (EGF) polymorphism, EGF serum levels, and esophageal adenocarcinoma risk and outcome. Clin Cancer Res *14*, 3216-3222.

Laufs, S., Schumacher, J., and Allgayer, H. (2006). Urokinase-receptor (u-PAR): an essential player in multiple games of cancer: a review on its role in tumor progression, invasion, metastasis, proliferation/dormancy, clinical outcome and minimal residual disease. Cell Cycle *5*, 1760-1771.

Lederberg, J., and McCray, A.T. (2001). 'Ome sweet 'omics - A genealogical treasury of words. Scientist *15*, 8-8.

Lehrbach, D.M., Cecconello, I., Ribeiro Jr, U., Capelozzi, V.L., Ab'saber, A.M., and Alves, V.A. (2009). Adenocarcinoma of the esophagogastric junction: relationship between clinicopathological data and p53, cyclin D1 and Bcl-2 immunoexpressions. Arq Gastroenterol *46*, 315-320.

Levine, A.J. (1997). p53, the cellular gatekeeper for growth and division. Cell *88*, 323-331.

Levine, A.J., Hu, W., and Feng, Z. (2006). The P53 pathway: what questions remain to be explored? Cell Death Differ *13*, 1027-1036.

Li, Y., Wo, J.M., Ray, M.B., Jones, W., Su, R.R., Ellis, S., and Martin, R.C. (2006). Cyclooxygenase-2 and epithelial growth factor receptor up-regulation during progression of Barrett's esophagus to adenocarcinoma. World J Gastroenterol *12*, 928-934.

Lipetz, L.E. (1984). A new method for determining peak absorbance of dense pigment samples and its application to the cone oil droplets of Emydoidea blandingii. Vision Res *24*, 567-604.

Liu, Y., Yeh, N., Zhu, X.H., Leversha, M., Cordon-Cardo, C., Ghossein, R., Singh, B., Holland, E., and Koff, A. (2007). Somatic cell type specific gene transfer reveals a tumor-promoting function for p21(Waf1/Cip1). EMBO J *26*, 4683-4693.

Locke, G.R., 3rd, Talley, N.J., Fett, S.L., Zinsmeister, A.R., and Melton, L.J., 3rd (1999). Risk factors associated with symptoms of gastroesophageal reflux. Am J Med *106*, 642-649.

Logan, C.Y., and Nusse, R. (2004). The Wnt signaling pathway in development and disease. Annu Rev Cell Dev Biol *20*, 781-810.

Louw, J.A., Kidd, M.S., Kummer, A.F., Taylor, K., Kotze, U., and Hanslo, D. (2001). The relationship between Helicobacter pylori infection, the virulence genotypes of the infecting strain and gastric cancer in the African setting. Helicobacter *6*, 268-273.

Ma, T., Van Tine, B.A., Wei, Y., Garrett, M.D., Nelson, D., Adams, P.D., Wang, J., Qin, J., Chow, L.T., and Harper, J.W. (2000). Cell cycle-regulated phosphorylation of p220(NPAT) by cyclin E/Cdk2 in Cajal bodies promotes histone gene transcription. Genes Dev *14*, 2298-2313.

Madani, K., Zhao, R., Lim, H.J., and Casson, A.G. (2010). Prognostic value of p53 mutations in oesophageal adenocarcinoma: final results of a 15-year prospective study. Eur J Cardiothorac Surg *37*, 1427-1432.

Maley, C.C., Galipeau, P.C., Li, X., Sanchez, C.A., Paulson, T.G., and Reid, B.J. (2004). Selectively advantageous mutations and hitchhikers in neoplasms: p16 lesions are selected in Barrett's esophagus. Cancer Res *64*, 3414-3427.

Marone, M., Scambia, G., Giannitelli, C., Ferrandina, G., Masciullo, V., Bellacosa, A., Benedetti-Panici, P., and Mancuso, S. (1998). Analysis of cyclin E and CDK2 in ovarian cancer: gene amplification and RNA overexpression. Int J Cancer *75*, 34-39.

Marshall, B.J., and Warren, J.R. (1984). Unidentified curved bacilli in the stomach of patients with gastritis and peptic ulceration. Lancet *1*, 1311-1315.

Masuda, Y., Tanaka, T., Inomata, N., Ohnuma, N., Tanaka, S., Itoh, Z., Hosoda, H., Kojima, M., and Kangawa, K. (2000). Ghrelin stimulates gastric acid secretion and motility in rats. Biochem Biophys Res Commun *276*, 905-908.

Mathe, E.A., Nguyen, G.H., Bowman, E.D., Zhao, Y., Budhu, A., Schetter, A.J., Braun, R., Reimers, M., Kumamoto, K., Hughes, D., *et al.* (2009). MicroRNA expression in squamous cell carcinoma and adenocarcinoma of the esophagus: associations with survival. Clin Cancer Res *15*, 6192-6200.

McMahon, B., and Kwaan, H.C. (2008). The plasminogen activator system and cancer. Pathophysiol Haemost Thromb *36*, 184-194.

Mercer, C.D., Rue, C., Hanelin, L., and Hill, L.D. (1985). Effect of obesity on esophageal transit. Am J Surg *149*, 177-181.

Metzger, R., Schneider, P.M., Warnecke-Eberz, U., Brabender, J., and Holscher, A.H. (2004). Molecular biology of esophageal cancer. Onkologie *27*, 200-206.

Miehlke, S., Yu, J., Schuppler, M., Frings, C., Kirsch, C., Negraszus, N., Morgner, A., Stolte, M., Ehninger, G., and Bayerdorffer, E. (2001). Helicobacter pylori vacA, iceA, and cagA status and pattern of gastritis in patients with malignant and benign gastroduodenal disease. Am J Gastroenterol *96*, 1008-1013.

Miller, C.T., Moy, J.R., Lin, L., Schipper, M., Normolle, D., Brenner, D.E., Iannettoni, M.D., Orringer, M.B., and Beer, D.G. (2003). Gene amplification in esophageal adenocarcinomas and Barrett's with high-grade dysplasia. Clin Cancer Res *9*, 4819-4825.

Mobius, C., Stein, H.J., Becker, I., Feith, M., Theisen, J., Gais, P., Jutting, U., and Siewert, J.R. (2003). The 'angiogenic switch' in the progression from Barrett's metaplasia to esophageal adenocarcinoma. Eur J Surg Oncol *29*, 890-894.

Mohammed, I., Cherkas, L.F., Riley, S.A., Spector, T.D., and Trudgill, N.J. (2005). Genetic influences in irritable bowel syndrome: a twin study. Am J Gastroenterol 100, 1340-1344.

Murray, L., Johnston, B., Lane, A., Harvey, I., Donovan, J., Nair, P., and Harvey, R. (2003). Relationship between body mass and gastro-oesophageal reflux symptoms: The Bristol Helicobacter Project. Int J Epidemiol *32*, 645-650.

Murray, L., Sedo, A., Scott, M., McManus, D., Sloan, J.M., Hardie, L.J., Forman, D., and Wild, C.P. (2006). TP53 and progression from Barrett's metaplasia to oesophageal adenocarcinoma in a UK population cohort. Gut *55*, 1390-1397.

Narikiyo, M., Tanabe, C., Yamada, Y., Igaki, H., Tachimori, Y., Kato, H., Muto, M., Montesano, R., Sakamoto, H., Nakajima, Y., *et al.* (2004). Frequent and preferential infection of Treponema denticola, Streptococcus mitis, and Streptococcus anginosus in esophageal cancers. Cancer Sci *95*, 569-574.

Nekarda, H., Schlegel, P., Schmitt, M., Stark, M., Mueller, J.D., Fink, U., and Siewert, J.R. (1998). Strong prognostic impact of tumor-associated urokinase-type plasminogen activator in completely resected adenocarcinoma of the esophagus. Clin Cancer Res *4*, 1755-1763.

Neuman, E., Ladha, M.H., Lin, N., Upton, T.M., Miller, S.J., DiRenzo, J., Pestell, R.G., Hinds, P.W., Dowdy, S.F., Brown, M., *et al.* (1997). Cyclin D1 stimulation of estrogen receptor transcriptional activity independent of cdk4. Mol Cell Biol *17*, 5338-5347.

Newman, J.V., Kosaka, T., Sheppard, B.J., Fox, J.G., and Schauer, D.B. (2001). Bacterial infection promotes colon tumorigenesis in Apc(Min/+) mice. J Infect Dis *184*, 227-230.

Nishida, M., Funahashi, T., and Shimomura, I. (2007). Pathophysiological significance of adiponectin. Med Mol Morphol *40*, 55-67.

Nwokolo, C.U., Freshwater, D.A., O'Hare, P., and Randeva, H.S. (2003). Plasma ghrelin following cure of Helicobacter pylori. Gut *52*, 637-640.

Nzeako, U.C., Guicciardi, M.E., Yoon, J.H., Bronk, S.F., and Gores, G.J. (2002). COX-2 inhibits Fas-mediated apoptosis in cholangiocarcinoma cells. Hepatology *35*, 552-559.

Ogunwobi, O., Mutungi, G., and Beales, I.L. (2006). Leptin stimulates proliferation and inhibits apoptosis in Barrett's esophageal adenocarcinoma cells by cyclooxygenase-2-dependent, prostaglandin-E2-mediated transactivation of the epidermal growth factor receptor and c-Jun NH2-terminal kinase activation. Endocrinology *147*, 4505-4516.

Ogunwobi, O.O., and Beales, I.L. (2008a). Globular adiponectin, acting via adiponectin receptor-1, inhibits leptin-stimulated oesophageal adenocarcinoma cell proliferation. Mol Cell Endocrinol *285*, 43-50.

Ogunwobi, O.O., and Beales, I.L. (2008b). Leptin stimulates the proliferation of human oesophageal adenocarcinoma cells via HB-EGF and Tgfalpha mediated transactivation of the epidermal growth factor receptor. Br J Biomed Sci *65*, 121-127.

Ong, C.A., Lao-Sirieix, P., and Fitzgerald, R.C. (2010). Biomarkers in Barrett's esophagus and esophageal adenocarcinoma: predictors of progression and prognosis. World J Gastroenterol *16*, 5669-5681.

Onwuegbusi, B.A., Aitchison, A., Chin, S.F., Kranjac, T., Mills, I., Huang, Y., Lao-Sirieix, P., Caldas, C., and Fitzgerald, R.C. (2006). Impaired transforming growth factor beta signalling in Barrett's carcinogenesis due to frequent SMAD4 inactivation. Gut *55*, 764-774.

Onwuegbusi, B.A., Rees, J.R., Lao-Sirieix, P., and Fitzgerald, R.C. (2007). Selective loss of TGFbeta Smad-dependent signalling prevents cell cycle arrest and promotes invasion in oesophageal adenocarcinoma cell lines. PLoS One *2*, e177.

Pandolfino, J.E., El-Serag, H.B., Zhang, Q., Shah, N., Ghosh, S.K., and Kahrilas, P.J. (2006). Obesity: a challenge to esophagogastric junction integrity. Gastroenterology *130*, 639-649.

Panwalker, A.P. (1988). Unusual infections associated with colorectal cancer. Rev Infect Dis *10*, 347-364.

Parkin, D.M., Bray, F., Ferlay, J., and Pisani, P. (2005). Global cancer statistics, 2002. CA Cancer J Clin *55*, 74-108.

Parsonnet, J., Friedman, G.D., Orentreich, N., and Vogelman, H. (1997). Risk for gastric cancer in people with CagA positive or CagA negative Helicobacter pylori infection. Gut *40*, 297-301.

Pasello, G., Agata, S., Bonaldi, L., Corradin, A., Montagna, M., Zamarchi, R., Parenti, A., Cagol, M., Zaninotto, G., Ruol, A., *et al.* (2009). DNA copy number alterations correlate with survival of esophageal adenocarcinoma patients. Mod Pathol *22*, 58-65.

Peek, R.M., Jr., and Blaser, M.J. (2002). Helicobacter pylori and gastrointestinal tract adenocarcinomas. Nat Rev Cancer *2*, 28-37.

Pei, Z., Bini, E.J., Yang, L., Zhou, M., Francois, F., and Blaser, M.J. (2004). Bacterial biota in the human distal esophagus. Proc Natl Acad Sci U S A *101*, 4250-4255.

Pei, Z., Yang, L., Peek, R.M., Jr Levine, S.M., Pride, D.T., and Blaser, M.J. (2005). Bacterial biota in reflux esophagitis and Barrettos esophagus. World J Gastroenterol *11*, 7277-7283.

Pellish, L.J., Hermos, J.A., and Eastwood, G.L. (1980). Cell proliferation in three types of Barrett's epithelium. Gut *21*, 26-31.

Peters, C.J., Rees, J.R., Hardwick, R.H., Hardwick, J.S., Vowler, S.L., Ong, C.A., Zhang, C., Save, V., O'Donovan, M., Rassl, D., *et al.* (2010). A 4-gene signature predicts survival of patients with resected adenocarcinoma of the esophagus, junction, and gastric cardia. Gastroenterology *139*, 1995-2004 e1915.

Petros, A.M., Gunasekera, A., Xu, N., Olejniczak, E.T., and Fesik, S.W. (2004). Defining the p53 DNA-binding domain/Bcl-x(L)-binding interface using NMR. FEBS Lett *559*, 171-174.

Polk, D.B., and Peek, R.M., Jr. (2010). Helicobacter pylori: gastric cancer and beyond. Nat Rev Cancer *10*, 403-414.

Pontiroli, A.E., and Galli, L. (1998). Duration of obesity is a risk factor for non-insulin-dependent diabetes mellitus, not for arterial hypertension or for hyperlipidaemia. Acta Diabetol *35*, 130-136.

Pounder, R.E., and Ng, D. (1995). The prevalence of Helicobacter pylori infection in different countries. Aliment Pharmacol Ther *9 Suppl 2*, 33-39.

Powell, E.L., Leoni, L.M., Canto, M.I., Forastiere, A.A., Iocobuzio-Donahue, C.A., Wang, J.S., Maitra, A., and Montgomery, E. (2005). Concordant loss of MTAP and p16/CDKN2A expression in gastroesophageal carcinogenesis: evidence of homozygous deletion in esophageal noninvasive precursor lesions and therapeutic implications. Am J Surg Pathol *29*, 1497-1504.

Preston-Martin, S., Pike, M.C., Ross, R.K., Jones, P.A., and Henderson, B.E. (1990). Increased cell division as a cause of human cancer. Cancer Res *50*, 7415-7421.

Raghunath, A., Hungin, A.P., Wooff, D., and Childs, S. (2003). Prevalence of Helicobacter pylori in patients with gastro-oesophageal reflux disease: systematic review. BMJ *326*, 737.

Ramel, S., Reid, B.J., Sanchez, C.A., Blount, P.L., Levine, D.S., Neshat, K., Haggitt, R.C., Dean, P.J., Thor, K., and Rabinovitch, P.S. (1992). Evaluation of p53 protein expression in Barrett's esophagus by two-parameter flow cytometry. Gastroenterology *102*, 1220-1228.

Raouf, A.A., Evoy, D.A., Carton, E., Mulligan, E., Griffin, M.M., and Reynolds, J.V. (2003). Loss of Bcl-2 expression in Barrett's dysplasia and adenocarcinoma is associated with tumor progression and worse survival but not with response to neoadjuvant chemoradiation. Dis Esophagus *16*, 17-23.

Rath, H.C., Herfarth, H.H., Ikeda, J.S., Grenther, W.B., Hamm, T.E., Jr., Balish, E., Taurog, J.D., Hammer, R.E., Wilson, K.H., and Sartor, R.B. (1996). Normal luminal bacteria, especially Bacteroides species, mediate chronic colitis, gastritis, and arthritis in HLA-B27/human beta2 microglobulin transgenic rats. J Clin Invest *98*, 945-953.

Rees, J.R., Onwuegbusi, B.A., Save, V.E., Alderson, D., and Fitzgerald, R.C. (2006). In vivo and in vitro evidence for transforming growth factor-beta1-mediated epithelial to mesenchymal transition in esophageal adenocarcinoma. Cancer Res *66*, 9583-9590.

Reid, B.J., Sanchez, C.A., Blount, P.L., and Levine, D.S. (1993). Barrett's esophagus: cell cycle abnormalities in advancing stages of neoplastic progression. Gastroenterology *105*, 119-129.

Rhead, J.L., Letley, D.P., Mohammadi, M., Hussein, N., Mohagheghi, M.A., Eshagh Hosseini, M., and Atherton, J.C. (2007). A new Helicobacter pylori vacuolating cytotoxin determinant, the intermediate region, is associated with gastric cancer. Gastroenterology *133*, 926-936.

Richter, J.E., Falk, G.W., and Vaezi, M.F. (1998). Helicobacter pylori and gastroesophageal reflux disease: the bug may not be all bad. Am J Gastroenterol *93*, 1800-1802.

Rocco, J.W., and Sidransky, D. (2001). p16(MTS-1/CDKN2/INK4a) in cancer progression. Exp Cell Res *264*, 42-55.

Rokkas, T., Pistiolas, D., Sechopoulos, P., Robotis, I., and Margantinis, G. (2007). Relationship between Helicobacter pylori infection and esophageal neoplasia: a meta-analysis. Clin Gastroenterol Hepatol *5*, 1413-1417, 1417 e1411-1412.

Roninson, I.B. (2002). Oncogenic functions of tumour suppressor p21(Waf1/Cip1/Sdi1): association with cell senescence and tumour-promoting activities of stromal fibroblasts. Cancer Lett *179*, 1-14.

Ronkainen, J., Aro, P., Storskrubb, T., Johansson, S.E., Lind, T., Bolling-Sternevald, E., Vieth, M., Stolte, M., Talley, N.J., and Agreus, L. (2005). Prevalence of Barrett's esophagus in the general population: an endoscopic study. Gastroenterology *129*, 1825-1831.

Roper, J., Francois, F., Shue, P.L., Mourad, M.S., Pei, Z., Olivares de Perez, A.Z., Perez-Perez, G.I., Tseng, C.H., and Blaser, M.J. (2008). Leptin and ghrelin in relation to Helicobacter pylori status in adult males. J Clin Endocrinol Metab *93*, 2350-2357.

Rubenstein, J.H., Dahlkemper, A., Kao, J.Y., Zhang, M., Morgenstern, H., McMahon, L., and Inadomi, J.M. (2008). A pilot study of the association of low plasma adiponectin and Barrett's esophagus. Am J Gastroenterol *103*, 1358-1364.

Rubenstein, J.H., Kao, J.Y., Madanick, R.D., Zhang, M., Wang, M., Spacek, M.B., Donovan, J.L., Bright, S.D., and Shaheen, N.J. (2009). Association of adiponectin multimers with Barrett's oesophagus. Gut *58*, 1583-1589.

Ruigomez, A., Rodriguez, L.A.G., Wallander, M.A., Johansson, S., Graffner, H., and Dent, J. (2004). Natural history of gastro-oesophageal reflux disease diagnosed in general practice. Aliment Pharmacol Ther 20,751-760.

Ruhl, C.E., and Everhart, J.E. (1999). Overweight, but not high dietary fat intake, increases risk of gastroesophageal reflux disease hospitalization: the NHANES I Epidemiologic Followup Study. First National Health and Nutrition Examination Survey. Ann Epidemiol *9*, 424-435.

Rygiel, A.M., Milano, F., Ten Kate, F.J., Schaap, A., Wang, K.K., Peppelenbosch, M.P., Bergman, J.J., and Krishnadath, K.K. (2008). Gains and amplifications of c-myc, EGFR, and 20.q13 loci in the no dysplasia-dysplasia-adenocarcinoma sequence of Barrett's esophagus. Cancer Epidemiol Biomarkers Prev *17*, 1380-1385.

Saad, R.S., El-Gohary, Y., Memari, E., Liu, Y.L., and Silverman, J.F. (2005). Endoglin (CD105) and vascular endothelial growth factor as prognostic markers in esophageal adenocarcinoma. Hum Pathol *36*, 955-961.

Sala, A., Kundu, M., Casella, I., Engelhard, A., Calabretta, B., Grasso, L., Paggi, M.G., Giordano, A., Watson, R.J., Khalili, K., *et al.* (1997). Activation of human B-MYB by cyclins. Proc Natl Acad Sci U S A *94*, 532-536.

Savage, D.C. (1977). Microbial ecology of the gastrointestinal tract. Annu Rev Microbiol *31*, 107-133.

Schauer, M., Janssen, K.P., Rimkus, C., Raggi, M., Feith, M., Friess, H., and Theisen, J. (2010). Microarray-based response prediction in esophageal adenocarcinoma. Clin Cancer Res *16*, 330-337.

Schober, F., Neumeier, M., Weigert, J., Wurm, S., Wanninger, J., Schaffler, A., Dada, A., Liebisch, G., Schmitz, G., Aslanidis, C., *et al.* (2007). Low molecular weight adiponectin negatively correlates with the waist circumference and monocytic IL-6 release. Biochem Biophys Res Commun *361*, 968-973.

Schulmann, K., Sterian, A., Berki, A., Yin, J., Sato, F., Xu, Y., Olaru, A., Wang, S., Mori, Y., Deacu, E., *et al.* (2005). Inactivation of p16, RUNX3, and HPP1 occurs early in Barrett's-associated neoplastic progression and predicts progression risk. Oncogene *24*, 4138-4148.

Scott, C.R., Smith, J.M., Cradock, M.M., and Pihoker, C. (1997). Characteristics of youth-onset noninsulin-dependent diabetes mellitus and insulin-dependent diabetes mellitus at diagnosis. Pediatrics *100*, 84-91.

Sellon, R.K., Tonkonogy, S., Schultz, M., Dieleman, L.A., Grenther, W., Balish, E., Rennick, D.M., and Sartor, R.B. (1998). Resident enteric bacteria are necessary for development of spontaneous colitis and immune system activation in interleukin-10-deficient mice. Infect Immun *66*, 5224-5231.

Shapiro, G.I., and Harper, J.W. (1999). Anticancer drug targets: cell cycle and checkpoint control. J Clin Invest *104*, 1645-1653.

Sherr, C.J. (2004). Principles of tumor suppression. Cell *116*, 235-246.

Shiff, S.J., Shivaprasad, P., and Santini, D.L. (2003). Cyclooxygenase inhibitors: drugs for cancer prevention. Curr Opin Pharmacol *3*, 352-361.

Shirvani, V.N., Ouatu-Lascar, R., Kaur, B.S., Omary, M.B., and Triadafilopoulos, G. (2000). Cyclooxygenase 2 expression in Barrett's esophagus and adenocarcinoma: Ex vivo induction by bile salts and acid exposure. Gastroenterology *118*, 487-496.

Somasundar, P., Riggs, D., Jackson, B., Vona-Davis, L., and McFadden, D.W. (2003). Leptin stimulates esophageal adenocarcinoma growth by nonapoptotic mechanisms. Am J Surg *186*, 575-578.

Song, F., Ito, K., Denning, T.L., Kuninger, D., Papaconstantinou, J., Gourley, W., Klimpel, G., Balish, E., Hokanson, J., and Ernst, P.B. (1999). Expression of the neutrophil chemokine KC in the colon of mice with enterocolitis and by intestinal epithelial cell lines: effects of flora and proinflammatory cytokines. J Immunol *162*, 2275-2280.

Sorberg, M., Nyren, O., and Granstrom, M. (2003). Unexpected decrease with age of Helicobacter pylori seroprevalence among Swedish blood donors. J Clin Microbiol *41*, 4038-4042.

Souza, R.F., Morales, C.P., and Spechler, S.J. (2001). Review article: a conceptual approach to understanding the molecular mechanisms of cancer development in Barrett's oesophagus. Aliment Pharmacol Ther *15*, 1087-1100.

Stamatakos, M., Palla, V., Karaiskos, I., Xiromeritis, K., Alexiou, I., Pateras, I., and Kontzoglou, K. (2010). Cell cyclins: triggering elements of cancer or not? World J Surg Oncol *8*, 111.

Stein, D.J., El-Serag, H.B., Kuczynski, J., Kramer, J.R., and Sampliner, R.E. (2005). The association of body mass index with Barrett's oesophagus. Aliment Pharmacol Ther *22*, 1005-1010.

Suerbaum, S. (2009). Microbiome analysis in the esophagus. Gastroenterology *137*, 419-421.

Sun, J. (2010). Matrix metalloproteinases and tissue inhibitor of metalloproteinases are essential for the inflammatory response in cancer cells. J Signal Transduct *2010*, 985132.

Suzuki, S., Wilson-Kubalek, E.M., Wert, D., Tsao, T.S., and Lee, D.H. (2007). The oligomeric structure of high molecular weight adiponectin. FEBS Lett *581*, 809-814.

Sydora, B.C., Tavernini, M.M., Doyle, J.S., and Fedorak, R.N. (2005). Association with selected bacteria does not cause enterocolitis in IL-10 gene-deficient mice despite a systemic immune response. Dig Dis Sci *50*, 905-913.

Tashiro, E., Tsuchiya, A., and Imoto, M. (2007). Functions of cyclin D1 as an oncogene and regulation of cyclin D1 expression. Cancer Sci *98*, 629-635.

Tatsuguchi, A., Miyake, K., Gudis, K., Futagami, S., Tsukui, T., Wada, K., Kishida, T., Fukuda, Y., Sugisaki, Y., and Sakamoto, C. (2004). Effect of Helicobacter pylori infection on ghrelin expression in human gastric mucosa. Am J Gastroenterol *99*, 2121-2127.

Thomadaki, H., and Scorilas, A. (2006). BCL2 family of apoptosis-related genes: functions and clinical implications in cancer. Crit Rev Clin Lab Sci *43*, 1-67.

Thrift, A.P., Pandeya, N., Smith, K.J., Green, A.C., Hayward, N.K., Webb, P.M., and Whiteman, D.C. (2011). Helicobacter pylori infection and the risks of Barrett's oesophagus: A population-based case-control study. Int J Cancer.

Traganos, F. (2004). Cycling without cyclins. Cell Cycle *3*, 32-34.

Trigg, M.E. (1998). Inoculation of a portion of marrow for transplant as a way to accelerate marrow recovery. Bone Marrow Transplant *22*, 616-617.

Tummuru, M.K., Cover, T.L., and Blaser, M.J. (1993). Cloning and expression of a high-molecular-mass major antigen of Helicobacter pylori: evidence of linkage to cytotoxin production. Infect Immun *61*, 1799-1809.

Vaezi, M.F., and Richter, J.E. (1996). Role of acid and duodenogastroesophageal reflux in gastroesophageal reflux disease. Gastroenterology *111*, 1192-1199.

Vaninetti, N.M., Geldenhuys, L., Porter, G.A., Risch, H., Hainaut, P., Guernsey, D.L., and Casson, A.G. (2008). Inducible nitric oxide synthase, nitrotyrosine and p53 mutations in the molecular pathogenesis of Barrett's esophagus and esophageal adenocarcinoma. Mol Carcinog *47*, 275-285.

Vieth, M., Schneider-Stock, R., Rohrich, K., May, A., Ell, C., Markwarth, A., Roessner, A., Stolte, M., and Tannapfel, A. (2004). INK4a-ARF alterations in Barrett's epithelium, intraepithelial neoplasia and Barrett's adenocarcinoma. Virchows Arch *445*, 135-141.

von Rahden, B.H., Stein, H.J., Feith, M., Puhringer, F., Theisen, J., Siewert, J.R., and Sarbia, M. (2006). Overexpression of TGF-beta1 in esophageal (Barrett's) adenocarcinoma is associated with advanced stage of disease and poor prognosis. Mol Carcinog *45*, 786-794.

Vousden, K.H. (2005). Apoptosis. p53 and PUMA: a deadly duo. Science *309*, 1685-1686.

Voutilainen, M., Sipponen, P., Mecklin, J-P., Juhola, M., and Färkkilä, M. (2000). Gastroesophageal Reflux Disease: Prevalence, Clinical, Endoscopic and Histopathological Findings in 1,128 Consecutive Patients Referred for Endoscopy due to Dyspeptic and Reflux Symptoms. Digestion 61 (1), 6-13.

Wang, C., Yuan, Y., and Hunt, R.H. (2009a). Helicobacter pylori infection and Barrett's esophagus: a systematic review and meta-analysis. Am J Gastroenterol *104*, 492-500; quiz 491, 501.

Wang, D., and DuBois, R.N. (2004). Cyclooxygenase 2-derived prostaglandin E2 regulates the angiogenic switch. Proc Natl Acad Sci U S A *101*, 415-416.

Wang, D., Mann, J.R., and DuBois, R.N. (2005). The role of prostaglandins and other eicosanoids in the gastrointestinal tract. Gastroenterology *128*, 1445-1461.

Wang, J.S., Guo, M., Montgomery, E.A., Thompson, R.E., Cosby, H., Hicks, L., Wang, S., Herman, J.G., and Canto, M.I. (2009b). DNA promoter hypermethylation of p16 and APC predicts neoplastic progression in Barrett's esophagus. Am J Gastroenterol *104*, 2153-2160.

Wang, K.L., Wu, T.T., Choi, I.S., Wang, H., Resetkova, E., Correa, A.M., Hofstetter, W.L., Swisher, S.G., Ajani, J.A., Rashid, A., *et al.* (2007). Expression of epidermal growth factor receptor in esophageal and esophagogastric junction adenocarcinomas: association with poor outcome. Cancer *109*, 658-667.

Wani, S., Puli, S.R., Shaheen, N.J., Westhoff, B., Slehria, S., Bansal, A., Rastogi, A., Sayana, H., and Sharma, P. (2009). Esophageal adenocarcinoma in Barrett's esophagus after endoscopic ablative therapy: a meta-analysis and systematic review. Am J Gastroenterol *104*, 502-513.

Ward, J.M., Anver, M.R., Haines, D.C., and Benveniste, R.E. (1994). Chronic active hepatitis in mice caused by Helicobacter hepaticus. Am J Pathol *145*, 959-968.

Webb, P.M., Law, M., Varghese, C., Forman, D., Yuan, J.M., Yu, M., Ross, R., Limberg, P.J., Mark , S.D., Taylor, P.R., *et al.* (2001). Gastric cancer and Helicobacter pylori: a combined analysis of 12 case control studies nested within prospective cohorts. Gut *49*, 347-353.

Whiteman, D.C., Sadeghi, S., Pandeya, N., Smithers, B.M., Gotley, D.C., Bain, C.J., Webb, P.M., and Green, A.C. (2008). Combined effects of obesity, acid reflux and smoking on the risk of adenocarcinomas of the oesophagus. Gut *57*, 173-180.

Wilkinson, N.W., Black, J.D., Roukhadze, E., Driscoll, D., Smiley, S., Hoshi, H., Geradts, J., Javle, M., and Brattain, M. (2004). Epidermal growth factor receptor expression correlates with histologic grade in resected esophageal adenocarcinoma. J Gastrointest Surg *8*, 448-453.

Wilson, K.T., Fu, S., Ramanujam, K.S., and Meltzer, S.J. (1998). Increased expression of inducible nitric oxide synthase and cyclooxygenase-2 in Barrett's esophagus and associated adenocarcinomas. Cancer Res *58*, 2929-2934.

Wren, A.M., Seal, L.J., Cohen, M.A., Brynes, A.E., Frost, G.S., Murphy, K.G., Dhillo, W.S., Ghatei, M.A., and Bloom, S.R. (2001). Ghrelin enhances appetite and increases food intake in humans. J Clin Endocrinol Metab *86*, 5992.

Wu, A.H., Wan, P., and Bernstein, L. (2001). A multiethnic population-based study of smoking, alcohol and body size and risk of adenocarcinomas of the stomach and esophagus (United States). Cancer Causes Control *12*, 721-732.

Wu, X., Gu, J., Wu, T.T., Swisher, S.G., Liao, Z., Correa, A.M., Liu, J., Etzel, C.J., Amos, C.I., Huang, M., *et al.* (2006). Genetic variations in radiation and chemotherapy drug action pathways predict clinical outcomes in esophageal cancer. J Clin Oncol *24*, 3789-3798.

Yang, L., Lu, X., Nossa, C.W., Francois, F., Peek, R.M., and Pei, Z. (2009). Inflammation and intestinal metaplasia of the distal esophagus are associated with alterations in the microbiome. Gastroenterology *137*, 588-597.

Yang, L., and Pei, Z. (2006). Bacteria, inflammation, and colon cancer. World J Gastroenterol *12*, 6741-6746.

Yarden, Y. (2001). The EGFR family and its ligands in human cancer. signalling mechanisms and therapeutic opportunities. Eur J Cancer *37 Suppl 4*, S3-8.

Ye, W., Held, M., Lagergren, J., Engstrand, L., Blot, W.J., McLaughlin, J.K., and Nyren, O. (2004). Helicobacter pylori infection and gastric atrophy: risk of adenocarcinoma and squamous-cell carcinoma of the esophagus and adenocarcinoma of the gastric cardia. J Natl Cancer Inst *96*, 388-396.

Ye, W., and Nyren, O. (2003). Risk of cancers of the oesophagus and stomach by histology or subsite in patients hospitalised for pernicious anaemia. Gut *52*, 938-941.

Yildirim, A., Bilici, M., Cayir, K., Yanmaz, V., Yildirim, S., and Tekin, S.B. (2009). Serum adiponectin levels in patients with esophageal cancer. Jpn J Clin Oncol *39*, 92-96.

Zhivotovsky, B., and Orrenius, S. (2006). Carcinogenesis and apoptosis: paradigms and paradoxes. Carcinogenesis *27*, 1939-1945.

3

Esophageal Motility and Gastroesophageal Reflux

Michele Grande, Massimo Villa and Federica Cadeddu
University of Rome Tor Vergata, Italy

1. Introduction

Gastroesophageal reflux disease (GERD) represents a real social problem in the western world. About 20% of population has at least once a week, typical symptoms of this disease (heartburn and acid regurgitation); this incidence is probably underestimated because many patients have symptoms referable to extra-esofageal locations (asthma, cough, hoarseness, , non cardiogenic chest pain). The Montreal consensus conference defined GERD as "a condition which develops when the reflux of gastric contents causes troublesome symptoms and/or complications" (Vakil et al.,2006) But this definition does not take into account all possible pathogenetic causes and their therapeutic implications. Therefore seems more relevant to the definition of Brazilian consensus conference who considered GERD to be "a chronic disorder related to the retrograde flow of gastro-duodenal contents into the esophagus and/or adjacent organs, resulting in a spectrum of symptoms, with or without tissue damage"(Moraes-Filho et al.,2002). This definition recognizes the chronic character of the disease, and acknowledges that the refluxate can be gastric and duodenal in origin, with important implications for the treatment of this disease (Herbella & Patti, 2010).

Gastric hydrochloric acid has long been recognized as harmful to the esophagus (Herbella et al. 2009). However, gastro-esophageal refluxate contains a variety of other noxious agents, including pepsin. Currently, it is recognized that this component of the refluxate (commonly called bile reflux and identified by the Bilitec bile reflux monitor using bilirubin as a marker) is composed of bile salts and pancreatic enzymes, and is also injurious to the esophageal mucosa (Tack, 2004). It causes symptoms, and could be linked to the development of Barrett's esophagus and esophageal adenocarcinoma (Herbella & Patti, 2010).

Besides the constituents of the refluxate, symptom perception and mucosal damage also appear to be linked to the patterns of esophageal exposure and the volume of the release. Individuals are more likely to perceive a reflux event if the refluxate has a high proximal extent and a large volume (Tack, 2004; Herbella & Patti, 2010).

A highly efficient barrier exists between the stomach and the esophagus formed by the lower esophageal sphincter (LES), the diaphragm, the His angle, the Gubaroff valve and the phrenoesophageal membrane (Herbella & Patti, 2010).

The most important factors at work in preventing reflux include, well the lower esophageal sphincter, esophageal clearance mechanisms that limit contact time with noxious substances, and mucosal protective factors intrinsic to the esophageal mucosa.

The LES, a 3- to 4-cm-long region of smooth muscle located at the esophagogastric junction, creates a zone of high pressure separating the esophageal and gastric compartments between swallows. The diaphragmatic crura assist the LES in the maintenance of a tonically closed sphincter. The hiatus hernia eliminates the contribution of the crural diaphragm to LES function and thereby promotes gastroesophageal reflux. The severity of reflux disease in patients with hiatal hernia has been positively correlated with the size of the hernia sac (Lowe,2006; Katz,2003).

The most common cause of gastroesophageal reflux is transient lower esophageal sphincter relaxation (TLESR) with an excessive exposure of the esophagus to gastric secretions as consequence of it. The initial event is in a sharp decrease in the tone pressure not triggered by swallowing or esophageal contractions. The duration of TLESR (about 10 seconds) is greater than those induced by swallowing (about 6-8 seconds) and is accompanied by gastroesophageal reflux.

Has been shown that TLESR occur with a frequency of 2-6 episodes for hour in normal subjects and increased in patients with GERD (3-8 episodes). In normal subjects, in fact, only 40-50% of such releases is followed by acid reflux while the percentage rises to 60-70% in patients with GERD (Mittal et al.,1995).

In healthy subjects showed reduced LES pressure in the postprandial period and during exercise; most reflux episodes (82%) occur during TLESR. The mechanism behind this release inappropriate is not yet clarified; some results suggest that this release occur in response to gastric distention and vagal stimulation.

The gastric distension is probably able to trigger such releases through the stimulation of mechanoreceptors located in the proximal stomach in the vicinity of the LES (Mittal et al.,1995).

Each time that gastric contents refluxing into the esophagus the extent of esophageal mucosal injury depends on several factors including the contact time between refluxate and the mucosa, the composition of refluxate and the intrinsic ability to resist damage the esophageal epithelium (Pope, 1994). As the capacity of the refluxate to cause inflammation and then symptoms depends on the time of contact between the esophageal mucosa and the acid content of the refluxate a prompt and speedy clearance of the refluxate is of primary importance. Acid clearance normally occurs as a two step process. At first most of the refluxed volume is cleared quickly by one or two peristaltic contractions, thereafter the remaining acid is neutralised by swallowed saliva (Timmer, 1994). Secondary peristalsis is triggered by oesophageal distension and contributes to oesophageal volume clearance after reflux (Schoeman & Holloway, 1995). It is the initial oesophageal motor event after most reflux episodes in normal subjects.

In fact, pH-metric studies in healthy subjects have shown that primary peristalsis is the most important mechanism of clearing after acid reflux in orthostatic position. When the subject is in supine position, however, most reflux is neutralized by means clearance produced by secondary peristalsis. The contact time between the esophageal mucosa and a acid reflux potentially damaging increase during sleep when esophageal clearance is greatly reduced due to the decrease in the number of swallowing, the volume and alkalinity of the saliva and the absence of gravity (Achem et al.,1997).

The esophageal acid clearance is a process that takes place in two stages. On one hand, the volume of the refluxate is removed by esophageal peristalsis, the other the acid pH is neutralized by bicarbonate rich saliva delivered by primary peristaltis.

Thus secondary peristalsis would not by itself be expected to restore oesophageal pH, but to complement and accelerate the effects of the primary peristalsis that follows (Schoeman & Holloway, 1995).

In normal subjects during concurrent ambulatory manometry and pH monitoring that while primary peristalsis was the most common initial oesophageal clearance event overall, secondary peristalsis was the important initial motor event when the subjects were supine or asleep, or both (Schoeman et al.,1995).

Several studies have shown that oesophageal function is impaired in patients with reflux oesophagitis, especially in high grade oesophagitis. Patients with reflux oesophagitis have reduced lower oesophageal sphincter pressures (figure 1), an increased incidence of failed peristalsis (figure 2), reduced distal peristaltic amplitudes, slower velocity of propagation and in some studies shorter duration of contractions (Timmer et al.,1994). Two groups have reported that healing of oesophagitis does not improve impaired oesophageal motility (Katz et al.,1986, Singh et al.,1992).

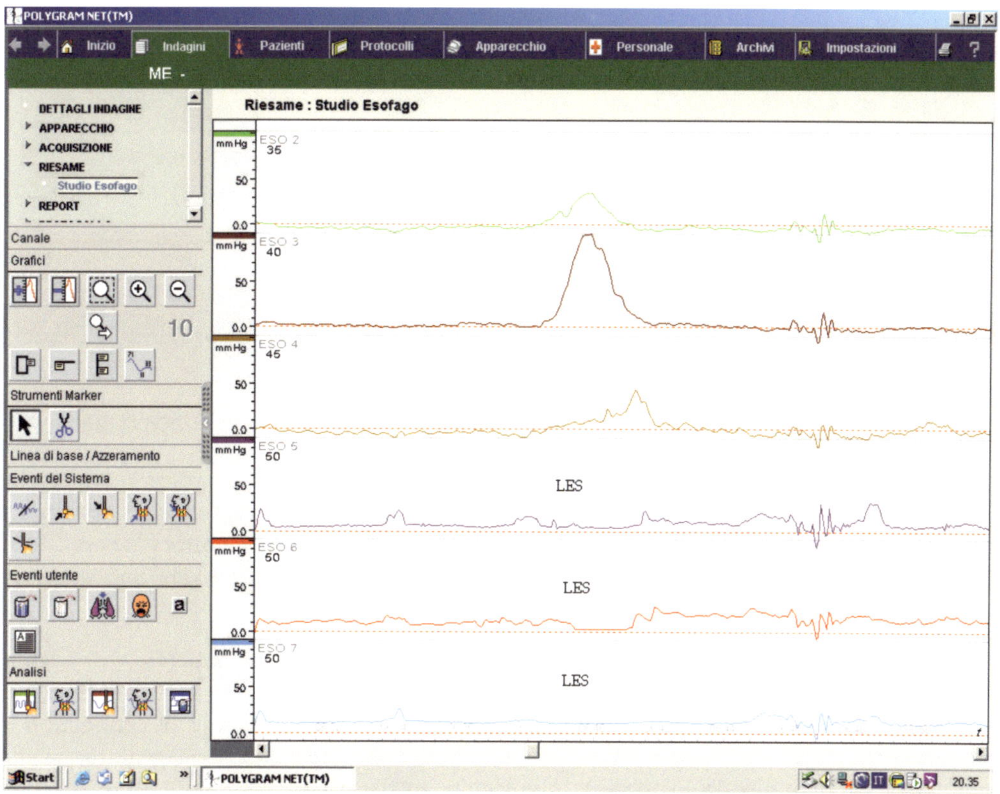

Fig. 1. Esophageal manometry in patients with gastroesophageal reflux with perfusion catheter to 6-way, three of which radial. Presence of low pressure LES and waves of low amplitude in the distal esofagus (45 cm).

An extension of the clearance time has been reported in about 50% of patients with esophagitis (Kahrilas, 1986). The frequency of abnormalities of peristalsis increases with the severity of reflux reaching 20% in patients with GERD without esophageal lesions, 25% in those with moderate esophagitis, and 48% in those with severe esophagitis (Kahrilas, 1986). A weak or ineffective peristalsis (waves of amplitude less than 30/40 mm Hg) is not able to eliminate acid reflux from the esophagus (Kahrilas, 1986).

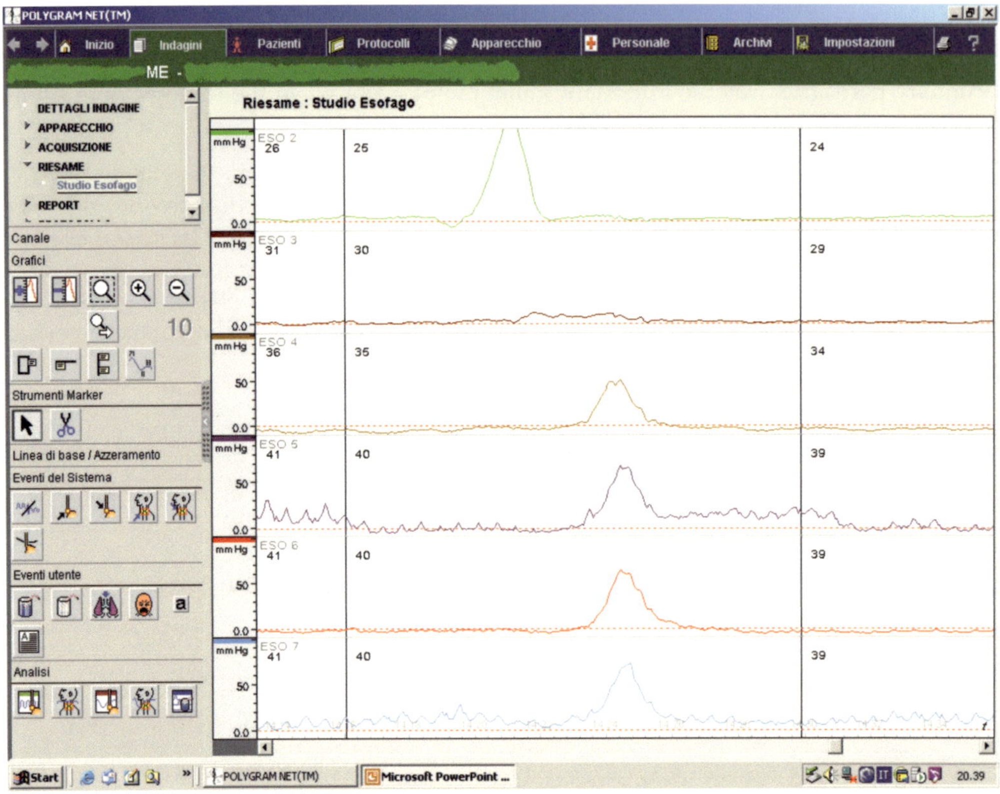

Fig. 2. Esophageal manometry with perfusion catheter to 6-way, three of which radial. Failed peristaltis in patients with gastroesophageal reflux.

Even lack of salivary function, characterized by reduced secretion or a reduced capacity for neutralization by saliva may result in a prolongation of esophageal clearance (Achem, 1997). For example, smokers have a reduced salivary secretion than nonsmokers and therefore have a higher incidence of GERD.

The velocity of propagation has been shown to be slower in patients with reflux oesophagitis. Gill et al have reported shorter durations of contraction in this condition (Gill et al.,1986). On the other hand, Singh et al have found a longer durations of contraction in patients with GERD compared with the controls (Singh et al.,1992). Oesophageal transit and acid clearance have also been shown to be slower in these patients (Singh et al.,1992). In agreement with those observations Timmer et al found, comparing oesophageal motility in patients with low grade oesophagitis with motility data obtained in a matched normal control group, reduced propagation velocity and duration of peristaltic contractions, with increase in the number of non transmitted contractions in patients with grade I and II oesophagitis. Peristaltic amplitude was not shown to be impaired (Timmer et al.,1994).

Defective peristalsis is associated with severe GERD, both in terms of symptoms and of mucosal damage (Diener et al.,2001). As matter of fact, the composite reflux score (DeMeester score) includes in its calculation two indirect measurements of esophageal clearance (number of reflux episodes longer than 5 min and length of the longest episode). In addition, the average esophageal clearance time can be calculated by dividing the total minutes the pH is below 4 by the number of reflux episodes (Johnson & DeMeester, 1974). This association also explains the high prevalence and severity of GERD in systemic diseases that affects peristalsis, such as connective tissue disorders (Patti et al.,2008).

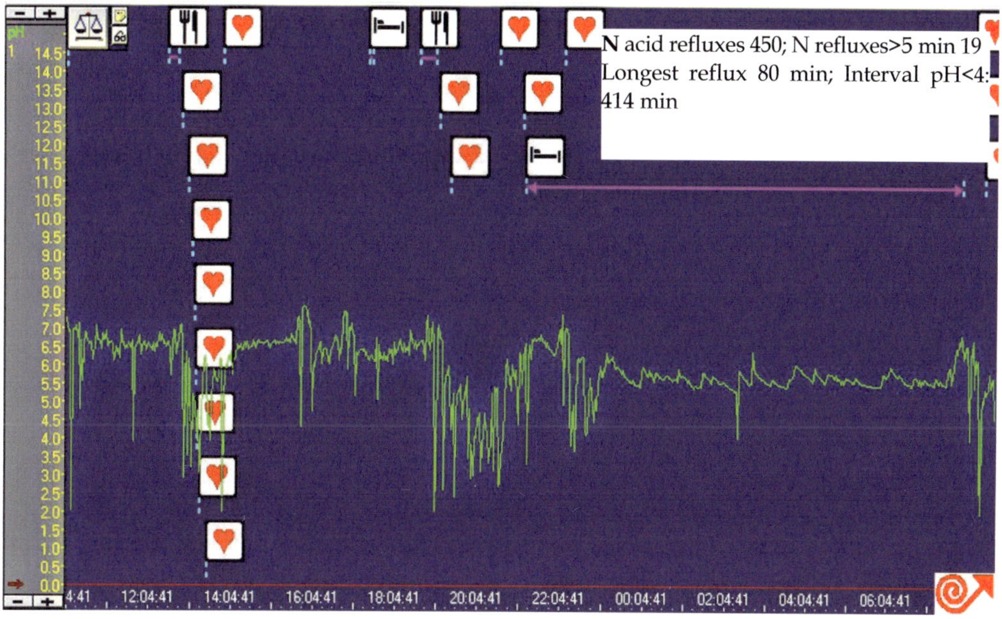

Fig. 3. Track condensed 24-hour pH-metry with antimony probe, the heart indicates the presence of reflux symptoms. Patients with pathological acid reflux (pH <4 lasting more than 5 minutes) in erect position (Number total reflux : 450; total reflux > 5 min : 19; duration of longest reflux : 80 min; total reflux time pH<4 : 414 min).

It is known that 40%-50% of patients with GERD have abnormal peristalsis (Diener et al.,2001). This dysmotility is particularly severe in about 20% of patients because of very low amplitude of peristalsis and/or abnormal propagation of the peristaltic waves (ineffective esophageal motility) (Patti & Perretta, 2003). Esophageal clearance is slower than normal, therefore, the refluxate is in contact with the esophageal mucosa for a longer period of time and it is able to reach more often the upper esophagus and pharynx (figures 3-5). Thus, these patients are prone to severe mucosal injury (including Barrett's esophagus) and frequent extra-esophageal symptoms such as cough (Herbella & Patti, 2010; Patti & Perretta, 2003; Meneghetti et al.,2005).

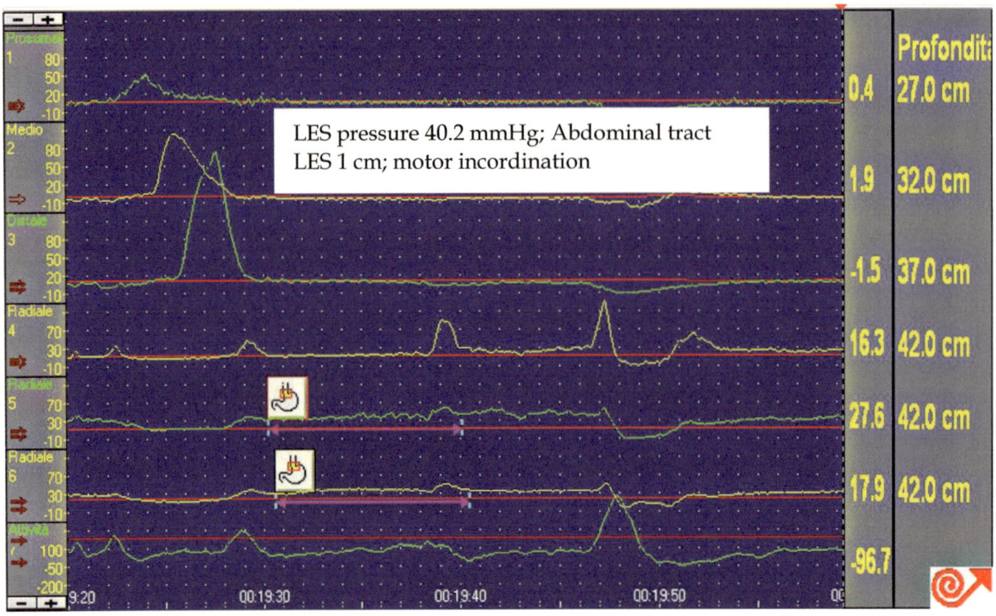

Fig. 4. Same case. Manometric examination shows reduced abdominal LES length (1 cm) with abnormal frequency of successful primary peristalsis, median response rate in this subject of only 33%.

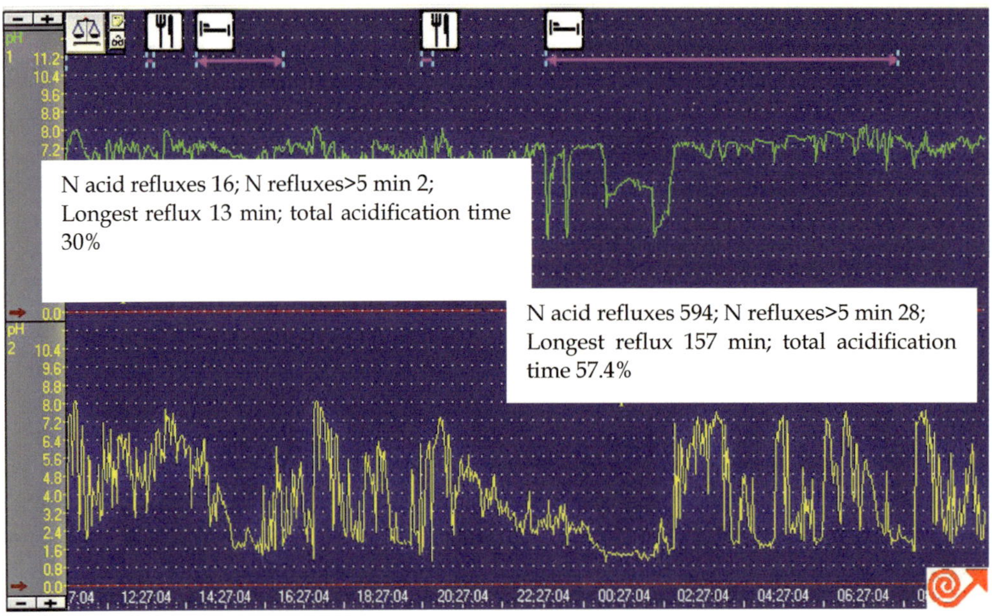

Fig. 5. Track condensed 24-hour pH-metry with antimony probe with two-way read points located 10 cm apart. The distal electrode is positioned 5 cm above the upper margin of the LES. Presence of reflux in erect and in supine position.

In addition to primary peristalsis alterations, patients with GERD have secondary peristalsis impairments and in most of them the esophageal distension is not capable of triggering secondary peristaltic contractions (Williams et al.,1992). As this deficit can occur even in subjects with normal primary peristalsis has been suggested that the phenomenon is due to an altered response to esophageal acid reflux and / or relaxing (Schoeman & Holloway, 1995).

Patients with reflux disease have considerably lower secondary peristaltic response rates than have aged matched controls with most patients failing to trigger any peristaltic response at all (Schoeman & Holloway, 1995). This finding supports and extends earlier findings on spontaneous reflux episodes, which showed that secondary peristalsis occurred less frequently after reflux in patients with reflux oesophagitis compared with normal subjects (Dodds et al.,1990).

Secondary peristalsis is a reflex response to oesophageal distension, the defect may lie in the oesophageal motor nerves or muscles oesophageal sensation, the central integrative mechanisms or a combination of these. Most patients with abnormal primary peristalsis also had abnormal secondary peristalsis and in these patients we postulate that the defect lies in the efferent limb of the motor pathway (Schoeman & Holloway, 1995). Most patients with abnormal secondary peristalsis, however, had normal primary peristalsis. Because secondary peristalsis seems to share a common motor pathway with primary peristalsis this side of the reflex would seem to be intact, implying that the defect in secondary peristalsis is due either to an abnormality of oesophageal sensation or in the integration of sensory information with the motor component of the reflex (Schoeman & Holloway, 1995). This hypothesis is supported by the findings of Williams et al who noted that the distension threshold required to trigger a motor response was higher in patients with oesophagitis than in healthy controls (Williams et al.,1992). Others, however, have found no difference in the threshold volume required to trigger oesophageal motor responses using slow (1 ml/s) infusions (Corazziari et al.,1986). Differences in the methods of these studies, however, make direct comparisons of these results difficult. Secondary peristalsis can effectively clear almost all of an injected acid bolus from the oesophagus leaving a negligible residual volume (Schoeman & Holloway, 1995). However, changes in oesophageal pH would be unlikely until neutralisation of the residual acid by bicarbonate rich saliva delivered by primary peristalsis (Schoeman & Holloway, 1995). Thus secondary peristalsis would not by itself be expected to restore oesophageal pH, but to complement and accelerate the effects of the primary peristalsis that follows. During the day when patients are awake, any effect of defective secondary peristalsis on acid clearance will be minimized by frequent primary peristalsis. Secondary peristalsis is likely to be more important, however, during sleep when the rate of primary peristalsis is substantially reduced (Orr et al.,1981).

While there is no doubt that these abnormalities are commonly present in patients with reflux oesophagitis, it's debated whether these are primary phenomena or the consequences of repetitive injury and inflammation caused by acid reflux. Currently, the most reliable data is that the abnormalities of oesophageal motor function in patients with reflux oesophagitis do not improve after complete healing of oesophagitis (Singh et al.,1992). This suggests that oesophageal dysmotility is a primary phenomenon and not a consequence of injury and inflammation. In that regard were detected an high prevalence of impairment of vagal cardiovascular reflexes in patients with gastro-oesophageal reflux disease (Cunningham et al.,1991).

A dysfunction of the parasympathetic system in the form of vagal neuropathy may help explain some of the changes found in the gastro-esophageal reflux disease (abnormalities of peristalsis, delayed esophageal transit, reduced LES pressure and delayed gastric emptying).

Other studies have shown that patients with reflux disease have a lower sensitivity threshold to esophageal distension compared with control subjects (Trimble et al.,1995). These patients have a normal acid exposure time but often complain of reflux symptoms. This suggests that some of them have a significantly increased esophageal sensitivity with a consequent increase in the perception of normal reflux.

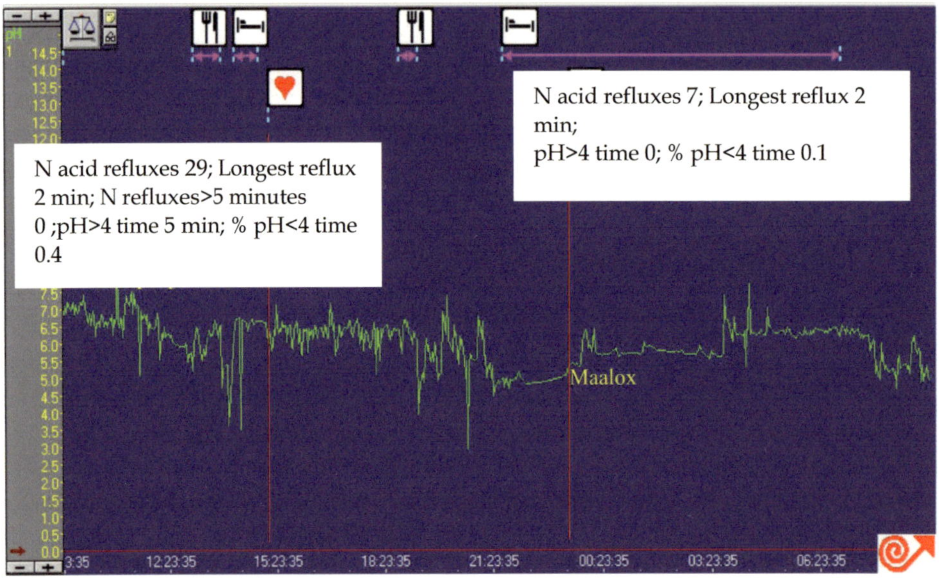

Fig. 6. 24-hour pH-metry probe with antimony. Patient that in the absence of acid reflux disease makes use of antacids. Functional heartburn ?

It is still unclear whether esophageal dysmotility is a primary condition that leads to GERD, or it is a consequence of esophageal inflammation. Medical therapy does not ameliorate esophageal peristalsis (McDougall et al.,1998; Xu et al.,2007).

However it has been shown that fundoplication improves the abnormal peristalsis in most patients (Herbella et al.,2007). The operation controls reflux because it improves esophageal motility, both in terms of LES competence and quality of esophageal peristalsis.

Proton pump inhibitors (PPIs), which potently inhibit gastric acid secretion, improve acid-reflux heartburn symptoms and esophageal mucosal breaks (figure 6). Meta-analyses of treatment for erosive GERD patients have shown that PPIs are much more effective in curing esophageal erosions and acid-reflux-related symptoms than are H2 receptor antagonists (H2RAs) or prokinetics (Sugimoto M et al, 2011). However, improvement of heartburn associated with NERD using standard PPI dosages are lower (around 30%-60%)

than for erosive GERD (Sugimoto M et al, 2011). NERD patients with typical symptoms, on average, show a smaller decrease in heartburn intensity also during 3-6 mo maintenance therapy with PPI compared with EE patients (Pace F et al, 2011). Again, it seems that the symptomatic response to PPI treatment is lower in NERD patients as compared to EE also during a maintenance regimen (Pace F et al, 2011). In patients with NERD or erosive esophagitis, a short period of high dose PPI (the so called PPI test) is a valuable tool for diagnosing suspected GERD symptoms as being acid-related, and thus for selecting those patients who will benefit from PPI therapy (Pace F et al, 2011). In the further management of these patients, 2 consecutive reductions in PPI dose are able to keep the vast majority of patients asymptomatic and to fully restore their quality of life (Pace F et al, 2011). The overall response to PPI therapy is lower in NERD patients than in EE patients.

In patients with GERD poorly responsive to standard PPI dose, laparoscopic Nissen-Rossetti fundoplication appears to be a safe and effective treatment of symptoms, esophageal damage, as well as both acid and bile reflux (Brillantino A et al, 2011).

In conclusion, application of the 24 hour ambulatory oesophageal pressure and pH monitoring technique did not show any differences in either pH profiles or motility variables before and after healing of reflux oesophagitis. The fact that oesophageal motility does not change after healing of oesophagitis supports the hypothesis that abnormalities in motility are pre-existent rather than the consequence of the inflammation. It could be argued, however, that the inflammation has caused irreversible changes in the oesophageal wall.

2. References

Achem, S. R.; Quigley, E. M. M.; Rao, S. S. C. & Snape W. J. Jr. (1997). Developments and controversies in gastrointestinal motility. *Digestive Disease and Sciences*, Vol. 15, suppl.1, ISSN 0163-2116

Brillantino A., Schettino M., Torelli F., Marano L., Porfidia R., Reda G., Grassia M., Braccio B., Di Martino N. (2011). Laparoscopic Nissen–Rossetti Fundoplication is a safe and effective treatment for both acid and bile gastroesophageal reflux in patients poorly responsive to proton pump inhibitor. *Surgical innovation* 1553350611409593, first published on July 7, 2011 as doi:10.1177/1553350611409593

Corazziari E.; Materia E, Pozzessere C.; Anzini F. &Torsoli A. (1986). Intraluminal pH and oesophageal motility in patients with gastro-oesophageal reflux. *Digestion*, Vol.35, N.3, 151-157, ISSN 0012-2823

Cunningham, K.M.; Horowitz, M,; Riddell P.S.; Maddern G.J.;Myers, J.C.; Holloway, R.H.; Wishart, J.M. & Jamieson, G.G. (1991). Relations among autonomic nerve dysfunction, oesophageal motility, and gastric emptying in gastro-oesophageal reflux disease. *Gut*, Vol.32, N.12, 1436-1440, ISSN 0017-5749

Diener, U.; Patti M.G.; Molena, D.; Fisichella, P.M. & Way, L.W. (2001). Esophageal dysmotility and gastroesophageal reflux disease. *Journal of Gastrointestinal Surgery*, Vol. 5, N.3: 260-265, ISSN 1091-255X

Dodds, W.J.; Kahrilas, P.J.; Dent, J.; Hogan, W.J.; Kern, M.K. & Arndorfer, R.C. (1990). Analysis of spontaneous gastroesophageal reflux and esophageal acid clearance in patients with reflux esophagitis. *Journal of Gastrointestinal Motility,*Vol 2, 79-89, ISBN 9783923022199

Gill, R.C.; Bowes, K.L.; Murphy, P.D. & Kingma, Y.J. (1986). Esophageal motor abnormalities in gastroesophageal reflux and the effects of fundoplication. *Gastroenterology,* Vol. 91, N.2, 364-369, ISSN 0016-5085

Herbella, F.A.; Nipominick, I. & Patti, M.G. (2009). From sponges to capsules. The history of esophageal pH monitoring. *Disease of the Esophagus*; Vol.22, N.2, 99-103, ISSN 1120-8694

Herbella, F.A. & Patti, M. G. (2010). Gastroesophageal reflux disease: From pathophysiology to treatment. *World Journal of Gastroenterology,* Vol.16, N.30, 3745-3749, ISSN 1007-9327

Herbella, F.A.; Tedesco, P.; Nipomnick, I.; Fisichella, P.M. & Patti, M.G. (2007). Effect of partial and total laparoscopic fundoplication on esophageal body motility. *Surgical Endoscopy,* Vol.21, N.2, 285-288, ISSN 0930-2794

Lowe, R. C. (2006). Medical management of gastroesophageal reflux disease. GI Motility online doi:10.1038/gimo54

Johnson, L.F. & Demeester, T.R. (1974). Twenty-four-hour pH monitoring of the distal esophagus. A quantitative measure of gastroesophageal reflux. *American Journal of Gastroenterology,* Vol.62, N.4, 325-332, ISSN 1948-9498

Kahrilas, P.J.; Dodds, W.J.; Hogan, W.J.; Kern, M.; Arndorfer, R.C. & Reece, A. (1986). Esophageal peristaltic dysfunction in peptic esophagitis. Gastroenterology, Vol.91, N.4, 897-904, ISSN 0016-5085

Katz, P.O. (2003). Optimizing medical therapy for gastroesophageal reflux disease: state of the art. *Reviews in Gastroenterological Disorders,* Vol.3, N.2, 59–69, ISSN 1533-001X

Katz, P.O.; Knuff, T.E.; Benjamin, S.B. & Castell, D.O. (1986). Abnormal esophageal pressures in reflux esophagitis: cause or effect? *American Journal of Gastroenterology,* Vol.81, N.9, 744-746, ISSN 0002-9270

McDougall, N.I.; Mooney, R.B.; Ferguson, W.R.; Collins, J.S.; Mc-Farland, R.J. & Love, A.H. (1998). The effect of healing oesophagitis on oesophageal motor function as determined by oesophageal scintigraphy and ambulatory oesophageal motility/pH monitoring. *Alimentary Pharmacology & Therapeutics,* 12, N.9, 899-907, ISSN 0269-2813

Meneghetti, A.T.; Tedesco, P.; Damani, T. & Patti, M.G. (2005). Esophageal mucosal damage may promote dysmotility and worsen esophageal acid exposure. *Journal of Gastrointestinal Surgery,* Vol.9, N.9, 1313-1317, ISSN 1091-255X.

Mittal, R.K.; Holloway, R.H.; Penagini, R.; Blackshaw, L.A. & Dent, J. (1995). Transient lower esophageal sphincter relaxation. *Gastroenterology,* Vol.109, N.2, 601-610, ISSN 0016-5085

Moraes-Filho, J.; Cecconello, I.; Gama-Rodrigues, J.; Castro, L.; Henry, M.A.; Meneghelli, U.G. & Quigley, E. (2002). Brazilian consensus on gastroesophageal reflux disease: proposals for assessment, classification, and management. *American Journal of Gastroenterology,* Vol.97, N.2, 241-248, ISSN 0002-9270

Orr, W.C.; Robinson, M.G. & Iohnson, L.F. (1981). Acid clearance during sleep in the pathogenesis of reflux esophagitis. *Digestive Diseases and Sciences,*Vol.26. N.5, 423-427, ISSN 0163-2116

Pace F, Riegler G, de Leone A, Dominici P, Grossi E, the EMERGE Study Group (2011). Gastroesophageal reflux disease management according to contemporary international guidelines: A translational study. *World J Gastroenterol*, Vol. 17, N. 9, 1160-1166, ISSN 1007-9327 (print) ISSN 2219-2840 (online)

Patti, M.G.; Gasper, W.J.; Fisichella, P.M.; Nipomnick, I. & Palazzo, F. (2008). Gastroesophageal reflux disease and connective tissue disorders: pathophysiology and implications for treatment. *Journal of Gastrointestinal Surgery*, 12(11): 1900-1906, ISSN 1091-255X

Patti, M.G. & Perretta, S. (2003). Gastro-oesophageal reflux disease: a decade of changes. *Asian Journal of Surgery*,Vol.26, N.1, pp. 4-6, ISSN 1015-9584

Pope, C. E. (1994). Acid-reflux disorders. *New England Journal of Medicine*, Vol.331, N.10, pp. 656-660, ISSN 0028-4793

Tack, J.; Koek, G.; Demedts, I.; Sifrim, D. & Janssens, J. (2004). Gastroesophageal reflux disease poorly responsive to single-dose proton pump inhibitors in patients without Barrett's esophagus: acid reflux, bile reflux, or both? *American Journal of Gastroenterology*, Vol. 99, N.6,pp. 981-988, ISSN 0002-9270

Schoeman, M.N. & Holloway, R.H. (1995). Integrity and characteristics of secondary oesophageal peristalsis in patients with gastro-oesophageal reflux disease. *Gut*, Vol.36, N.4, pp. 499-504, ISSN 0017-5749

Schoeman, M.N.; Tippett, M.D.; Akkermans, L.M.; Dent, J. & Holloway, R.H. (1995). Mechanisms of gastroesophageal reflux in ambulant healthy human subjects. *Gastroenterology*, Vol.108, N.1, pp. 83-91, ISSN 0016-0012

Singh, P.; Adamopoulos, A.; Taylor, R.H. & Colin-Jones, D.G. (1992). Oesophageal motor function before and after healing of oesophagitis. *Gut*, Vol.33, N.12, pp.1590-1596, ISSN 0017-5749

Sugimoto M.; Nishino M.; Kodaira C.; Yamade M.; Uotani T.; Ikuma M.; Umemura K.; Furuta T. (2011). Characteristics of non-erosive gastroesophageal reflux disease refractory to proton pump inhibitor therapy. World J Gastroenterol, Vol. 17, N. 14: 1858-1865, ISSN 1007-9327 (print) ISSN 2219-2840 (online)

Timmer, R.; Breumelhof, R.; Nadorp, J.H. & Smout, A.J. (1994). Oesophageal motility and gastro-oesophageal reflux before and after healing of reflux oesophagitis. A study using 24 hour ambulatory pH and pressure monitoring. *Gut*, Vol.35, N.11, 1519-1522, ISSN 0017-5749

Trimble, K.C.; Pryde, A. & Heading, R.C. (1995). Lowered oesophageal sensory thresholds in patients with symptomatic but not excess gastro-oesophageal reflux: evidence for a spectrum of visceral sensitivity in GORD. *Gut*, Vol.37, N.1, 7-12, ISSN 0017-5749.

Vakil, N.; van Zanten, S.V.; Kahrilas, P.; Dent, J. & Jones, R. (2006). The Montreal definition and classification of gastroesophageal reflux disease: a global evidence-based consensus. *American Journal of Gastroenterology*, Vol.101, N.8, pp. 1900-1920, ISSN 0002-9270

Williams, D.; Thompson, D.G.; Marples, M.; Heggie, L.; O'Hanrahan, T.; Mani, V. & Bancewicz, J. (1992). Identification of an abnormal esophageal clearance response to intraluminal distention in patients with esophagitis. *Gastroenterology*, Vol.103, N.3, pp. 943-953, ISSN 0016-0012

Xu, J.Y.; Xie, X.P.; Song , G.Q. & Hou, X.H. (2007). Healing of severe reflux esophagitis with PPI does not improve esophageal dysmotility. *Diseases of the Esophagus*, Vol.20, N.4, pp. 346-352, ISSN 1120-8694

4

Dental Erosions – Extraesophageal Manifestation of Gastroesophageal Reflux

Ivana Stojšin and Tatjana Brkanić
University of Novi Sad, Serbia

1. Introduction

Dentists are often the first healthcare line that can - diagnose certain systemic diseases through their oral manifestations. One of such diseases is the gastroesophageal reflux disease (GERD) which may be recognised through its extraesophageal manifestation in the form of dental erosions (Howeden, 1971; Myllarniemi & Saario, 1985; Jarvinen et al., 1988; Bartlett & Smith.1996; Lazarchik &Filler, 1997; Lussi, 2006). The exact cause of dental erosion is the gastro-esophago-pharyngeal reflux, also called proximal reflux, which takes place in a minority of patients with GERD. Usually, the gastroesophageal reflux is confined to the lower portion of the esophagus, where it may cause esophagitis.

Erosion comes from the Latin verb erodere, erosi, erosum, meaning gnaw, corrode and it is described as a process of gradual degradation of a surface by an electrolytic or chemical process. In clinical terms, dental erosions are defined as a physical result of pathological, chronic, localised, painless loss of dental hard tissue, the outer surface of which is chemically destroyed by acid or chelates. Acids that come into contact with tooth surfaces and cause these changes are not products of intra-oral bacterial flora (Pintborg, 1970; Eccles, 1982; Imfeld, 1996). Dental erosions are of multifactorial aetiology and each factor has a significant role not only in the formation of a defect but also its prevention. The interaction of all factors may cause a synergistic effect. They are usually described as a surface phenomenon, although the process may enter the subsurface structure (Young & Tenuta, 2011). According to the depth of the lesions they may be divided into surface and deep ones. According to the localisation they may be divided into generalized and localised, while according to pathogenic activities, into on manifesting and latent ones. According to the origin of the acid they may be divided into endogenous, exogenous and idiopathic. Idiopathic erosive changes are those which, based on medical history and objective findings, we are not in the position to define the origins of the erosive agent. Exogenous erosive changes have occurred as a consequence of acidulous reaction on dental hard tissues, when the acid enters the oral cavity from an external environment. Exogenous acids, originally, may be dietary, medicational or environmental (Allan, 1967; Gandara&Truelove, 1999). Endogenous ones develop under the influence of gastric hydrochloric acid. This acid comes to the oral ecosystem by recurrent vomiting, regurgitation or reflux (Imfeld, 1996). Psychosomatic disorders (neurotic vomiting, anorexia nervosa, bulimia) are common causes of regurgitation and vomiting, which are self-induced (Klein&Walsh, 2004). On the other hand, there are somatic causes. These include pregnancy, alcoholism and the antabuse therapy for alcohol abuse (Robb & Smith, 1990). This group also comprises gastrointestinal disorders such as gastric dysfunctions (Holst&Lange, 1939), chronic constipation (Bargen &Austin, 1937), hiatus hernia (Howeden, 1971), duodenal and peptic ulcer (Allan, 1969) and the gastroesophageal reflux disease (Gregory-Head & Curtis, 1997).

GERD is a usual condition that encompasses 65% of the population of highly developed countries in a certain period of their lives (Lussi, 2006). On average, 7% of patients have daily problems, and 36%, once a month (Nebel, Fornes&Castell, 1976).

GERD was for the first time connected to dental erosions in the case study presented by Howden (Howeden, 1971) and the hypothesis that it might become a diagnostic mark of an earlier acidulous reflux in the mouth cavity was formulated by Myllarniemi and Saario (Myllarniemi & Saario, 1985). Numerous scientific papers, both case studies and epidemiological studies, published in the past thirty-five years, point to GERD as a risk factor in the formation of erosive changes on hard tooth tissue, as well as to the possibility of using this tooth defect as a diagnostic marker of this gastrointestinal disorder (Jarvinen et al., 1988; Bartlett & Smith.1996; Lazarchik &Filler, 1997; Lussi, 2006).

Dental erosions associated with GERD also occur in children until their teenage years, they especially often occur in children with cerebral palsy (Goncalves et al., 2008). In adults, the value of the prevalence of dental erosion in patients diagnosed with the disease observed is in the range of 5-28%, while the prevalence of GERD in patients with erosive changes is in the range of 21-83%. In children, the prevalence of dental erosion in patients diagnosed with the reflux disease ranges from 17-87% (Vahil et al., 2006). The diversity of the percentages of dental erosion among the subjects covers a very wide range due to the non-standardised scales, estimates of examined surfaces, specificity of the population tested and the subjective factors - assessment capabilities of examiners.

The connection between this common medical condition and the erosive changes on teeth is not absolute because not everyone with a diagnosed reflux disease has them (Bartlett, Evans&Smith, 1996). On the other hand, there are those that have no subjective problems, but have changes on a specific location that proves the existence of regurgitation and reflux (Dene, 2002). GERD may be a risk factor for the appearance of dental erosions only if it is in combination with regurgitation (Addy, Embery&Edgar, 2000). The refluxate is composed of gastric acid, a small quantity of undigested food, pepsin, and in cases of duodenogastric reflux may contain bile acid and trypsin. The intensity of erosive changes is determined by the content and the pH value of the regurgitated material, number of regurgitation episodes, by the length of time this content stayed in the mouth, which is in direct connection with the quantity of secreted saliva, its pH value, its buffer capacity and its ionic content. To all the above mentioned we must add the influence of habits in terms of oral hygiene maintenance (Gilmour&Beckelt, 1993).

2. Pathophysiology of change appearance

Erosion is a disorder in which the characters such as: structural characteristics of teeth, physiological characteristics of saliva and dental pellicle, characteristics of acids and habits act as very important factors in their development and, therefore, must be carefully analysed. The seriousness of erosive changes is determined by the sensitivity of dental tissue to dissolution. Enamel is mineralised with less soluble minerals than dentine, therefore its surface is eroded more slowly (Lussi et al., 2011).

Minerals, protein, lipids and water are the basic constituents of the hard dental tissue. They are of similar chemical composition and different morphology. Table 1.

COMPONENTS	VOL % enamel	WEIGHT % enamel	VOL % dentine	WEIGHT % dentine
Carbonate hydroxyapatite	85	96	47	70
water	12	3	20	12
Proteins and lipids	3	1	33	18

Table 1. Chemical composition of enamel and dentine in per cents

2.1 Enamel

Enamel represents the hardest tissue in the human organism. Regardless of the high percentage of mineral phases in its structure in the form of hydroxyapatites, enamel is semi-permeable. It is the consequence of the organic matrix that forms the interprismatic and intercristaline coats which are morphologically defined as enamel pores (Roberson, Heymann&Swift,2002). Semi-permeability is the consequence of both the existence of enamel cavities and not adequately mineralised enamel prisms that form the defects. This fine net of macro and micro pores enables the process of enamel diffusion. Water passes with diluted ions and small molecules through the organic part between enamel crystals and establishes a fluid flow which is directly dependent on the tooth morphology and the age of the patient. Permeability decreases with age because organic channels are sealed by deposition of crystals as well as by the formation of a biofilm on its outer surface (Vulović, 2005)

The mineral phase is presented by hydroxyapatite $Ca_{10} (PO_4)_6 (OH)_2$. Pure, natural hydroxyapatite is a very stable and poorly soluble compound. However, apatite of the human enamel is not absolutely pure, it contains about 2-4% of carbonates and 1% of other chemical elements, therefore this apatite is called carbonated. Its solubility is greater than that of pure hydroxyapatite. Certain calcium ions may be substituted by other metal ions, such as sodium, magnesium and potassium. Certain OH ions may be substituted by fluoride ions when fluorapatite is created. The formula of pure fluorapatite is $Ca_{10} (PO_4)_6 F_2$. Fluorides affect hardness, chemical reactivity and the stability of apatite crystals. This type of hydroxyapatites is a less soluble mineral. Phosphate ions are replaced by carbonate ones, but not in a one to one ratio, therefore, the formula of such hydroxyapatite is $Ca_{10-x} Na_x (PO_4)_{6-y}(CO_3)_z (OH)_2$. The sensitivity of carbonated apatite depends on the orientation of crystals. The presence of various "impurities", especially carbonates and magnesium in the crystal petals of hydroxyapatite crystals and it increases its solubility, while the presence of fluoride, strontium and other elements are stabilise enamel (Roberson, Heymann&Swift, 2002; Vulović, 2005) The density and hardness of the enamel tissue decreases with the increase of the distance from the tooth surface (He & Swain, 2009) and solubility increases (Theuns et al., 1986).

2.2 Dentine

Dentine differs from enamel not only by its morphology but also by its chemical structure. The mineral composition is much smaller while the organic one is much greater than in enamel Table 1. The organic component is represented by type I collagen and the non-collagen protein component is represented by phosphoproteins, glycoprotein, proteoglycanes (Lussi et al., 2011). In terms of weight 1% goes to lipids (Odutuga & Prout, 1974). The mineral phase is here also represented by hydroxyapatite crystals, but these are much smaller. The percentage of carbonate is greater in dentine than in enamel (Lussi, 2006) therefore it is sensitive to acidulous solutions. The mineral composition of dentine grows with age.

Acid as an erosive agent, in order to demineralise the crystals on the tooth surface, must be in direct contact with the tooth substance and this is only possible if it gets through plaque or the dental pellicle and by passing through the protein lipid layers of prisms and crystals through processes of diffusion, it reaches the single crystals.

2.3 Dental pellicle

Dental pellicle represents a cellular organic material from saliva which is deposited on the surfaces of the clinical crown (Eisenburger et al., 2001). The pellicle is formed a couple of seconds after exposure of the tooth surface to the oral environment, by sedimentation of salivary proteins and glycoprotein's and contains lipids and some enzymes. It continuously regenerates during the life cycle of a tooth. It is believed that the function of pellicle is: the protection of enamel as a terminal tissue, reduction of friction between teeth and providing the matrix for the re-mineralization of the enamel surface. The build-up of the pellicle from salivary proteins enables the third function because the some components have a base group through which they absorb phosphate ions, and others, which have acidulous proteins, absorb calcium ions. The composition, thickness and maturation time affect the protective properties of the pellicle. This membrane demonstrates continuously selective potential (semi-permeable membrane) and they suppressively influence the diffusion of acids and thereby reduce the dissolution rate of hydroxyapatite (Hanning, Hanning&Attin, 2005). In situ studies have shown that the thinnest pellicle is formed on the palatal surface of the upper front teeth (0.3-0.38 micrometers) and the thickest on the lingual surfaces (0.96-1.06 micrometers) after one hour of intraoral exposure (Amaechi et al., 1999).Tooth surfaces with the thickest pellicular formations show the lowest percentage of erosive changes 1.7 -2% (Young & Khan,2002)

2.4 Saliva

Saliva is considered the most important biological factor in the prevention of erosive changes by both its indirect, the formation of dental pellicle, and direct effects. It affects directly the dissolution, elimination, neutralization of acidulous compounds, and, at the same time, reduces the level of demineralisation and remineralisation with its ionic composition of calcium, phosphate and fluoride.

Saliva is a complex secretion of three pairs of major salivary glands and numerous minor mucous glands. The total average amount of saliva secreted varies within 0.5 to 1 l per day (according to some authors even up to 1.5 l per day). The total quantity of saliva depends on the individual characteristics of each person, as well as on the type, length and intensity of stimuli. It can be non-stimulated and stimulated.

Un-stimulated saliva represents a mixture of secretions of the parotid, sub-mandibular, sublingual and other minor mucosa glands. It also contains gingival cervical liquid, desquamated epithelial cells, bacteria, viruses, leucocytes, food residues and blood. The average quantity of secrete saliva is 0.3 ml per minute, while the individual column may range between 0.01 -1.9 ml per minute. Un-stimulated saliva of subject with reflux disease has a significantly lower pH and calcium concentration. Phosphate and urea concentrations were lower but not statistically significantly lower (Stojšin, 2009).

Stimulated saliva is a secretion product of the parotid salivary gland as a direct response to a stimulus and enables physiological functions during the periods of intensified activities as well as protection of the oral tissue integrity. The quantity of this kind of saliva secretion varies from 0.5 - 7.0 millilitres per minute (Vulović, 2005).

Saliva contains water (99 %) and the rest (1%) comprises organic molecules (proteins, glycoproteins and lipids), small organic molecules (glucose and urea) and electrolytes (sodium, calcium, chlorine and phosphorus).

The acidity of the oral environment directly depends on the level of acidic products, speed of elimination and the ability to neutralise acids. The speed of eliminating acids is conditioned by the speed of salivation and the quantity of saliva. At lower speed of saliva pH synthesis it may be 5.3, and at higher speed of synthesis in the parotid glands it may be up to 7.8 (Anđić,2000).

Saliva represents an ionic reservoir of chemical elements which compose hydroxyapatite. It is oversaturated by ions of calcium, phosphates and hydroxyl ions, which enable the remineralisation of teeth, but also disable the dissolution of tooth tissue in saliva with pH values below 7 and down to the critical value. The picture clearly shows normal morphological characteristics of enamel, the enamel dentine border and dentine after one hour exposure to artificial saliva with pH 7. Oversaturation with ions that compose hydroxyapatite is present even in the extracellular liquid phase of dental plaque which is in direct contact with the tooth surface. Such state of the saliva decreases only when the pH value in the plaque drops low enough so that the concentration of hydroxyl and phosphate ions reduces below the critical value by binding phosphate ions PO_4 in HPO_4(Anđić, 2000).

Numerous salivary proteins (staterin, acidic proteins rich with prolines and many phosphoproteins) help remineralisation of the sub-surface lesion of the enamel. These proteins are capable of binding calcium and preventing calcium salts from precipitation in an oversaturated solution such as saliva and plaque. With the increase of saliva secretion, staterin secretion increases as well.

The chemical protection of saliva is reflected in maintaining certain acidity in the mouth. The control of the optimal acidity in the mouth is based on physical effects (dilution and rinsing) and on the buffering abilities of the saliva. The buffering system consists of bicarbonates, phosphates, proteins and urea (Edgar, 1992; Edgar & O'Mullane, 1996).

3. Chemical aspects of demineralisation

The basic cause of enamel demineralisation is the existence of the critical pH value, which, in case of enamel, is 5.5. The critical pH value is the value when the solution (saliva or the liquid component of plaque) is saturated with relevant mineral particles that enamel is composed of. If the pH value of the solution is above the critical value, the solution is oversaturated and it causes precipitation. If the pH value of the solution is below 5.5, the solution us not saturated and it causes demineralisation. In people with a low concentration of calcium and phosphate in the saliva and in the plaque liquid, the critical pH value may be even 6.5(Daves, 2003).

Hydroxyapatite dissolves because there are products of solubility marked by Ksp (*product of solubility*) and it is $[Ca]^{10}[PO_4]^6[OH]^2$. The value within the brackets shows the effective concentration, i.e. the activity of component ions. The product of concentration of component ions is labelled with mol/L and for hydroxypatite it is 10^{-117}. Ksp is a constant concentration for each component individually. In any kind of liquid, saliva, liquid component of plaque, a refreshment beverage, gastric juice and hydroxyapatite dissolves into its *ionic products* (Ip)[1].

$$Ca_{10}(PO4)_6(OH)_2 \_\_\_\_ 10\,Ca^{2+} + 6\,PO_4^{3-} + 2\,OH^- \qquad (1)$$

If Ip = Ksp, then the solution is saturated with elements constituting hydroxyapatite and there is a balance between the concentration of ions and the concentration of products. If Ip less than Ksp, the solution is not saturated and demineralisation takes place, and if Ip is larger than Ksp, the solution is oversaturated and remineralisation or precipitation take place. There are two basic reasons for dissolution of enamel in acids. Hydrogen ions of acid react with the ionic product (OH) and water is created. By disrupting the concentration of products of hydroxyapatite the stability of the concentration of products is also disrupted and demineralisation takes place. The other reasons are inorganic phosphates that appear in saliva and the liquid component of plaque in four different forms, such as H_3PO_4, $H_2PO_4^-$, HPO^{2-} and $PO43^-$. Their proportion directly depends on the pH values of the environment. Low pH value causes low values of PO_4^{3-} which influences Ip of hydroxyapatite. As soon as Ip < Ksp, demineralisation takes place (Daves, 2003; Lussi, 2006)

The chemical process of development of the erosive process is complex. Hydrochloride acid of the regurgitated stomach content reduces the pH value within the mouth. It undergoes electrolytic dissociation in a water environment of the oral ecosystem. The increased concentration of hydrogen ions in the saliva contributes to ionic exchange between saliva and the pellicular or plaque liquid. Disharmony in the ionic concentration starts a chemical reaction[2]

$$Ca_{10-x}Na_x(PO4)_{6-y}(CO_3)_z(OH)_{2-u}F_u + 3H^+ \_\_\_\_\_\_$$

$$(10-x)\,Ca^{2+} + x\,Na^+ + (6-y)(HPO_4^{2-}) + z\,(HCO_3^-) + H_2O + u\,F^- \qquad (2)$$

Hydrogen ions directly react with the mineral component of tough tooth tissue; it dissolves them, reacts with carbonate ions and phosphates as the chemical equation shows. Ions of chlorine have no effect in the process of demineralisation.

The non-ionised form of acid passes through the interprismatic area and dissolves the minerals under the surface layer. This causes the calcium and phosphate ions to mobilise and consequently, the pH value rises within the salivary pellicle, i.e. the saliva on the contact surface (Featherstone & Rodgers, 1981; Ganss, Klimek & Starck, 2004). The process halts if there is no new inflow of acid. The next regulating phase or sipping sour beverages or transfer of liquid from side of the mouth to the other again lowers the pH value and a new demineralisation cycle takes place.

Identical processes take place in the dentine as well; they are just much more complex because of the larger quantity of organic matter in this tissue. Structural characteristics of dentine influence the possible penetration of hydrogen ions, demineralisation and evacuation of elements formed during demineralisation (Kleter et a., 1994)

Erosive changes may appear on primary teeth as well. The mineral content of deciduous teeth enamel is lower than in permanent ones. In situ, the enamel of primary teeth is much more sensitive to acidic influence than the enamel of permanent teeth (Johanson et al., 2001). while the dentine of milk teeth is less sensitive to acidic influence than in case of permanent teeth (Hunter et al., 2000).

Hipersalivation which is a reflex occurring before vomiting represents the response of the vomiting centre in the brain (Feldman, Scharschmidt & Sleisenger, 1998) which significantly reduces the process of erosion. Such reactions may be noticed in eating disorders, rumination and chronic alcoholism. Patients with gastroesophageal reflux disease cannot expect the protective effect of hypersalivation before the episode of reflux because the reflux of the gastric juice is an involuntary event and therefore there is no coordination with the autonomous nervous system (Lussi, 2006). From the aspect of dental erosions, the daily rhythm of salivation is especially significant, according to which saliva secretion practically cease from midnight to six o'clock in the morning and then there is a spontaneous increase until 6 p.m., when non-stimulated salivation reaches its maximum, and then it goes on to decrease until cessation at midnight (Anđić, 2000). Night regurgitations episodes are especially important risk factors for the occurrence of erosive changes because there is no protective effect of saliva.

Erosive demineralisation of the tooth crown is characterised by initial softening of the enamel surface in a nanoscopic scale which, in the course of time, grows into microscopically observable morphological changes, which through prolonged exposition lead to macroscopic defects. The erosive defect is determined by the depth of the cavities and the thickness of the demineralised substrate. The level of demineralisation is determined by the immersion time and acid. The thickness of the initial demineralisation ranges between 0.2 and 3 micrometers (Amaechi & Higham, 2001; Lussi et al., 2011). Partial loss of superficial minerals affects the reduction of the superficial hardness, which makes enamel vulnerable against physical forces. Cheeks, tongue, abrasive food, tooth brushes, as well as ultrasound processing of dental tissue may lead to the elimination of the demineralised organic filling of hard dental tissues (Eisenburger, Shellis &Addy, 2004). Enamel remains sensitive to abrasive forces even one hour after having been exposed to acid (Lussi et al., 2011).

4. Pathohystology of erosive changes

The specific morphology of hard dental tissues affects the formation of the characteristic pathohystological images of erosive changes.

4.1 Enamel

The basic structural unit of enamel is enamel prism with its crystals of apatite which show signs of inclination towards the edge of the prism. Enamel prisms are in strings lining from the enamel-dentine border towards the surface of the tooth. In the outer-most surface layers as well as in the region of the enamel-dentine border the presence of aprismatic enamel can be observed. Enamel prisms from the neighbouring lines are linked because their shape resembles a keyhole. They tend to gather into groups. They are radially placed around the tooth axis, which can clearly be seen in the photographs made by an electronic microscope Figure 1. Each prism consists of a head and a tail. The head of one prism is joined with two tails of the two neighbouring prisms and vice versa (Roberson,Heymann&Swift, 2002.) Each enamel prism has its coating and it represents the entrance of the aggressive noxious, so the process of demineralisation goes from the outer surface of the prism towards the central part and the emerging defects remind of honeycombs (Meurman & Frank, 1991), which can clearly be seen in the central part Figure 2. Ultra-structural examinations (scanning electron microscopy - SEM, atomic force microscope - AFM) have shown that demineralisation causes changes both in the prismatic and the aprismatic enamel, both on prisms and in the interprismatic region (Amaechi &Higham, 2001; Meurman & ten Cate, 1996). In the aprismatic enamel, demineralisation is irregular and zones of changed mineral content in different places are formed.

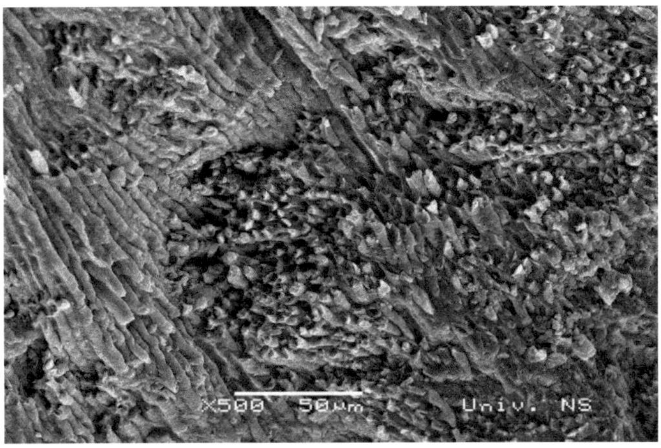

Fig. 1. SEM photographs of tooth enamel enlarged 500 x. Enamel prisms are in strings lining from the enamel-dentine border towards the surface of the tooth. Enamel prisms are grouped in bundles.

4.2 Dentine

Dentine makes the largest part of the dental tissue. The basic structural unit is a dentine tubule. The system of dentine tubules starts at the enamel-dentine border in the form of very thin branches, then they change into broader little channels and in the region of pulp they end as wider tubules. Between the numerous tubules, there is the intertubular dentine. Within the tubules themselves, there is a stem of dentine productive cells - odontoblast, the activity of which produces a new type of dentine called peritubular dentine (Roberson, Heymann & Swift, 2002).Figure 3.

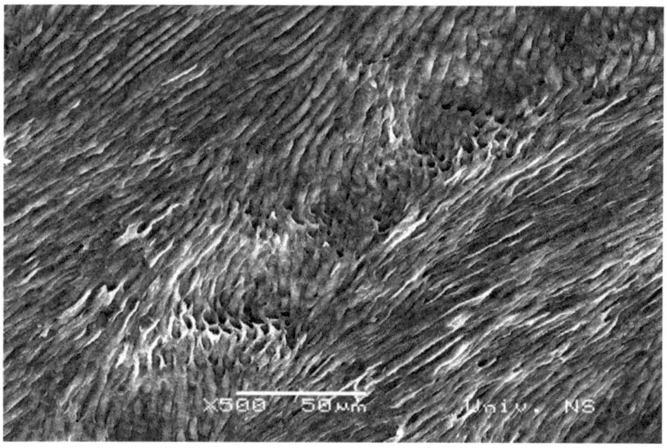

Fig. 2. SEM microphotograph of enamel after 15 minutes of exposure to the solution of HCL pH 1.Enlarged 500 x. The cross section of enamel prisms resembling honeycomb. It is recognizable rounded lines of fracture.

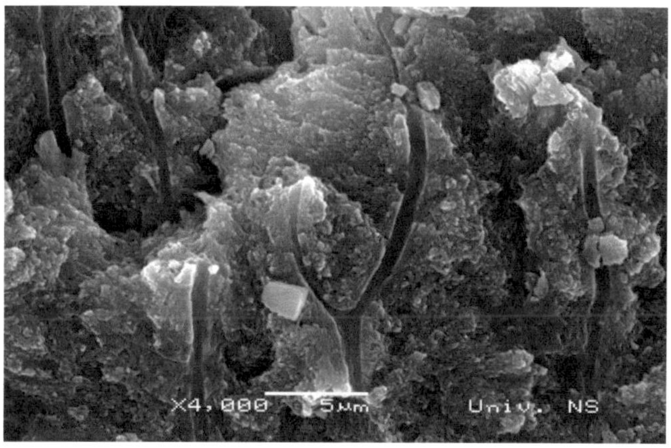

Fig. 3. SEM photographs of tooth dentine enlarged 4000x. Present dentine tubules are lined with peritubular dentin. Between the tubules is intertubular dentin.

When dentine is exposed to acid, the first signs of demineralisation are observable at the border of the peritubular and intertubular dentine, after which loss of peritubular dentine follows and widening of the lumen of dentine tubules and eventually a superficial layer of demineralised collagen matrix is, formed (Schlueter et al., 2011). In the initial period, this layer of collagen matrix protects the down lying tissue from further demineralisation, but it is very sensitive to the effects of mechanical forces and proteolytic enzymes and is fast eliminated and dentine tubes become exposed. Continuous exposure to acids causes' reduction of the demineralisation rate and at a certain thickness, the mineral loss is much less (Lussi et al., 2011), which may be explained by the buffering characteristic of collagen. The organic matrix may be degraded by specific and non-specific proteolytic enzymes (Schluter et al., 2010). Figure four depicts in the scanned electronic microphotograph the image of dentine at a longitudinal crosscut, exposed to the effects of pure hydrochloric acid pH 1 within 15 minutes. After only fifteen minutes the edges of the breakage become rounded and slowly the image of normal morphology is lost. Figure 4.

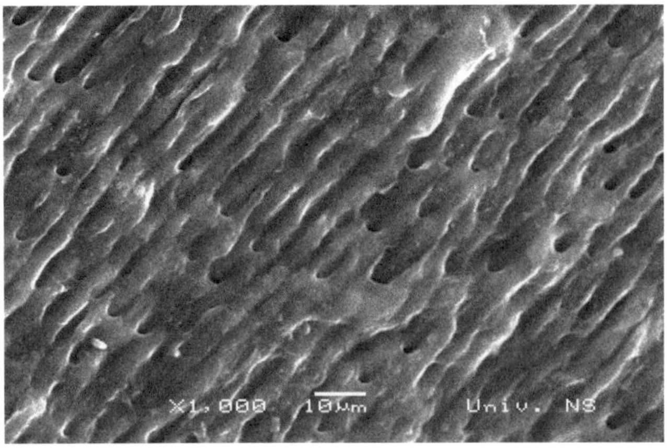

Fig. 4. SEM of dentine exposed to HCL pH1 for 15 min. After only fifteen minutes the edges of the breakage become rounded and the extent of dentinal tubules entrance.

Scanning electronic microphotography (SEM) of the exposed enamel, the enamel-dentine border and dentine in artificial saliva during a period of one hour shows no changes of dental structure and clearly defined morphological characteristics, however, if we submerge the sample of dental tissue into a centrifugal filtrate of stomach content within the same time interval, then the microphotograph is completely different Figure 5. Intensive erosions of the exposed surfaces with loss morphological characteristics prove the aggressive effect of stomach content on hard dental tissue (Stojšin, 2009).

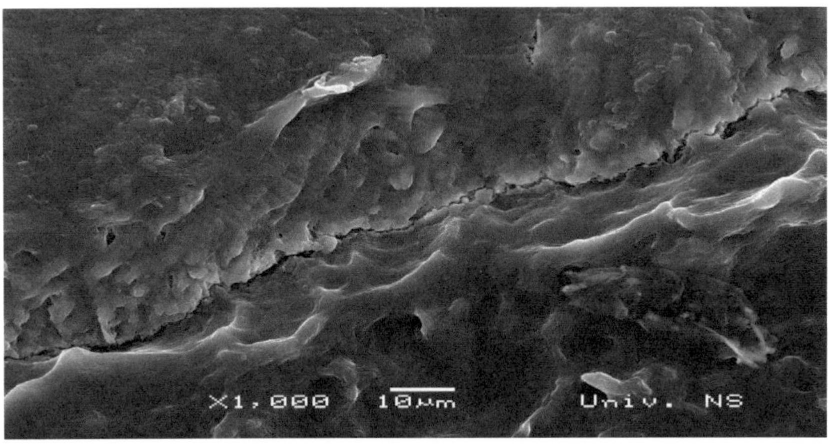

Fig. 5. SEM photograph of enamel, enamel-dentine border and dentine after one-hour exposure to centrifugal filtrate of stomach content. Clearly visible histo-morphological total loss characteristics observed tissue. Rounded bearing ameloblasts in the dentine.

Continuous erosive demineralisation with loss of hard dental tissue and exposure of dentine affects the activation of protective activities of pulp cells - of odontoblast and the synthesis of reactive and reparatory dentine which causes obturation of dental tubules themselves. It is a biological compensatory response. If the process continues the reparatory capacities wear off, pulp cavum exposes, inflammatory processes on the pulp disuse develop as well as necrosis and periapical pathology. Chronic inflammatory processes in the perapical region may be focal points with consequences to overall health.

5. Clinical assessment

Diagnosing dental erosions is difficult because there is not a single method or a procedure that would indicate early detection and quantification of these changes. In the early stadium, the changed surface of the enamel is smooth, shiny, without macroscopic defects (Amaechi & Higham, 2005). Sometimes it may be dull and without emphasised coloured lines as well as clearly established borders towards the changed part of the dental tissue.

In patients with the reflux disease, the defects are observable on the palatal surface of upper anterior teeth. The palatal surface becomes smooth, shiny and hard and the vestibule-oral diameter shrinks. The incisal edge seems thinned, translucent and slashed. In the gingival region existence of enamel collar may be detected. With loss of enamel, the tooth becomes yellowish, because of the bare dentine. The oral surfaces of the upper premolar and molar lose their morphology. Palatal lumps are becoming rounded or in their places cuplike dents occur and in advanced stadium a steep plane is formed, i.e. a complete loss of morphology Figure 6.

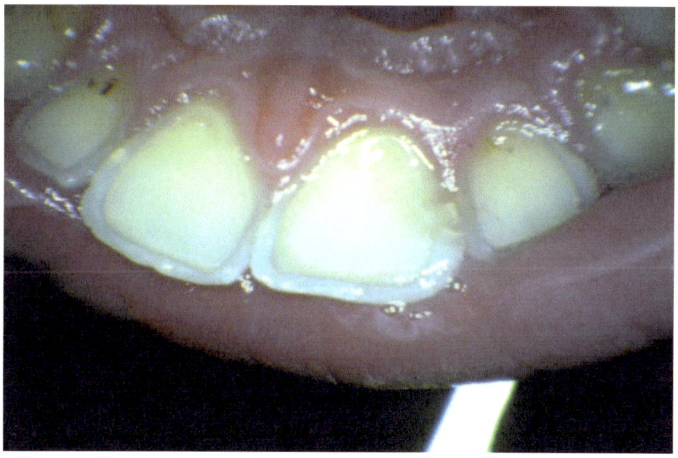

Fig. 6. Palatal surfaces of upper anterior teeth. The surface becomes smooth, shiny and hard and the vestibule-oral diameter shrinks. The incisal edge seems thinned, translucent and slashed

If the defect is localised on the lower anterior teeth, the incisal edge becomes a surface and later a groove is formed with its bottom in the dentine Figure 7.

The changes are much more often observable on the occlusal and vestibular surfaces of lower side teeth than in the anterior ones, because the lower anterior teeth bathe in excretions of the sublingual and submandibular saliva gland. The dorsum of the tongue directs the regurgitated content into the side region of the mandible, therefore, on the occlusal surfaces, the morphology is lost and cuplike defects are formed. On the vestibular surfaces, the changes are manifested through wide concavities. If the changes appear on the vestibular surfaces of the bottom anterior teeth then the direction of flow of the regurgitated content may clearly be seen Figure 8.

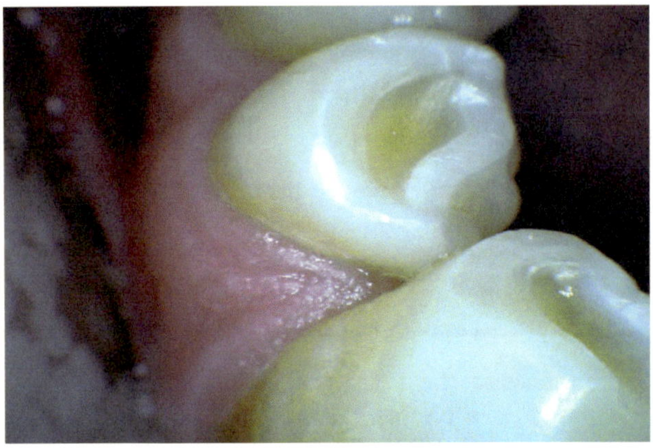

Fig. 7. Incisal surface of the lower anterior teeth with a groove in the dentine

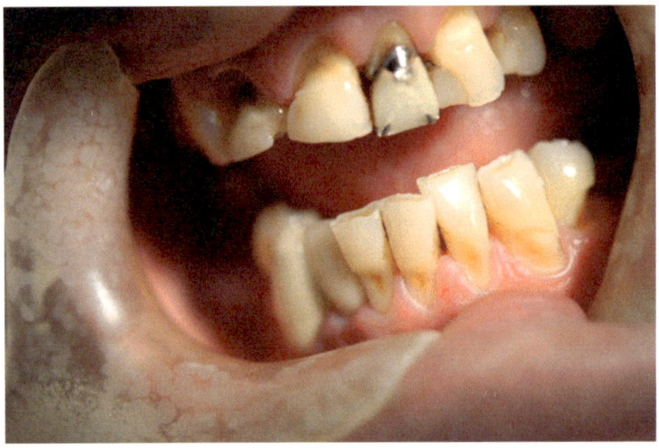

Fig. 8. Vestibular surfaces of the bottom anterior teeth. The gingival part of the vestibular surfaces of teeth has the defects that are wider than deep.

Amalgam or composite fillings on such teeth seem as grown and are located above the tooth structure Figure 9.

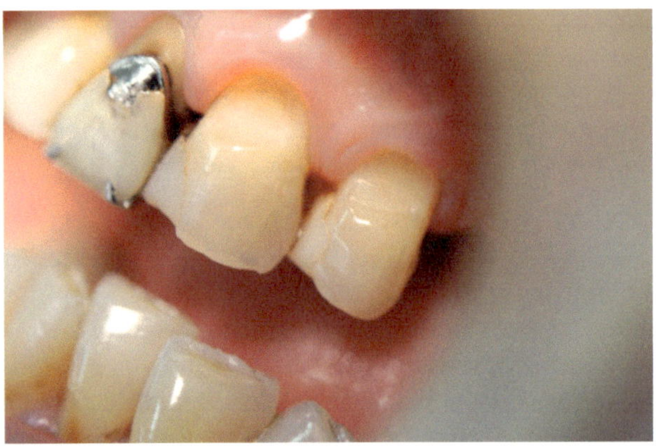

Fig. 9. Definitive fillings have "grown" from the dental tissue

Loss of enamel leads to the opening of dentine tubules and a consecutive phenomenon of dentine hypersensitivity as one of the symptoms. The pain is manifested as a shooting sensation to physical, chemical, thermal and evaporative triggers. Exogenous erosions are characterised by spherical defects on the occlusal surfaces. The vestibular surfaces may have defects of different shapes with the basic characteristic that they are rather wide than deep, but in all above mentioned shapes, there is loss of dental tissue (Lussi, 2006). The synergic effect of endogenous and exogenous agents brings about generalised changes that disturb the function of the masticatory apparatus.

It is even more difficult to diagnose erosive changes on primary teeth (Show &Sullivan, 2000). Enamel and dentin are thinner, less mineralised and more porous, so the aggressive effect of acid is even more expressed. The defects are smooth, shiny and rather wide than deep. In children, the changes are most often localised on the occlusal surfaces of molars and the incision edges of anterior teeth, which leads to loss of morphology, dentine hypersensitivity as well as complete loss of the crown of the tooth. All this leads to pulp inflammation and premature extraction of a milk tooth with all its consequences. When it is about defects on primary teeth they always have to be observed from the aspect of cumulative multifactoriality. Attrition of incisal edges in deciduous dentition is frequent during exfoliation and it is very difficult to assess then what the cause of the change is (Lussi, 2006).

In order to diagnose dental erosion, we need a thorough anamnesis, objective examination, analysis and assessment. Therefore a good questionnaire is needed with precisely defined questions which would enable easy diagnostics of the etiological factors as well as saliva analysis (determining the daily quantity of saliva, ph value, quantity of calcium and phosphate, the buffer capacity).

After an established diagnosis, it is necessary to follow the progress dynamics and a silicon index is used for this purpose, as well as the index of dental erosions, study models by Wicken and photographs (Daves, 2003).

Erosive effects of acids are only one of the mechanisms for the occurrence of dental defects. Numerous indices can be found in literature and they are mainly modifications of indices suggested by Eccles, Smith and Knight. The indices often used are also those suggested by the British Children's National Health, National Diet and Nutrition Surveys as well as the index suggested by Lussi (Lussi, 2006). All of them include diagnostic criteria for differentiating erosive changes from other forms of dental defects and criteria for the qualification of hard dental tissue loss.

6. Differential diagnosis

Erosions as causes of dental tissue loss are part of a much broader picture of dental defects, such as attrition, abrasion and abfraction.

Attrition is a defect of both dental tissue and restoration, and is caused by tooth to tooth contact during mastication or para-functions. Occlusal surfaces are smooth, shiny, evened and hard and on amalgam fillings facets are observable. The bottom of the defect may be located both in enamel and in dentine (Gandara&Truelove, 1999).

Abrasions occur with direct contact between the tooth and an alien substance (tooth whitening paste, anti-nicotine, soda...). The changes are usually localised in the cervical region of premolars and molars, always rather wide that deep (Roberson, Heymann & Swift, 2002).

Abfraction is a defect which is characterised by loss of dental tissue in the cervical region. It is caused by compression and stretching forces which take place during dental flexure. At inadequate occlusal relation, the changes are localised mainly vestibularly and they are of a wedged shape (Attin et al., 2004).

7. Prevention of erosive changes

The first step in every prevention is the identification of the etiological factor and its elimination. Many general medical diseases and conditions have repercussions in the mouth, both on soft tissue as well as on teeth. Therefore, an adequate therapy requires cooperation between experts of different specialties - gastroenterologists, oncologists, psychiatrists and dentists. Good prevention should include pharmacists who must, when issuing medication to patients, indicate the side effects of certain medications such as xerostomia (antihistamines, antidepressants, appetite suppressors ...). Some drugs directly express a high degree of erosiveness (chewing vitamin C, acetylsalylic acids ...) and it is necessary to inform patients how to minimize this effect (rinsing with re-mineralising agents) (Amaechi & Higham, 2005; Toumba, 2001).

If, after taken anamnesis, it is confirmed that the acid source is of exogenous source, education and consultation take a dominant role along with long-term examination of the health status of hard dental tissue (Gandara&Truelove, 1999).

All prevention measures may be divided into:

7.1 Measures that regulate the frequency of inflow and quantity of aggressive noxious factors

The first preventive measure is the regulation of regurgitation and reflux and that is the duty of physicians and specialists in gastroenterology. The proton pump inhibitors (PPI) represent the most effective therapy for gastroesophageal reflux. The dietetic measures include the reduction in the amount of intake of food and drink that are known to have erosive potential, change in the manner of their intake, especially beverages, is an important preventive factor for avoiding cumulative effects of acid of endogenous and exogenous origin in patients diagnosed with the reflux disease. It is better to consume the beverages through a straw and swallow them right away rather than shake them in the mouth (Gandara&Truelove, 1999). It is a known fact that cold beverages have much less erosive effect than beverages at room temperature (Amaechi & Higham, 2001). Dentists may suggest increased consumption of milk, cheese, almond in order to neutralize acidity in the mouth (Gedalia et al., 1992) as well as rinsing the mouth with soda solution. However, the aforementioned dietetic measures have no sense without the appropriate pharmacological therapy with proton pump inhibitors (PPI) and that basically, without it; the war against dental erosions is lost in advance.

7.2 Measures of enhancing the defence mechanism (salivary flow and pellicular formation)

This measure implies establishing hyper-salivation in the mouth which would intensify the protective characteristics of saliva. Consuming pastilles without sugar initiates salivation. A significant effect may be achieved by rinsing the mouth with artificial saliva in order to eliminate potential causes. Chewing gums, which are regularly prescribed to patients with exogenous erosions, are not advisable for patients with the reflux disease because of the effects on gastric secretion (Deshpande & Hugar, 2004). With expressed xerostomia it is necessary to prescribe pilocarpine –Salargan (Gandara&Truelove, 1999).

7.3 Measures of enhancing resistance and remineralisation of hard dental tissue

Increase of resistance and remineralisation of hard dental tissue may be achieved by preparations based on fluorine in the form of 2% solution of sodium fluoride and fluoride pastilles, jellies and lacquer.

Pastilles have the most positive effect because on the one hand they contain fluorides, and on the other they cause hyper-salivation (Jarvinen, Rytoma & Heinonen 1992; Stojšin, 2006). In all patients with observable changes on hard dental tissue, the application of fluorine in dental practice twice a year is necessary.

7.4 Measures of achieving mechanical protection

In patients with an evident gastroesophageal reflux it is advisable that they wear overnight occlusal protectors with applied fluorine preparations (Gandara & Truelove, 1999; West, 2011).

7.5 Measures of decreasing the effects of abrasive forces

The softened hard dental tissue is susceptible to the effects of aggressive tooth brushes and abrasive tooth pastes. Inadequate application of oral hygiene maintenance agents as well as the technique cause increase in the incidence and prevalence of other types of non carious dental tissue defects. That is why it is necessary to engage dentists more intensely in the dental health education. After waking up, the mouth should be first rinsed and then, after 30-60 minutes, the teeth should be cleaned. People with the reflux disease should use a soft toothbrush and non-abrasive pastes and brushing movements should be moderate and not too rough, whilst retaining the Bass methodology of brushing the teeth. Low pH value tooth pastes should be avoided.

8. Therapy

The detection of erosive changes either by patients or by a dentist is not easy. The patient turns for help only when it comes to short sharp pain sensations to thermal, evaporative, tactile, osmotic stimuli or with the occurrence of major defects that disrupt the aesthetics and function. General indications for restorative treatment are:

- Presence of dentine hypersensitivity
- Bad aesthetics
- Loss of vertical dimension of occlusion
- Endangered pulp - dentine complex
- Necessary rehabilitation of toothless areas.

The choice of treatment in dentine hypersensitivity depends on the type of patient's personality, history of the disease and an objective diagnosis (Amaechi & Higham, 2001).

There are two basic principles of medication effects and they are closure of dentinal tubules, or desensitisation of teeth. Desensitisation is achieved by preparations that contain potassium nitrate. The greatest success may be achieved by a 15% solution, 10% gel or toothpastes containing 10% potassium nitrate (Colgate R). Desensitization is achieved by the use of low-energy lasers (Kargul & Bakkal, 2009).

The therapeutic procedure in which the obliteration of dentinal tubules is emphasised may go in two directions. The agents that mimic the natural processes are fluorine preparations (sodium fluoride, sodium monofluorophosphate, tin fluoride) strontium chloride, calcium hydroxide and oxalates. The second group comprises the agents and procedures for closing the dentinal tubules and are represented by materials that mechanically or chemically bind to tooth surfaces, which are primers Copalit, Duraphat), adhesives (Gluma adhesive, Micro prima) and finally, composites and glass ionomer used in the case of dental defects of more extensive dental defects (Jarvinen et al., 1988; Živković, 1998).

The reconstruction of defects localised on non-occlusive surfaces is not problematic. If the bottom of the defect is localised in the enamel, the use of composites with micro-fillers is recommended with previous acid treatment of enamel. In cases where the bottom of the lesions is localised in the dentin or event the cement has been affected, it is necessary to use of dentin bonding systems in combination with composites or glass ionomers. For deeper defects, a layered technique is used with the use of adhesive systems, glass ionomer cement and the last generation of composites, compomers (Kargul & Bakkal, 2009; Jarvinen et al., 1988). Of all the composites, it would be the best to use a Nano DCPA - Whisker composite, which is capable of emitting calcium and phosphate ions [DCPA - Dicalcium Phosphate Anhydrate] (Show & Sullivan, 2000). The defects may be reconstructed also with ceramic facets, but more rarely because they are considered to be sensitive to acidic fluoride gels (Kargul & Bakkal, 2009; Mahoney & Kilpatrick, 2003).

The reconstruction of erosive defects on palatal surfaces of anterior teeth may be achieved with facets where the metal base is made of nickel-chrome alloy or gold. Preparation of the dental tissue is minimal and consists only of evening the enamel collar in the gingival third of the palatal surface of the eroded tooth and roughens the contact surface. In patients with the defected vertical dimension of the occlusion, first the Dahl's apparatus is placed in order to intrude an antagonist or a facet is constructed which is higher than necessary (Lussi et al., 1991). The binding mass for the facet may be resin or glass ionomer cement. Extensive defects of the palatal surface of the tooth may be reconstructed with purely metal facets. Vestibular defects and defects of the incisal edge may be reconstructed with non-metal ceramic facets or composites, but here, we must note that the same effect may be achieved with classical crowns.

The erosive effects in the side region in most cases are localised on the occlusal surfaces in the form of cuplike cavities. The deformed occlusal surfaces may be reconstructed with composites with micro-fillers or gold onlays with minimal tooth preparation and in absolutely dry working area. Conventional glass ionomer cements are not suggested because they have low resistance to wear and sensitivity in acidic environments. In cases when the defects are more extensive and encompass both occlusal and proximal surfaces of the tooth or they extend as far as cement, a good reconstruction is established with ceramic or conventional metallic crowns. In cases of generalised erosion of the side region, the reconstruction of the eroded dental tissue may be achieved with adhesive or ceramic onlays, metal, metal-ceramic crowns or non-metal ceramics with or without extension of the clinical crown (Lussi et al., 1991).

9. Conclusion

Dental erosion has to be recognized as extra esophageal manifestation of gastroesophageal reflux disease. It can result in tooth sensitivity, poor esthetic, loos of occlusal vertical dimension and functional problems. Clinicians must have thorough understanding of the causes of dental erosion as identification of the cause is the first step in its management. The inspection of the oral cavity in search for dental erosion should become a routine maneuver in patients who have GERD.

10. Acknowledgment

The authors thank Mr. Miloš Bokorov,Mr. Karlo Poljaković and Mr. Marko Stojšin for assistance with manuscript preparation. I would also like to thank our beloved family and friends for their understanding and support.

11. References

Addy, M. et al.,(2000). Tooth wear and sensitivity: clinical advances in restotative dentistry. *Martin Dunitz Ltd.* ISBN 1-85317-826-8, London, Engleska

Allan, D.N.,(1967). Enamel erosion with lemon juice, *British Dental Journal,* Vol. 122, No. 7.pp.300-2,(April 1967). ISSN 0007-0610

Allan,D.N.,(1969). Dental erosion from vomiting: a case report. *British Dental Journal,* Vol.126, pp 311-2, ISSN 0007-0610

Amaechi,B.T.et al.,(1999).Thickness of acquired salivary pellicle as a determinant of the sites of dental erosion. *Journal of Dental Research,* Vol. 78. pp.1821- 8. ISSN 0022-0345

Amaechi,B.T.& Higham,S.M.,(2001). In vitro remineralisation of eroded enamel lesions by saliva. *Journal of Dentistry.* Vol.29, No.5, pp.371-6. ISSN 0300-5712

Amaechi,T.B. & Higham, M.S.,(2001). Eroded lesion remineralisation by saliva as a possible factor in situ-specificity of human dental erosion. *Archives of Oral Biology.* (August 2001), Vol.46, No.8, pp.697-703, ISSN 0003 -9969

Amaechi,T.B. & Higham, M.S., (2005). Dental erosion: possible approaches to prevention and control. Journal of Dentistry,(March 2005), Vol. 33, No.(3), pp. 243-52

Anđić, J., (2000). Oral homeostasis, Second edition, *Nauka,* Beograd.

Attin, T. et al.(2004) Brushing Abrasion of Softened and Remineralised Dentin: an in situ, *Caries Research,* (Jan-Feb 2004), Vol.38, No.1, pp.62-6, ISSN (printed) 0008 -6568, (electronic) 1421-976x

Bargen, J.A. & Austin, L.T., (1937). Decalcification of teeth as a result of obstipation with long continued vomiting: report of a case, *The Journal of American Dental Association,* (Jan 1937), Vol. 24, pp. 1271-3, ISSN 0375 - 8451

Bartlett,D.W.; Evans,D.F. & Smith,B.G.,(1996). The relationship between gastroesophageal reflux disease and dental erosion. *Journal of Oral Rehabilitation,* Vol. 23, No. 5, pp. 289-97, (May 1996), ISSN (printed)0305 -182x,(electronic)1365-2842

Bartlett,D. & Smith,B., (1996), The dental relevance of gastro-oesophageal reflux part 2, *Dent Update,* Vol. 23, pp. 250-3, (Julay - August 1996), ISSN (print)0305 - 182x,(electronic)1365-2842

Daves, C., (2003). What is the Critical pH and Why Does a Tooth Dissolve In Acid. *Journal of the Canadian Dental Association*, Vol. 69, No. 11, pp.722-4, ISSN 0008-3372

Dena, A. Ali. et al., (2002). Dental erosion caused by silent gastroesophageal refluks disease. *The Journal of American Dental Association*, Vol. 133, No. 6, pp. 734-7, ISSN 0002 - 8177

Deshpande, S.D. & Hugar, S.M., (2004). Dental erosion in children: An increasing clinical problem. *Journal of Indian Society and Pedodontics and Preventive Dentistry,* Vol. 22, No. 3, pp.118-27, ISSN 0970-4388

Eccles,J.D.,(1982). Tooth surface loss from abrasion, attrition and erosion. *Dent Update, Vol.* 9, No. 7, pp.373-81,(August 1982),

Edgar, M.W. & O'Mullane, M.D., (1990). Saliva and oral health. *British Dental Journal.* Vol. 169, No. 3-4, pp.96-8,(August 1990), ISSN 0007-0610

Edgar,A., (1992). Saliva its secretion, composition and functions. *British Dental Journal.* Vol. 172, No. 8, pp.305-12, (April 1992), ISSN 0007-0610

Eisenburger,M. et al., (2001). Effect of time on the remineralisation of enamel by synthetic saliva after citric acid erosion. *Caries Research.* Vol. 35, pp. 211-5. *ISSN* (printed): *0008-6568. ISSN* (electronic): 1421-976X.

Eisenburger,M.; Shellis,R.P. & Addy., (2004). Scanning electron microscopy of softened enamel. *Caries Research.* Vol. 38, No. 1, pp.67-74, (Jan-Feb 2004). *ISSN* (printed): *0008-6568. ISSN* (electronic): 1421-976X.

Featherstone,J.D.B. & Rodgers,B.E., (1981). Effect of acetic, lactic and other organic acids on the formation of artificial carious lesion. *Caries Research.* Vol. 15, pp. 377-85. *ISSN* (printed): *0008-6568. ISSN* (electronic): 1421-976X.

Feldman,M.; Scharschmidt,B. & Sleisenger,M.,(1998. Gastrointestinal and Liver Disease: Pathophysiology, Diagnosis, Management. Edition 6, *Saunders,* pp 117-27, Philadelphia.

Gandara,B. & Truelove,E., (1999). Diagnosisi and Management of Dental Erosion. *The Journal of Contemporary Dental Practice,* Vol. 1, No. 1, pp. 16-23, (November 1999). ISSN 1526-3711.

Ganss,C.; Klimek,J. & Starck,C., (2004). Quantitative analysis of the impact of the organic matrix on the fluoride effect on erosion progression in human dentin using longitudinal microradiograph. *Archives of Oral Biology.* Vol. 49, Issue 11. pp.931-5. ISSN 0003-9969.

Gedalia et al., (1992). Effect of hard cheese exposure with and without fluoride prerinse, on the rehardening of softened human enamel. *Caries Research.* Vol 26. No. 4, pp.290-2, ISSN (printed): *0008-6568. ISSN* (electronic): 1421-976X.

Gilmour,A.G. & Beckelt,H.A.,(1993). The voluntary reflux phenomenon. *British Dental Journal.* Vol. 175, No. 10, pp.368-72. ISSN 0007-0610.

Gregory-Head,B.L. & Curtis,D.A.,(1977). Erosion caused by gastroesophageal reflux: diagnosis considerations. *Journal of Prosthodontics.* Vol. 6, No. 4, pp. 278-85. ISSN 1059-941x.

Hanning,C.; Hanning,M. & Attin T.,(2005). Enzyms in the acquired enamel pellicle. *European Journal of Oral Sciences.* Vol. 113, pp. 2-13, ISSN 0909-8836

He,L.H. & Swain,M.V.,(2009). Enamel – a functionally graded natural coating. *Journal of Dentistry.* Vol. 37, No. 8, pp.596-603, ISSN 0300-5712

Holst,J.J. & Lange,F.,(1939). Perimolysis:a contribution towards the genesis of tooth wasting from non-mechanical causes. *Acta Odontologica Scandinavica.* Vol. 1, No. 1, pp.36-48, ISSN 0001-6357

Howden,G.F.,(1971). Erosion as the representing symptom in hiatus hernia. *British Dental Journal.* Vol. 131, Issue. 10, pp. 455-6. ISSN 0007-0610

Hunter,M.L. et al., (2000). Erosion of deciduous and permanent hard tissue in the oral environment. *Journal of Dentistry*. Vol. 28, No.4, pp.257-63. ISSN 0300-5712

Imfeld,T.,(1996). Dental erosion. Definition, classification and links. Eurpean *Journal of Oral Sciences*. Vol. 104, Issue 2, pp. 151-5. ISSN 0909-8836

Jarvinen, V.(1988). Dental erosion and upper gastrointestnal disorders. *Oral Surgery Oral Medicine Oral Pathology Oral Radiology and Endodonttology*. Vol. 65, No. 3, pp.298-303, ISSN 0012-3692.

Jarvinen,V.K.; Rytoma,I.I. & Heinonen,O.P.,(1992). Location of dental erosion in a referred population. *Caries Research*. Vol. 26, No. 5, pp. 391-6. ISSN 0008-6568

Johanson,A.K. et al., (2001.) Dental erosion in deciduous teeth - an in vivo and in vitro study. *Journal of Dentistry*. Vol. 29, No. 5, pp.333-40. ISSN 0300-5712

Kargul,B. & Bakkal,M.,(2009).Prevalence,Etiology,Risk Factors,Diagnosis and preventive strategies of Dental eosion.Literature Review(Part I & Part II), *Acta Stomatologica Croatica,*Vol. 43, No. 3, 165-87. ISSN(print) 0001-7019

Klein,D.W. & Walsh,B.T.,(2004). Eating disorders: clinical features and pathophysiology. *Physiology & Behavior*. Vol. 81, No. 2, pp. 359-74. ISSN 0031-9384.

Kleter,G.A. et al.,(1994).The influence of the organic matrix on demineralization of bovine root dentin in vitro. *Journal of Dental Research*. Vol. 73, No. 9, pp 1523-39, ISSN(print) 0022-0345, ISSN(on line)1544-0591

Lazarchik,D. & Filler,S.,(1997). Effects of gastroesophageal reflux on the oral cavity. *The American Journal of Medicine*. Vol. 103, Issue 5a, pp. 107-13, ISSN 0002-9343

Lussi,A. et al.,(1991). Dental erosion in population of Swiss adults. *Community Dentistry and Oral Epidemiology*. Vol. 19, No. 5, pp.286-290, ISSN (print) 0301 -5661, ISSN (online) 1600 - 0528

Lussi,A.(2006). Dental Erosion From Diagnosis to Therapy. Monogr In Oral Sci, II Series, Karger AG, ISBN 3-8055-8097-5 , Basel, Switzerland.

Lussi,A. et al. (2011).Dental erosion - An Overview with Emphasis on Chemical and Histopathological Aspects. *Caries Research*. Vol. 45, Suppl. 1, pp. 2-12. , ISSN (printed): *0008-6568. ISSN* (electronic): 1421-976X.

Mahoney,E.K. & Kilpatrick,N.M.,(2003). Dental erosion part 1 Etiology and prevalence of dental erosion. *New Zealand Dental Journal*. Vol. 99, No. 2, pp.33-41, ISSN 0028 - 8047

Meurman,J.H. & Frank,R.M.,(1991). Scanning electron microscopy study of the effect of salivary pellicle on enamel erosion. *Caries Research*. Vol. 25, No. 1, pp. 1-6, ISSN (printed): *0008-6568. ISSN* (electronic): 1421-976X.

Meurman,J.H. & ten Cate, J.M.,(1996). Pathogenesis and modifying factors of dental erosion. *European Journal of Oral Sciences*. Vol. 104, Issue 2, pp. 199-206, ISSN 0909-8836.

Myllarniemi,H. & Saario,I. (1985) A new type of sliding hiatus hernia. Annals of Surgery. Vol. 202, Issue 2, pp.159-161, ISSN 0003-4932

Nebel,O.T.;Fornes,M.F. & Castell,D.O., (1976).Symptomatic gastroesophageal reflux: incidence and precipitating factors. *The American Journal of Digestive Diseases*. Vol. 21, No. 11, pp. 953-956, ISSN 0002-9211.

Odutuga,A.A. & Prout,R.E.S.,(1974). Lipid analysis of human enamel and dentine. *Archives of Oral Biology*. Vol. 19, pp. 729-31, ISSN 0003-9969

Pindborg,J.J.,(1970). Pathology of the dental hard tissues. *W.B.Saunders Co.*,First edition, ASIN B00138LVQU, Philadelphia, U.S.A.

Rios,D. et al.,(2008). Scanning electron microscopy study of the in situ effect of salivary stimulation on erosion and abrasion in human and bovine enamel. *Brazilian Oral Research*. Vol. 22, No. 2, pp. 132-8. ISSN (print) 1806 - 8324

Robb,N.D. & Smith,B.G.N.,(1990). Prevalence of pathological tooth wear in patients with chronic alchoholism. *British Dental Journal*. Vol. 169, pp.367-9. Published online, doi:10.1038/sj.bdj.4807386

Schlueter,N.et al., (2010). Influence of the digestive enzymes trypsin and pepsin in vitro on the progression of erosion in dentin. *Archives of Oral Biology*. Vol. 55, Issue 4, pp. 294-9. ISSN 0003 - 9969.

Goncalves,G.K., et al.(2008). Dental erosion in cerebral palsy patients. *Journal of Dentistry for Children*, Vol. 25, No. 2, May-August 2008, pp. 117 -20. ISSN 0022 - 0353

Schlueter,N.et al.,(2011). Methods for the Measurement and characterization of Erosion in Enamel and Dentin. *Caries Research*. Vol. 45, Supp. 1, pp. 13-23 ISSN (printed): *0008-6568. ISSN* (electronic): 1421-976X.

Show,L.O. & Sullivan,E.U.K., (2000). National Clinical Guidelines in Paediatric Dentistry Diagnosis and prevention of dental erosion in children. *International Journal of Paediatric Dentistry*. Vol. 10, Issue 4, pp.356-65, ISSN (print) 0960 -7439, ISSN (online) 1365 -263X.

Stojšin,I., Blažić,L. & Brkanić,T.,(2006). Therapy of dentine hypersensitivity, *Stomatološki Informator* . Val .V, No. 18, pp. 7-12, ISSN 1451-3439.

Stojšin,I.,(2009).Dental manifestation of gastroesophageal reflux disease. *PhD thesis*, Novi Sad, Srbija.

Roberson, M.T., Heymann,O.H. & Swift J.E., (2002). Sturtevant's Art & Science of operative dentistry. Four editions, *Mosby Inc.* ISBN 0-323-01087-3, U.S.A.

Theuns, H.M. et al.,(1986). Experimental evidence for a gradient in the solubility and in the rate of dissolution of human enamel. *Caries Research*. Vol. 20, No. 1, pp. 24-31, ISSN (printed): *0008-6568. ISSN* (electronic): 1421-976X.

Toumba,J.K.(2001). Slow release devices for fluoride delivery to high-risk individuals. *Caries Research*. Vol. 35, Suppl. 1, pp. 10-13. , ISSN (printed): *0008-6568. ISSN* (electronic): 1421-976X.

Vakil,N.(2006). The Montreal definition and clasiffication of gastro-esophageal reflux disease: a global evidence - based consens. *The American Journal of Gastroenterology*. Vol. 101, No. 8, pp. 1900-1920. ISSN 0002-9270.

Vulović,M. et al.(2005): Preventive Dentistry. Second revised and updated edition, *Draslar*, Belgrade, ISBN 86-7614-026-x,Srbija.

Young,W.G. & Khan,F.(2002), Sites of dental erosion are saliva-dependent. *Journal of Oral Rehabilitation*, Vol. 29, Issue 1, pp.35-43, ISSN(online) 1365 - 2842.

Young,A. & Tenuta,L.M.A.(2011). Initial Erosion Models. Caries Research, Vol. 45, No. 1, pp. 33-41.

Živković, S.(1998). Dentin adhesivna sredstva u stomatolgiji. First edition, *Balkanski Stomatološki forum*, Beograd, Srbija.

West,X.N.;Davies,M & Amaechi,T.B.(2011). In vitro and In situ Erosion Models for Evaluating Tooth Substance Loss. *Caries Researcs*. Vol. 45, Supp. 1, pp. 43-52. , ISSN (printed): *0008-6568. ISSN* (electronic): 1421-976X.

5

Analysis of Symptoms in Patients with Minimal Change Esophagitis Versus Those with Reflux Esophagitis and Peptic Ulcer

Yasuyuki Shimoyama[1], Motoyasu Kusano[2] and Osamu Kawamura[1]

[1]Gunma University Graduate School of Medicine, Department of Medicine and Molecular Science,
[2]Gunma University Hospital, Department of Endoscopy and Endoscopic Surgery, Japan

1. Introduction

According to the 2006 Montreal globally acceptable definition and classification of gastroesophageal reflux disease (GERD), this condition develops when the reflux of gastric contents causes symptoms or complications (Vakil et al., 2006). Because reflux esophagitis is defined as occurring when reflux of gastric acid into the esophagus causes mucosal breaks, erosions and/or ulcers, this condition requires endoscopic diagnosis. Non-erosive reflux disease (NERD) is defined by occurrence of reflux symptoms in patients without any endoscopic mucosal breaks. Thus, NERD includes prominent erythema without clear demarcation or whitish cloudiness of the lower esophageal mucosa obscuring the longitudinal blood vessels, which used to be known as the "discoloring" type of reflux esophagitis in Japan. In the present study, we characterized the symptoms and pathophysiology of patients with minimal change esophagitis (MC esophagitis), who had prominent erythema and whitish cloudiness of the esophageal mucosa.

2. Subjects and methods

The subjects were 347 patients who attended the Gastroenterology Outpatient Department of Gunma University Hospital with symptoms of upper abdominal pain or discomfort. All of them underwent upper gastrointestinal endoscopy to rule out organic disorders. The endoscopic diagnosis was determined by reviewing the endoscopic findings documented for each patient (Table 1). The endoscopists were unaware of the results of the patient questionnaire when they performed endoscopy, and only experienced endoscopists (who had carried out more than 3,000 endoscopic procedures) performed examinations in the present study. The modified Los Angeles (LA) classification was used for endoscopic diagnosis of GERD (Hongo, 2006). This classification employs the term "mucosal break" to describe mucosal lesions of the esophagus, with a mucosal break being defined as an area of slough or erythema that is clearly demarcated from the adjacent normal-looking mucosa. According to the original LA classification, GERD is divided into four grades from A to D. Grade A means one or more mucosal breaks no longer than 5 mm, none of which extends between the tops of two mucosal folds. Grade B is one or more mucosal breaks>5 mm long, none of which extends between the tops of two mucosal folds. Grade C means mucosal breaks that extend between the tops of two or more mucosal folds, but are not circumferential, while Grade D indicates one or more circumferential mucosal breaks (Armstrong et al., 1996). Before Grade A, we added Grade M (minimal change), which was defined as prominent erythema without clear demarcation or whitish cloudiness of the lower esophageal mucosa obscuring the longitudinal blood vessels (Fig. 1). This corresponds to the so-called "discoloring" type of reflux esophagitis in Japanese terminology. A diagnosis of peptic ulcer (gastric or duodenal ulcer) was made if a lesion with definite plaque was identified. Endoscopic gastritis was classified as erosive (frank erosions), superficial (redness, edema, and adherent mucus in the gastric body), or atrophic (distal migration of the border between the pyloric and fundic glands in the gastric body, as well as clearly visible vessels). When a patient had two or more diagnoses, the following order of priority was employed: GERD, gastric ulcer, duodenal ulcer, gastritis (erosive, superficial, or atrophic), or normal. Patients who were endoscopically normal or had gastroduodenitis were classified into a non-esophagitis and non-ulcer (NE-NU) group. There were 39 patients with MC esophagitis, 85 with GERD (LA grade≥A), 195 in the NE-NU group, and 28 with gastric ulcer or duodenal ulcer (GU+DU).

	MC esophagitis (n = 39)	GERD (n = 85)	NE-NU (gastritis,duodenitis,or normal) (n = 195)	GU + DU (n = 28)
Sex (men, women)	19, 20	52, 33	81, 114	19, 9
Mean age (years)±SD	59.7 ± 13.1	60.9 ± 14.1	58.6 ± 14.2	55.2 ± 18.9
Endoscopic severity (n)				
Grade M	39	0	0	0
Grade A + B	0	74	0	0
Grade C + D	0	11	0	0

Table 1. Demographic data of the subjects

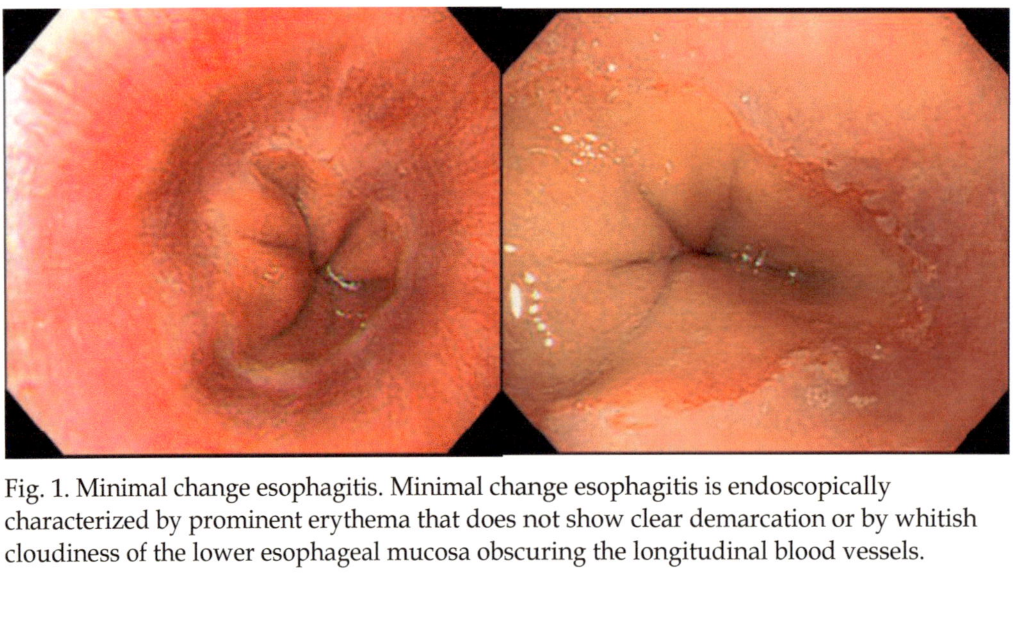

Fig. 1. Minimal change esophagitis. Minimal change esophagitis is endoscopically characterized by prominent erythema that does not show clear demarcation or by whitish cloudiness of the lower esophageal mucosa obscuring the longitudinal blood vessels.

Each subject completed a 37-item self-administered questionnaire that covered gastroesophageal reflux symptoms, dysmotility-like symptoms, ulcer-like symptoms, and psychosomatic symptoms. The questions were randomly arranged and each question could be answered as "yes" or "no") (Table 2). There were 12 questions dealing with gastroesophageal reflux. In particular, heartburn was assessed from multiple perspectives, including the actual symptoms, timing of onset, and influence of posture: "Do you get heartburn?"; "Do you subconsciously rub your chest with your hand?"; "Do you get a stinging sensation in your chest?"; "Do you mainly get heartburn after meals?"; and "Do you get heartburn if you bend forward?". In addition, 10 questions related to dysmotility and 4 questions related to ulcers were used to examine accessory symptoms of GERD. The questions related to dysmotility included: "Does your stomach get bloated?"; "Does your stomach ever feel heavy after meals?"; "Do you feel full right after meals?"; and "Do you get nausea?". The questions relating to ulcer symptoms included: "Do you get pain in the stomach after you eat?"; "Do you get pain in the stomach at night?"; and "Do you get pain when you have an empty stomach?". Furthermore, 11 questions dealt with psychosomatic symptoms, including: "Do you feel sick?", "Are you anxious?" and "Do you feel languid?". Subjects completed the questionnaire prior to endoscopy. An explanation of the questions was not provided, but information was given if a subject had any queries. The frequency of "yes" answers was calculated for each question. The χ^2 test was used to compare data among the MC esophagitis, GERD, and NE-NU groups, with $P<0.05$ being considered statistically significant.

3. Results

Figures 2-5 displays the symptoms in each category that showed significant differences ($p<0.05$ by the χ^2 test) among the four groups (MC esophagitis, GERD, NE-NU, and GU+DU groups).

Question
Gastroesophageal reflux symptoms
Do you get heartburn?
Do you subconsciously rub your chest with your hand?
Do you cough?
Do you get a stinging sensation in your chest?
Do you mainly get heartburn after meals?
Do you get pain in the throat?
Do you get heartburn if you bend forward?
Do some things get stuck when you swallow?
Do you get heartburn when lying down?
Do you feel a burning sensation from the pit of the stomach to the lower chest?
Do you get acidic liquid coming up into your mouth?
Do you get pain in the chest?

Dysmotility-like symptoms
Do you get nausea on waking?
Does your stomach get bloated?
Does your stomach ever feel heavy after meals?
Do you feel sick and heavy after fatty meals?
Do you feel sick and heavy after you overeat?
Do you feel full right after meals?
Do you burp a lot?
Are you unable to eat immediately after waking in the morning?
Do you get nausea?
Does your stomach ever feel heavy when it is empty?

Ulcer-like symtoms
Do you get pain in the stomach after you eat?
Do you have dark feces?
Do you get pain in the stomach at night?
Do you get pain in the stomach when it is empty?

Psychosomatic symptoms
Do you fall asleep unpleasantly?
Do you wake up unpleasantly?
Do you get frustrated?
Do you feel like taking a break?
Do you have change in the sense of taste?
Have you lost the desire to eat?
Do you feel sick?
Are you anxious?
Are you unable to sleep long enough?
Do you easily get tired?
Do you feel languid?

Did you experience any of these symptoms during the previous 2 weeks?
Please circle "yes" or "no".

Table 2. The 37-item questionnaire

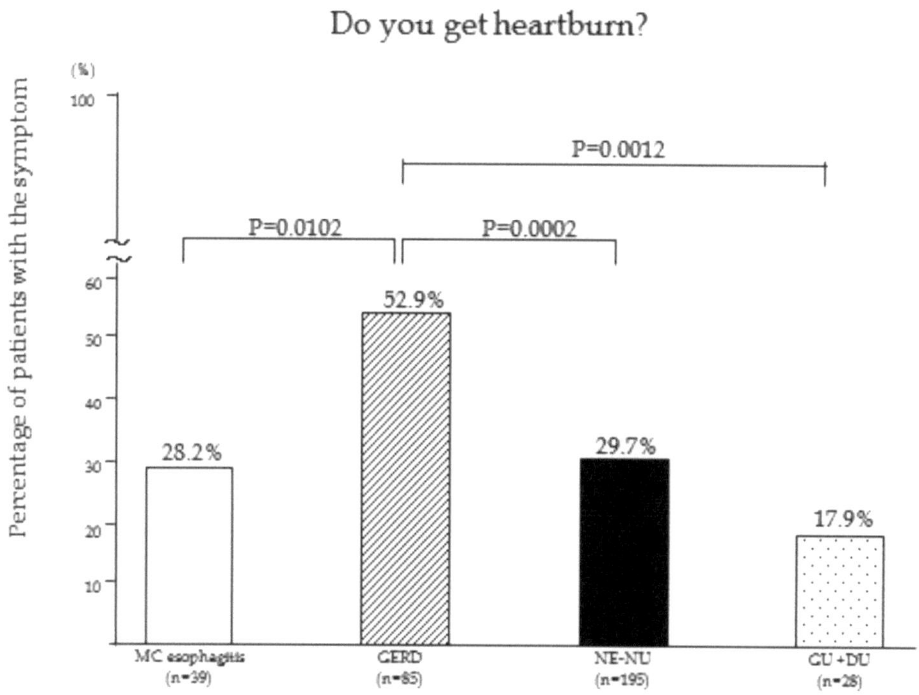
Do you get heartburn?
Percentage of patients with the symptom
(%)
100
60
50
40
30
20
10
P=0.0012
P=0.0102
P=0.0002
28.2%
52.9%
29.7%
17.9%
MC esophagitis
(n=39)
GERD
(n=85)
NE-NU
(n=195)
GU+DU
(n=28)

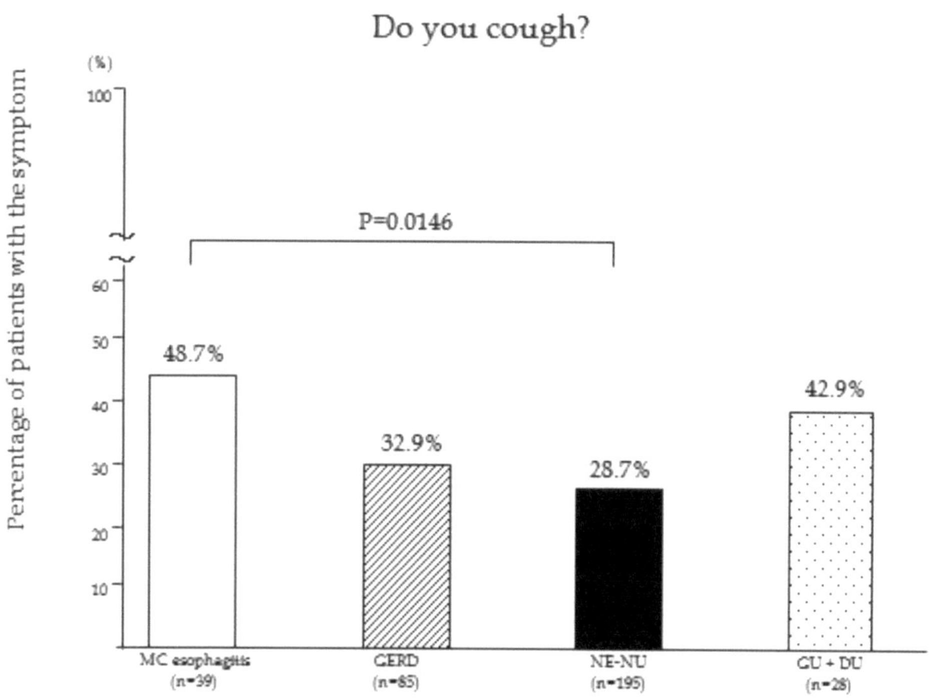
Do you cough?
Percentage of patients with the symptom
(%)
100
60
50
40
30
20
10
P=0.0146
48.7%
32.9%
28.7%
42.9%
MC esophagitis
(n=39)
GERD
(n=85)
NE-NU
(n=195)
GU+DU
(n=28)

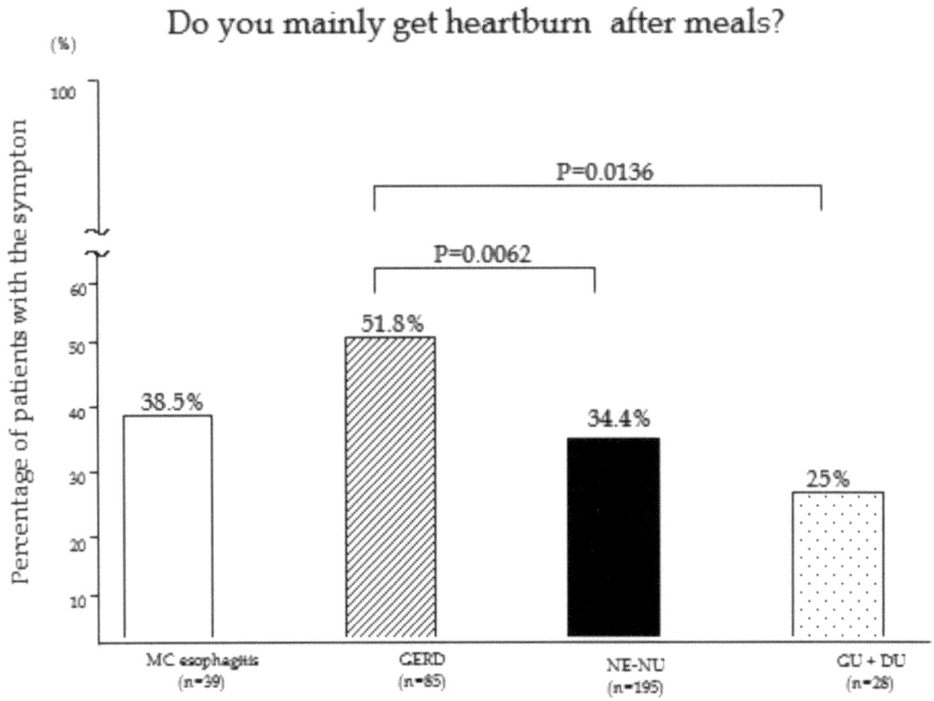
Do you mainly get heartburn after meals?
(%)
100
60
50
40
30
20
10
Percentage of patients with the sympton
P=0.0136
P=0.0062
51.8%
38.5%
34.4%
25%
MC esophagitis (n=39)
GERD (n=85)
NE-NU (n=195)
GU + DU (n=28)

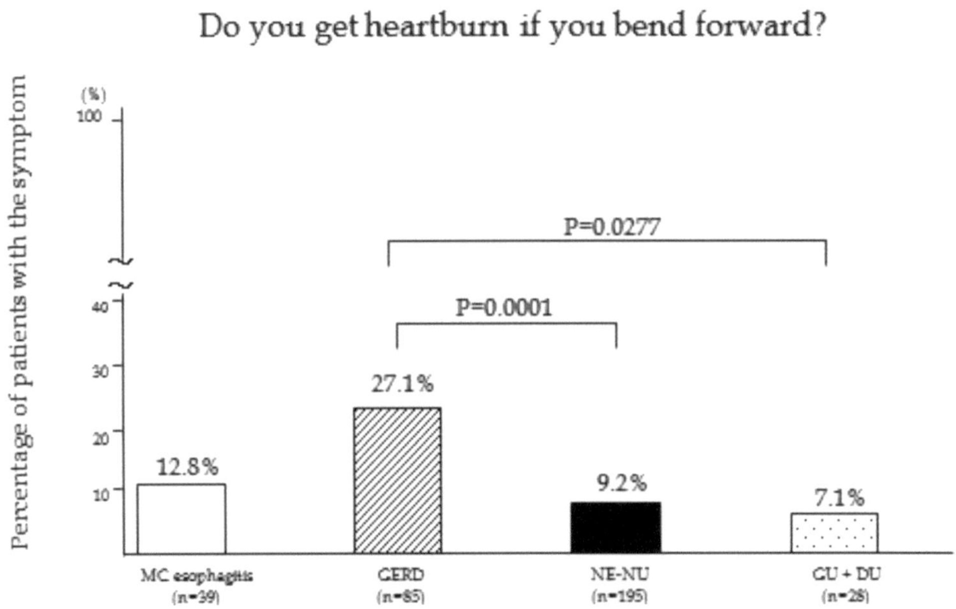
Do you get heartburn if you bend forward?
(%)
100
40
30
20
10
Percentage of patients with the symptom
P=0.0277
P=0.0001
27.1%
12.8%
9.2%
7.1%
MC esophagitis (n=39)
GERD (n=85)
NE-NU (n=195)
GU + DU (n=28)

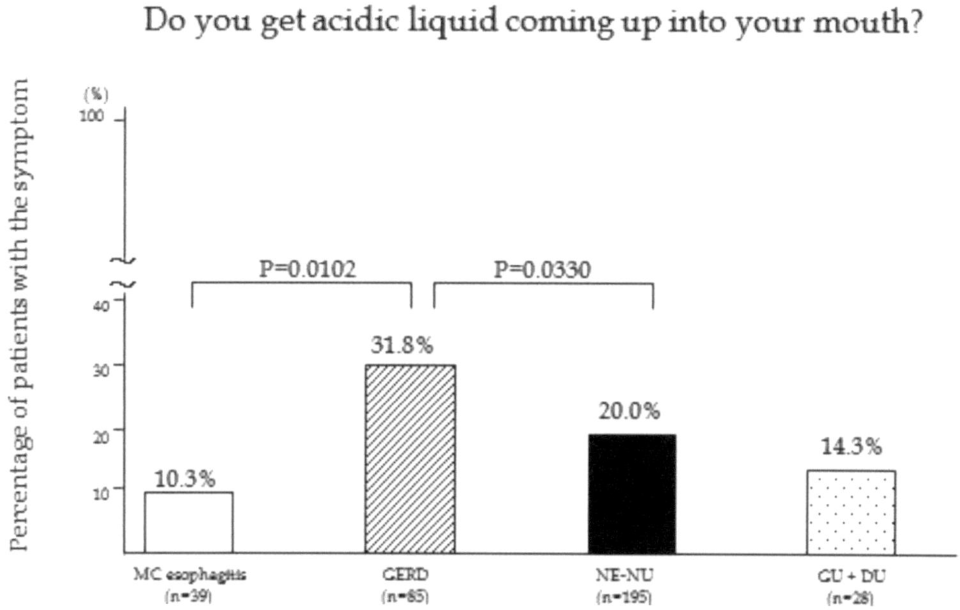

Fig. 2. Gastroesophageal reflux symptoms showing significant differences among the groups Comparison was done among the MC esophagitis, GERD, NE-NU, and GU+DU groups by the χ^2 test.

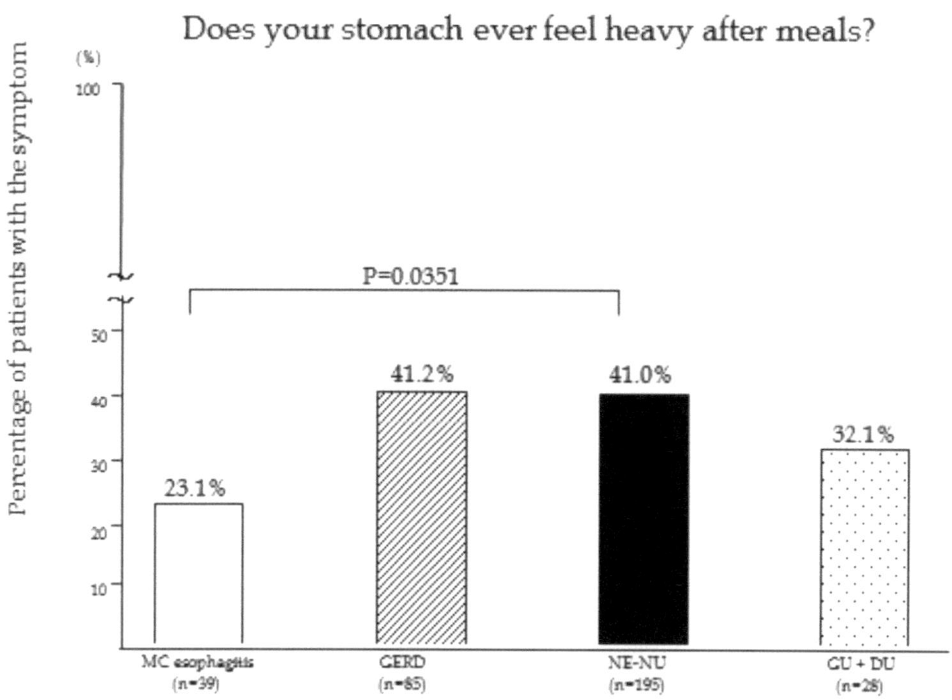

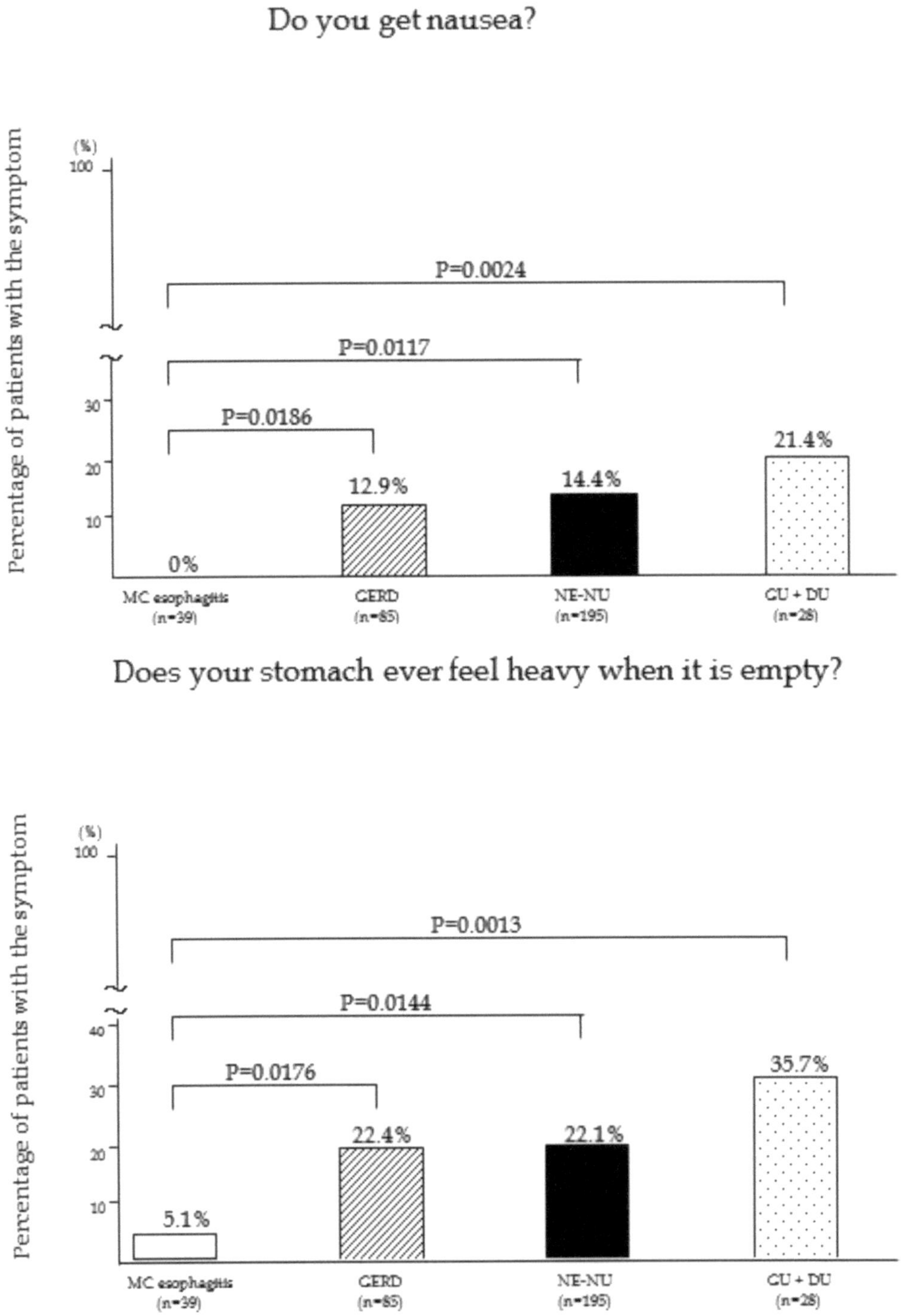

Fig. 3. Dysmotility-like symptoms showing significant differences among the groups Comparison was done among the MC esophagitis, GERD, NE-NU, and GU+DU groups by the χ^2 test.

Do you get pain in the stomach at night?

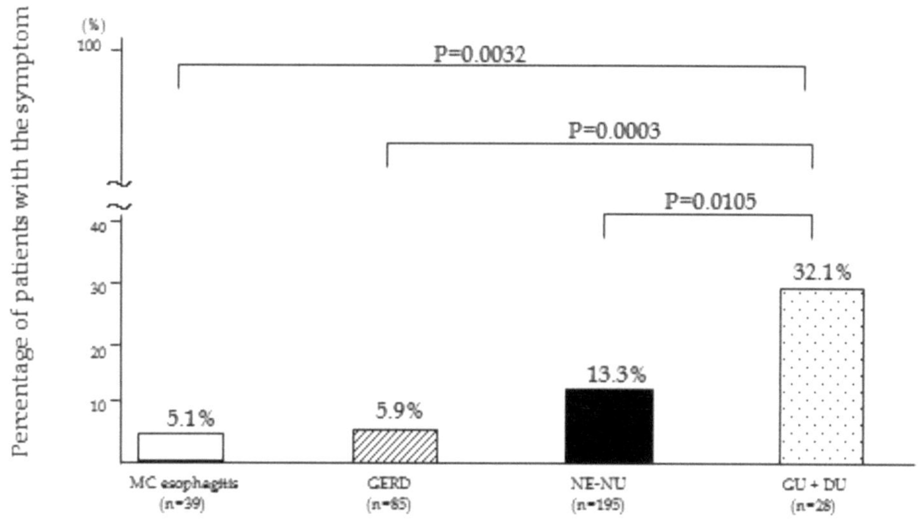

Do you get pain in the stomach when it is empty?

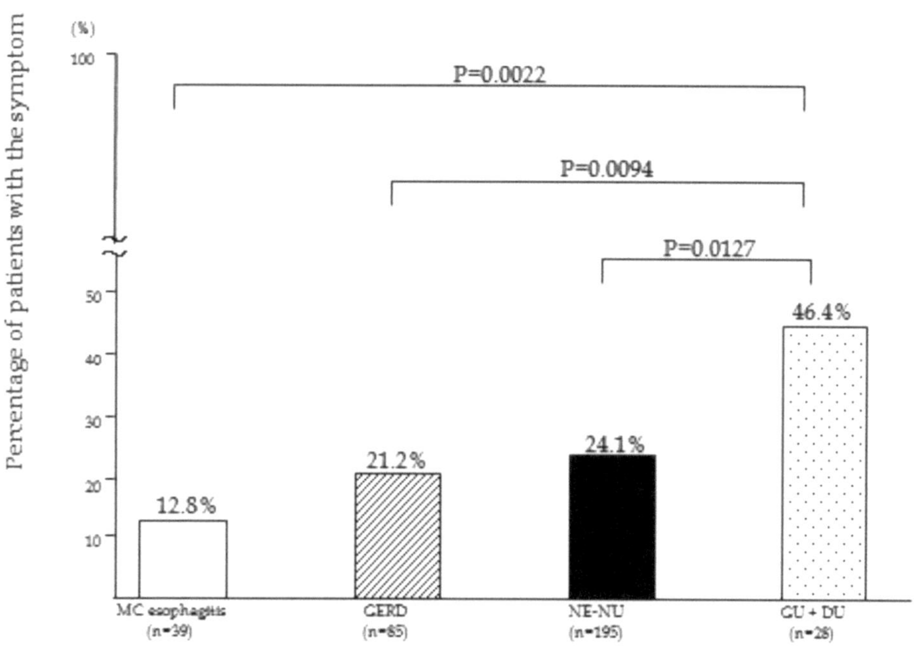

Fig. 4. Ulcer-like symptoms showing significant differences among the groups
Comparison was done among the MC esophagitis, GERD, NE-NU, and GU+DU groups by the χ^2 test.

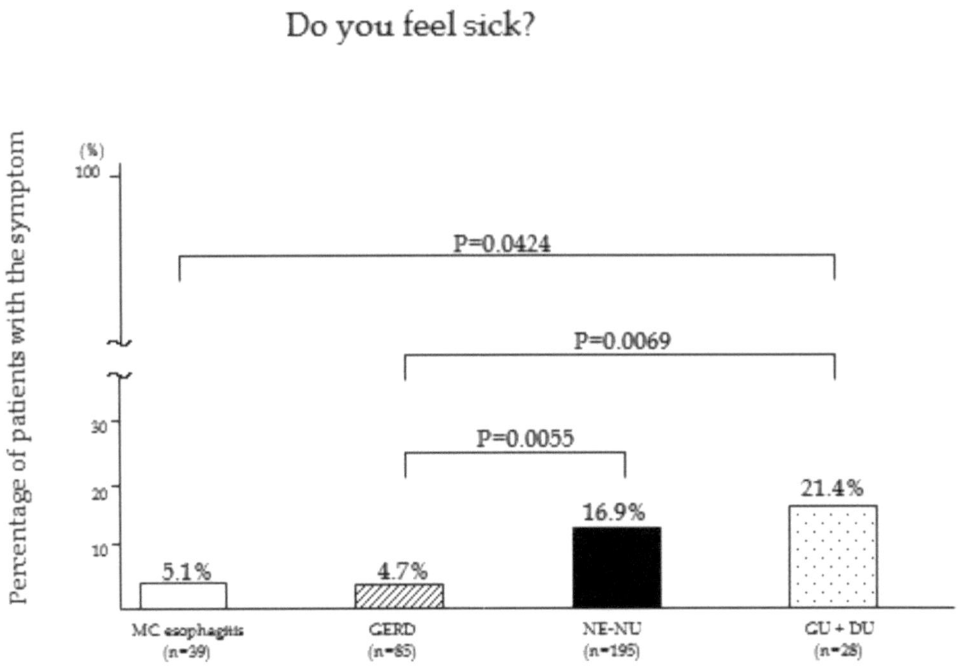
Do you feel sick?
Percentage of patients with the symptom
(%)
100
30
20
10
P=0.0424
P=0.0069
P=0.0055
5.1%
4.7%
16.9%
21.4%
MC esophagitis
(n=39)
GERD
(n=85)
NE-NU
(n=195)
GU + DU
(n=28)

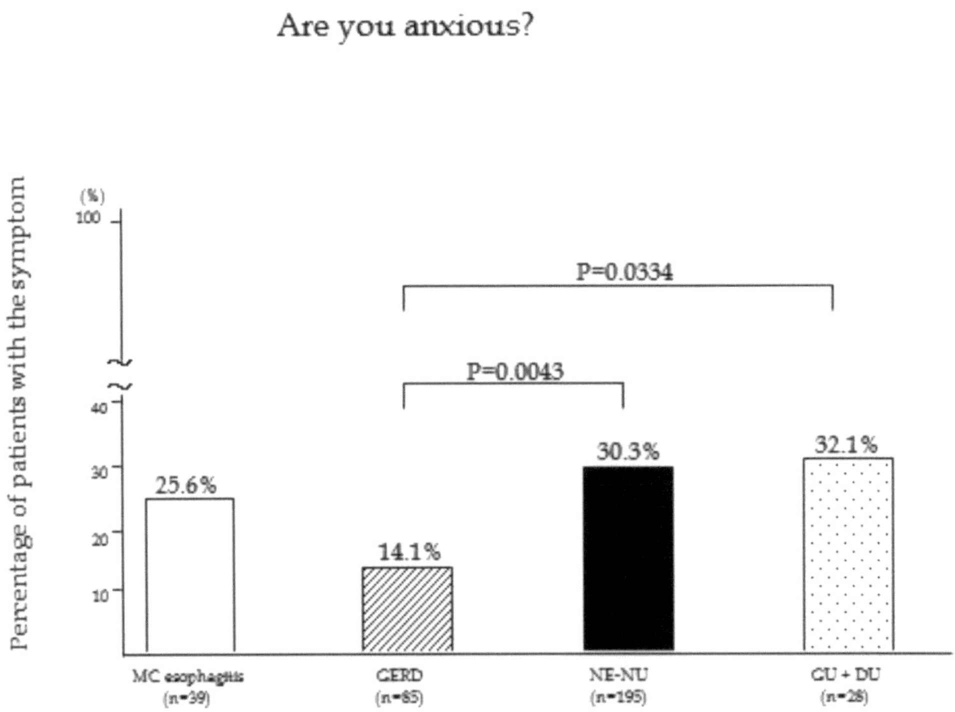
Are you anxious?
Percentage of patients with the symptom
(%)
100
40
30
20
10
P=0.0334
P=0.0043
25.6%
14.1%
30.3%
32.1%
MC esophagitis
(n=39)
GERD
(n=85)
NE-NU
(n=195)
GU + DU
(n=28)

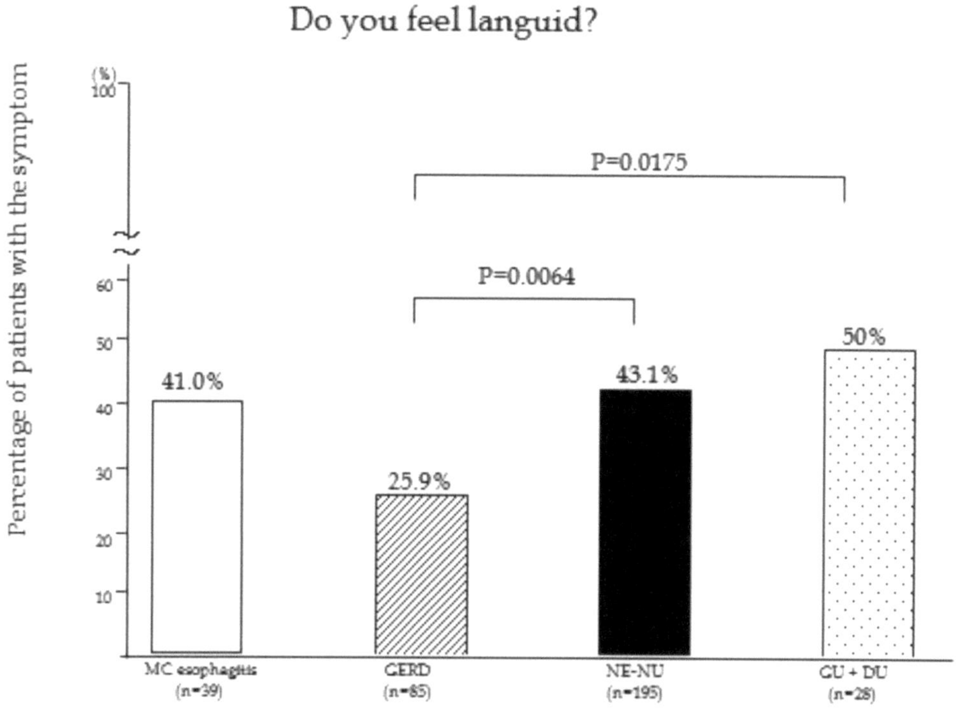

Fig. 5. Psychosomatic symptoms showing significant differences among the groups
Comparison was done among the MC esophagitis, GERD, NE-NU, and GU+DU groups by the χ^2 test.

With regard to gastroesophageal reflux symptoms, significant intergroup differences were seen for the following questions (Fig. 2): "Do you get heartburn?", "Do you mainly get heartburn after meals?", "Do you get heartburn if you bend forward?", "Do you get acidic liquid coming up into your mouth?", and "Do you cough?". Heartburn was significantly more frequent in the GERD group (52.9%) than in the MC esophagitis group (28.2%, P=0.0102), the NE-NU group (29.7%, P=0.0002), or the GU+DU group (17.9%, P=0.0012). Cough was significantly more common in the MC esophagitis group (48.7%) than in the NE-NU group (28.7%, P=0.0146). Occurrence of heartburn mainly after meals was significantly more frequent in the GERD group (51.8%) than in the NE-NU group (34.4%, P=0.0062) or the GU+DU group (25%, P=0.0136). Heartburn on bending forward was also significantly more common in the GERD group (27.1%) than in the NE-NU group (9.2%, P=0.0001) or the GU+DU group (7.1%, P=0.0277). Moreover, acid liquid reflux showed a significantly higher prevalence in the GERD group (31.8%) than in the MC esophagitis group (10.3%, P=0.0102) or the NE-NU group (20%, P=0.0330). Among dysmotility-like symptoms, significant intergroup differences were noted for the following questions (Fig. 3): "Does your stomach ever feel heavy after meals?", "Do you get nausea?", and "Does your stomach ever feel heavy when it is empty?". In the MC esophagitis group, a heavy stomach after meals was significantly less frequent than in the NE-NU group (23.1% vs. 41%, P=0.0351). In addition, nausea was significantly less common in the MC esophagitis group (0%) than in the GERD group (12.9%, P=0.0186), the NE-NU group (14.4%, P=0.0117), or the GU+DU group (21.4%,

P=0.0024). Furthermore, heaviness of an empty stomach was significantly less frequent in the MC esophagitis group (5.1%) than in the GERD group (22.4%, P=0.0176), the NE-NU group (22.1%, P=0.0144), or the GU+DU group (35.7%, P=0.0013). Questions about ulcer-like symptoms showed significant intergroup differences for the following items (Fig. 4): "Do you get pain in the stomach at night?" and "Do you get pain in the stomach when it is empty?". Nocturnal gastralgia was significantly more frequent in the GU+DU group (32.1%) than in the MC esophagitis group (5.1%, P=0.0032), the GERD group (5.9%, P=0.0003), or the NE-NU group (13.3%, P=0.0105). The frequency of gastralgia between meals was significantly higher in the GU+DU group (46.4%) than in the MC esophagitis group (12.8%, P=0.0022), the GERD group (21.2%, P=0.0094), or the NE-NU group (24.1%, P=0.0127). Psychosomatic symptoms showed significant intergroup differences for the following items (Fig. 5): "Do you feel sick?", "Are you anxious?", and "Do you feel languid?". There was a significantly lower frequency of nausea in the GERD group (4.7%) than in the NE-NU group (16.9%, P=0.0055) or the GU+DU group (21.4%, P=0.0069). Nausea was also significantly less common in the MC esophagitis group (5.1%) than in the GU+DU group (21.4%, P=0.0424). The frequency of anxiety was significantly lower in the GERD group (14.1%) than in the NE-NU group (30.3%, P=0.0043) or the GU+DU group (32.1%, P=0.0334). A languid feeling was also significantly less common in the GERD group (25.9%) than in the NE-NU group (43.1%, P=0.0064) or the GU+DU group (50%, P=0.0175).

4. Discussion

In Japan, a modified version of the Los Angeles (LA) classification with the addition of Grade N (normal esophageal mucosa) and Grade M (minimal change esophagitis) is widely accepted (Hongo, 2006). In the first report about the original LA classification, seven items related to minimal change were included: (1) localised area(s) of erythema in one or more segment at the mucosal junction, (2) indistinctness or blurring of all or part of the mucosal junction, (3) friability at the mucosal junction, (4) diffuse erythema of the distal esophagus, (5) patchy erythema of the distal esophagus, (6) increased vascularity of the distal esophagus, and (7) edema/accentuation of mucosal folds (Armstrong et al., 1996). Agreement between experienced endoscopists was acceptable to good for recognition of 3 out of 7 items (erythema, Kappa value (K)=0.77; friability, K=0.55; and increased vascularity, K=0.83). However, agreement between inexperienced endoscopists was poor for recognition of 4 items (blurring, K=0.22; friability, K=0.19; increased vascularity, K=0.39; and edema, K=0.19), so the category of minimal change was not adopted. K statistics can be used for interpretation of results as follows. When Po is the observed proportion of agreement and Pc is the expected (chance) agreement, the equation is obtained: K=Po-Pc/1-Pc (K=-1: complete disagreement, K=0: chance agreement, $0<K<0.4$: poor agreement, $0.4\leq K<0.7$: acceptable agreement, $0.7\leq K<1$: good, K=1: complete agreement). MC esophagitis has been reported to feature prominent erythema without clear demarcation or whitish cloudiness, but the original LA classification does not mention whitish cloudiness. Despite this, MC esophagitis is commonly accepted as part of the spectrum of reflux esophagitis in Japan. In the present study, a 37-item self-administered questionnaire covering questions on gastroesophageal reflux symptoms, dysmotility symptoms, ulcer symptoms and psychosomatic symptoms was used to assess the symptoms of MC esophagitis patients in comparison with GERD patients, NE-NU patients, and GU+DU patients. With regard to gastroesophageal reflux, positive answers to "Do you get heartburn?", "Do you mainly get heartburn after meals?", "Do you get heartburn if you bend forward?", and "Do you get acidic liquid coming up into your mouth?" were significantly more frequent for GERD patients than for NE-NU patients, while the positive rates were similar for MC esophagitis patients and NE-NU patients. "Do you cough?" was significantly more likely to receive a positive answer from MC esophagitis patients than from NE-NU patients. Thus, "cough" was a characteristic symptom of MC esophagitis compared with NE-NU in the present study. With regard to dysmotility-like symptoms, "Does your stomach ever feel heavy after meals?", "Do you get nausea?" and "Does your stomach ever feel heavy when it is empty?" were significantly more likely to receive positive answers from NE-NU patients than from MC esophagitis patients. These dysmotility-like symptoms were characteristic of NE-NU in the present study. "Nausea" and "heavy stomach" are typical symptoms of functional dyspepsia (FD), suggesting that some NE-NU patients may have FD. This may be the reason why such symptoms were significantly more likely to be positive in the NE-NU group than in the MC esophagitis group. However, it is unclear how closely NE-NU patients conform to the definition of FD established by the Rome III global diagnostic criteria for Functional Gastrointestinal Disorders in 2006 (Galmiche et al., 2006). With regard to ulcer-like symptoms, "Do you get pain in the stomach at night?" and "Do you get pain in the stomach when it is empty?" were significantly more likely to be positive among GU+DU patients than among MC esophagitis patients or NE-NU patients. These ulcer-like symptoms were characteristic of GU+DU patients in the present study, but were uncommon among both MC esophagitis and NE-NU patients. With regard to psychosomatic symptoms, "Do you feel sick?", "Are you anxious?" and "Do you feel languid?" were positive significantly less often in GERD patients than NE-NU patients or GU+DU patients, while positivity for these questions was similar among MC esophagitis and NE-NU patients. Thus, both MC esophagitis and NE-NU patients had similar gastroesophageal reflux symptoms ("heartburn"), ulcer-like symptoms ("pain in the stomach"), and psychosomatic symptoms ("sick", "anxious", and "languid"), although they had differing dysmotility-like symptoms ("nausea" and "heavy stomach"). With regard to the pathophysiology of MC esophagitis, the total number of reflux episodes was greater in MC esophagitis patients compared with normal controls and MC esophagitis was similar to reflux esophagitis (Kusano, 2004). Patients with pathological reflux ($pH<4$ for $\geq 4\%$ of the time) were significantly less likely to be in grade N (11.8%) than to have MC esophagitis (57.1%), a finding which suggested the clinical significance of classifying NERD as grade N or MC esophagitis (Joh et al., 2007). According to the 2006 Montreal definition, reflux cough syndrome is an extraesophageal manifestation of GERD (Vakil et al., 2006). In patients with chronic cough and gastroesophageal reflux, esophageal acid reflux leads to a significant increase of cough frequency (Ing et al., 1994), while the pathogenesis of chronic cough and gastroesophageal reflux are associated (Ing et al., 1994). Most of the patients whose chronic cough responds to proton pump inhibitor (PPI) therapy have weakly acidic esophagopharyngeal gas reflux (Kawamura et al., 2011). In this study, the characteristic symptom of MC esophagitis was "cough", indicating that the pathophysiological basis of some of the MC esophagitis is GERD.

5. Conclusion

Patients with some MC esophagitis can be pathophysiologically classified as having GERD. Therefore, PPI therapy should be tried as their initial treatment, although the symptomatology of **some** MC esophagitis patients is similar to that of NE-NU patients with respect to ulcer-like and psychosomatic symptoms.

6. References

Armstrong, D., Bennett, J.R., Blum, A.L., et al. (1996). The endoscopic assessment of esophagitis: a progress report on observer agreement. *Gastroenterology*, Vol. 111, No. 1, pp. 85-92

Galmiche, J.P., Clouse, R.E., Balint, A., et al. (2006). Functional esophageal disorders. *Gastroenterology*, Vol. 130, No. 5, pp. 1459-1465

Hongo, M. (2006). Minimal changes in reflux esophagitis: red ones and white ones. *Journal of Gastroenterology*, Vol. 41, No. 2, pp. 95-99

Kawamura, O., Shimoyama, Y., Hosaka, H., et al. (2011). Increase of weakly acidic gas esophagopharyngeal reflux (EPR) and swallowing-induced acidic/weakly acidic EPR in patients with chronic cough responding to proton pump inhibitors. *Neurogastroenterology and motility*, Vol.23, No.5, pp. 411-e172

Ing AJ, Ngu MC, Breslin AB. (1994). Pathogenesis of chronic persistent cough associated with gastroesophageal reflux. *American Journal of respiratory and critical care medicine*, Vol. 149, No.1,pp. 160-167

Joh, T., Miwa, H., Higuchi, K., et al. (2007). Validity of endoscopic classification for non-erosive reflux disease. *Journal of Gastroenterology*, Vol. 42, No. 6, pp. 444-449

Kusano, M. (2004). Diagnosis and investigation of gastro-oesophageal reflux disease in Japanese patients. *Alimentary Pharmacology Therapeutics*, Vol. 20, suppl. 8, pp. 4-18

Vakil, N., van Zanten, S.V., Kahrilas, P., et al. (2006). The Montreal definition and classification of gastroesophageal reflux disease: a global evidence-based consensus. *American Journal of Gastroenterology*, Vol. 101, No. 8, pp. 1900-1920

Part 2

Medical and Surgical Treatment

6

Treatment of GERD

Bojan Tepeš
AM DC Rogaška,
Slovenia

1. Introduction

Gastroesophageal reflux disease (GERD) is a condition that develops when the reflux of stomach contents causes troublesome symptoms and/or complications (Vakil, et al , 2006a). GERD results from the combination of excessive gastroesophageal reflux of gastric juice and impaired esophageal clearance of the refluxate. The three dominant pathophysiologic mechanisms causing gastroesophageal junction incompetence are: transient lower esophageal sphincter relaxations (tLESRs), a hypotensive lower esophageal sphincter (LES), and anatomic disruption of the gastroesophageal junction, often associated with a hiatal hernia. The dominant mechanism varies as a function of disease severity with tLESRs predominating with mild disease and mechanisms associated LES dysfunction and hiatus hernia predominating with more severe disease (Bardham CP, et al, 1995).

According to Montreal classification we divide GERD into esophageal and extraesophageal syndromes, with extraesophageal syndromes divided into established and proposed associations (Vakil,et al. 2006; figure 1,2).

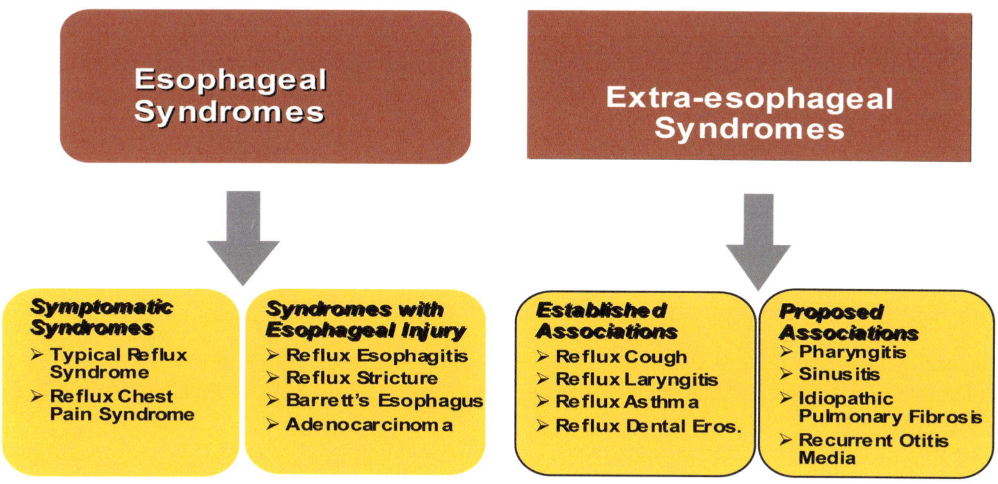

Fig. 1. Montreal classification of GERD

The prevalence of GERD is the greatest in developed world from 10 % in UK and Spain to 29 % in the USA (Dent, et al, 2005). Nonerosive reflux disease (NERD) is the most prevalent form of GERD with prevalence between 50 % and 70 % (Johansson KE, et al 1986 ; Jones RH, et al.1995).According to Rome III. criteria NERD is further subdivided to thrue NERD and functional heartburn (Drossman D, 2006; figure 2).

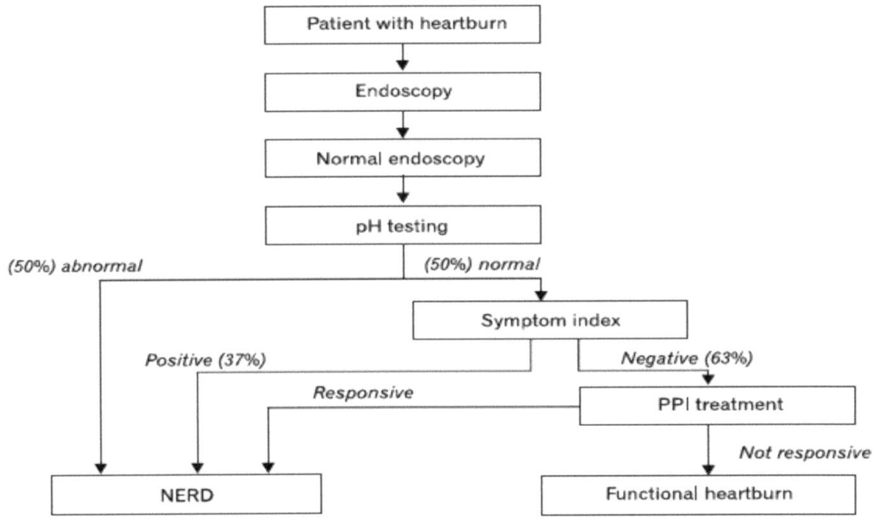

Fig. 2. Diagnostic algorithm for NERD

With medical therapy we can act on the acidity of refluxat (proton pump inhibitors - PPI, H2 blockers, antacids) or with surgery on mechanical reasons for reflux (laparascopic or open surgical technics). At the moment we don't have medicines in routine clinical practice that can correct the basic reasons for pathologic gastric reflux into the esophagus. In this chapter I would like to address some questions about GERD therapy in different subtypes of GERD and in some specific conditions (gravidity) as well as about long term therapy of GERD and potential side effects of long term PPI therapy.

2. GERD therapy

In the medical management of GERD we can use a "step up" approach (beginning with lifestyle and dietary measures and increasing the treatment from antacids to H 2 blockers and finally to proton pump inhibitors or a "step down" approach (beginning with potent antisecretory agents- PPIs to achieve rapid symptom control and then incrementally decreasing the intervention until patients remain in remission).

We always have to inform patients about necessary lifestyle modifications and about use of antacids and alginates for acid breakthrough symptoms. PPIs are the therapy of choice for GERD patients.

2.1 Lifestyle modifications

GERD is a chronic disease with frequent relapses. Patients should be informed about preventive measures - lifestyle modifications that can have an important influence on their GERD symptoms (Kahrilas, et al, 2008).

Head of bed elevation for 6-8 inches is important for individuals with nocturnal or Extraesophageal syndromes. Patients should refrain from assuming a supine position after meals and avoid having meals three hours before bedtime, both of which will minimize reflux. Obesity is a risk factor for GERD, erosive esophagitis, and esophageal adenocarcinoma. However, improvement in symptoms following weight loss is not uniform. Nevertheless, because of a possible benefit, and because of its other positive effects on human health , weight loss should be recommended (Hampel H, et al, 2005). Patients should be informed that alcohol use and smoking should be stopped, because of its harmful effect on mucosa and because smoking diminishes salivation.

Other measures includes avoidance of reflux-inducing foods (fatty foods, chocolate, peppermint, and excessive alcohol) which may reduce lower esophageal sphincter pressure. Patient should selectively avoid food known to cause symptoms like colas, red wine, and orange juice (pH 2.5 to 3.9).

A systematic review of the articles published on lifestyle modification concluded that at the moment, data support only positive impact of weight loss and head of bed elevation. (Kaltenbach T, et al , 2006).

2.2 Medical therapy of GERD and NERD

The severity of symptoms does not correlate with the presence or with severity of subtypes of GERD (Smout AJPM, 1997).

Treatment of GERD should aime at the relief of symptoms and healing of mucosal injury. There is no difference in therapeutic approach to erosive esophagitis (ERD) or nonerosive esophagitis (NERD) patients.

Antacides and alginate antacids provide only temporal benefit and are ineffective in healing of esophageal mucosal injury. They can be used alone only in case of infrequent postprandial symptoms.

Prokinetic drugs enhance gastrointestinal motility. These drugs can theoretically be useful adjuncts in the treatment of GERD by increasing lower esophageal sphincter pressure, enhancing gastric emptying, or improving peristalsis.They can be used only in some special circumstances: in case of delayed gastric emptying or duodenogastroesophageal reflux (Kahrilas PJ,et al,2008).

H 2 receptor antagonists (H 2 blockers) inhibit acid secretion by blocking histamine H 2 receptors on the parietal cell. H 2 blockers heal 52 % of patients with esophagitis compared to 8% with placebo. (NNT is 5 for H2 blockers compared to placebo in healing of GERD) (Khan M , et al 2007, Moayyedi P & Talley NJ, 2006).The problem of H 2 blockers is tachyphylaxis (reduction in therapeutic effect) after one week of therapy. The therapeutic effect of H2 blockers drop to approximately 50 % after 7 days of therapy (Sachs et al 2006).

Proton pump inhibitors (PPIs) are prodrugs which are activated in the stomach by a two step process. First step is conversion of PPI to its sulfenamide derivative and in the second step sulfenamid is protonated to benzimidazole , which binds irreversible to the H/K ATPase. That blocks the H/K ecxhange and prevent parietal cell from producing acid. PPIs concentrate in the parietal cell secretory canaliculus , where pH is approximately 1,0 (the second step in PPI activation needs pKa close to 1). Renal medulla and resorbtive surface of bone (osteoclasts have proton pump) do not have a low pH enough to permit the second step of PPI activation. Elsewhere in the body PPIs follow first-order kinetics. Blood levels of PPIs decrease as the drugs are metabolized in the liver and then excreted primarily in the urine or stool (Shi S&Klotz U, 2008, Shin JM,&Sachs G, 2008, Sachs G, et al. 1995, Sachs G, et al 2006).

We have several PPIs with different daily doses recomended by manufacturer (table 1) NNT is 2 for PPI compared to placebo in healing of GERD (Khan M , et al 2007, Moayyedi P & Talley NJ, 2006).

• Delayed release:	Omeprazole	20 mg qd
	Lansoprazole	30 mg qd
	Rabeprazole	20 mg qd
	Pantoprazole	40 mg qd
	Esomeprazole	40 mg qd
• Immediate release:	Omeprazole + bicarbonate	40 mg qd
• Dual delayed release:	Dexlansoprazole	60 md qd

Table 1. Different Proton pump inhibitors and recommended daily doses

PPIs inhibit only active pumps. A single dose of a PPI does not inhibit all pumps and does not result in profound inhibition of acid secretion. Acid production is inhibited with subsequent PPI doses, taking 5-7 days to achieve a steady state. Acid inhibition is never complete because of continued synthesis of new proton pumps. When PPIs are given twice daily, more active proton pumps are exposed to drug, and steady-state inhibition of gastric acid secretion is achieved more rapidly and more complete (Bell NJV, et al 1992).

PPIs are usually prescribed once daily, usually in the morning. Food affects the bioavailability of each molecule, so it is our practice to recommend that all PPIs should be given prior to meals for optimal efficacy. Results of intragastric pH studies showed that superior daytime pH control (time intragastric pH>4) was seen when the PPI was taken before breakfast compared to after meal. PPIs are responsible for inhibiting gastric acid secretion, thereby decreasing potential damage to the esophageal mucosa. In addition, by raising gastric pH, the conversion of pepsinogen to pepsin, another player of mucosal damage, is inhibited. (Hatlebakk JG,et al , 2000).

In a large meta analysis of 136 randomized controlled trials involving 35 978 patients with esophagitis, the healing rate among those patients treated with PPIs was 83 %. In all trials antacids were used to treat breakthrough symptoms. There were no major differences in efficacy among standard dose of various PPI.

PPIs are better in healing erosive esophagitis than in controlling GERD symptoms. In a large patient unmeat needs survey, patients on PPIs reported the highest level of satisfaction (57,9 %) , followed by H-2 blockers (46,1 %; Crawley MS&Schmitt CM, 2000).

FDA approved dosing of PPIs in GERD patients is once daily. In our daily practice we know that substantial number of patients (32 %) on once daily PPI continue to demonstrate abnormal distal esophageal acid exposure and this proportion can be lowered to less than 10 % by increasing standard therapy of PPI to BID (Charbel S, et al , 2006). There is no supporting data for the use of nocturnal dose of a H 2 blocker to twice daily PPI therapy (Vakil N, et al , 2006b). Dosing a PPI before dinner is significantly more effective for nocturnal acid control than dosing before breakfast (Hatlebakk JG,et al, 1998) .The American College of Gastroenterology currently recommends dosing PPIs before evening meal if nighttime acid controlled is needed (DeVault KR& Castell DO , 2005) Because of the short plasma half-life of the PPIs, loss of nocturnal acid control occurs approximately 7 hours after evening dose (Peghini PL,et al 1998).

Patients with GERD (erosive or nonerosive) should be treated with standard dose of PPIs for at least 2-3 months.

The proportion of NERD patients responding to a standard dose of PPI is approximately 20-30% lower than what has been documented in patients with erosive esophagitis. In a systematic review of the literature, PPI symptomatic response pooled rate was 36.7% (95% CI: 34.1-39.3) in NERD patients and 55.5% (95% CI: 51.5-59.5) in those with erosive esophagitis.(Dean BB , et al , 2004). The greater the distal esophageal acid exposure, the higher the proportion of NERD patients reporting symptom resolution.(Lind T, et al, 1997) Patients with NERD also demonstrate longer lag time to sustained symptom response when compared to patients with erosive esophagitis (2 to 3-fold). Furthermore, patients with NERD demonstrate similar symptomatic response to half and full standard dose of PPI, unlike patients with erosive esophagitis who demonstrate an incremental increase in healing and symptom resolution with standard dose compared to half dose of PPIs (Richter JE,et al , 2000). The reason for the differences in therapeutic response between NERD and erosive esophagitis is primarily due to the common inclusion of functional heartburn subjects in the NERD group. However, because most NERD patients demonstrate only modest abnormal esophageal acid exposure, even after excluding functional heartburn patients, the NERD symptomatic response rate to PPI remains lower that what has been observed in erosive esophagitis patients (Hershovici T & Fas R, 2010).

The most common side effects of proton-pump inhibitors are headache, diarrhea, constipation, and abdominal pain. Although in clinical trials these symptoms were not significantly more common with proton-pump inhibitors than with placebo, they have been confirmed in some patients with a test–retest strategy.

2.3 GERD and pregnancy

The smooth muscle relaxation as well as the increased intraabdominal pressure that occurs during pregnancy predisposes to gastroesophageal reflux (Katz PO& Castell DO, 1998). The greatest experience with pharmacologic acid-suppressive therapy in pregnant women has been with the H2 receptor antagonists ranitidine and cimetidine, which appear to be safe during pregnancy (Larson JD, et al, 1997). There is less experience using proton pump inhibitors during pregnancy, but they are probably safe. A meta-analysis of seven studies (involving a total of 1530 exposed and 133,410 non-exposed pregnant women) found no significant difference in the risk for major congenital birth defects, spontaneous abortions, or preterm delivery (Gill SK,et al, 2009).

2.4 Medical therapy of extraesophageal syndromes

Astma, cronic cough, laryngitis and non cardial chest pain (esophageal syndrome) are among the conditions where an association with GERD is well established. On the other side GERD can be just one of possible ethiologic factors for that diseases. The causal relationship of GERD with with this nonspecific syndromes in absence of a concomitant esophageal GERD syndrome remains controversial and unproven.

In the pro-GERD study that included 6215 patients in Europe 34,9 % of patients with GERD and 30,5 % of patients with NERD have some Extraesophageal Syndromes (Jaspersen D, et al. 2003).

In patients with chronic cough, asthma and laryngeal symptoms PPI standard dose BID is usally prescribed. With this approach likelihood of normalizing esophageal acid exexposure is 93% - 99 % (Charbel S, et al, 2005). Therapy is usually prescribed for 3 months. Studies to support this approach are open label and uncontrolled (Kahrilas Pa, et al, 2008; Tepeš B, 2006). Patients with extraesophageal syndromes can be treated with PPIs only if concomitant esophageal GERD syndrome is present.

2.5 NCCP

Chest pain indistinguishable from ischemic cardiac pain can be caused by GERD – noncardiac chest pain / NCCP (Vakil, et al, 2006a). Community prevalence rates of NCCP are from 23% to 33% (Locke GR, et al, 1997; Eslick GD, et al, 2003). In patients with chest pain ischemic heart disease must be excluded first, GERD is the next most likely pathology. PPIs BID for 8 weeks are recommended in patients with NCCP.Those patients with a good therapeutic response need maintenance therapy with PPIs. If patients do not response to PPIs manomety testing is necessary and specific therapy for motility disorders if proven are needed.

2.6 Maintenance therapy of GERD

Patients with erosive esophagitis have up to 80 % chance of recurrence within 12 months of treatment discontinuation (Johnson DA, et al, 2001; Vakil NB, et al, 2001). GERD recurrence is dramatically decreased by PPI treatment (*Donnellan C, et al, 2005, Tepeš , et al, 2009*). A systematic review of 17 studies (15 of which were randomized controlled trials) showed that subjects with either nonerosive or uninvestigated GERD did well with on-demand regimens (Pace F, et al, 2007). In study where patients with known erosive esophagitis after being healed with PPI therapy were randomized to either continuous or on-demand therapy, recurrence of erosive disease was higher in subjects treated with on-demand compared continuous therapy (42% vs 19% at 6 months; $P < .00001$). On-demand therapy cannot be recommended for maintaining healing of erosive esophagitis (Sjostedt S, et al ,2005).

In our experience patients with GERD LA C and LA D need standard PPI dose or even higher dose as a maintenance therapy, patients with GERD LA B need standard dose of PPI and in those with GERD A can be put on half a standard dose of PPI (Figure 3,4 Tepeš, et al 2009).

Maintenance therapy should be prescribed to all patients with Barrett oesophagus. Some uncontrolled studies showed that PPI therapy can in part prevent progression of Barrett esophagus to dysplasia and adenocarcinoma (El Serag HB, et al, 2004).

Recommendations regarding maintenance therapy in group of patients with Extraesophageal syndromes are based on expert opinion , because we do not have data from prospective control trials. Step-down therapy should be attempted in all patients with extraesophageal reflux syndromes after empirical twice-daily three months PPI therapy. Continuing maintenance PPI therapy should be predicated on either the requirements of therapy for concomitant esophageal GERD syndromes or extraesophageal syndrome symptoms. In both cases, maintenance therapy should be with the lowest PPI dose necessary (Kahrilas PJ, et al, 2008) .

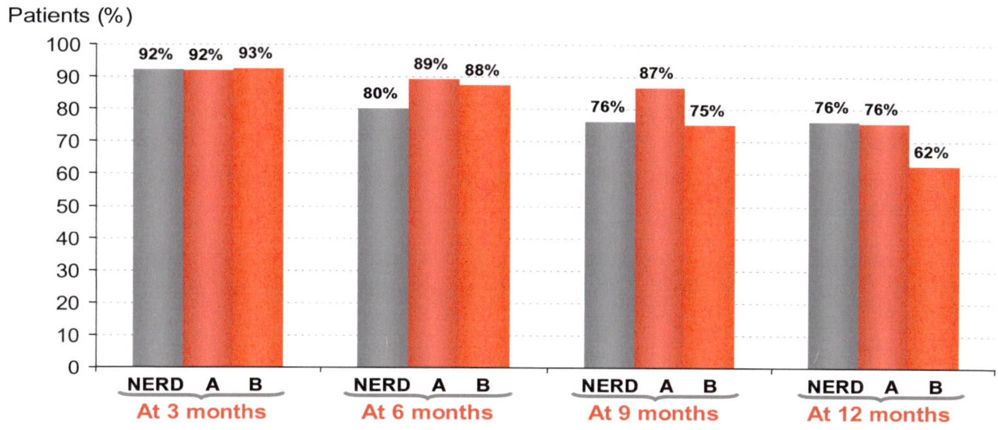

Fig. 3. Cumulative percent of patients in remission in group A2 (omeprazole 10 mg daily) at 3, 6, 9, and 12 months of maintenance therapy by baseline number of patients with a specific grade of disease (intention-to-treat, ITT)

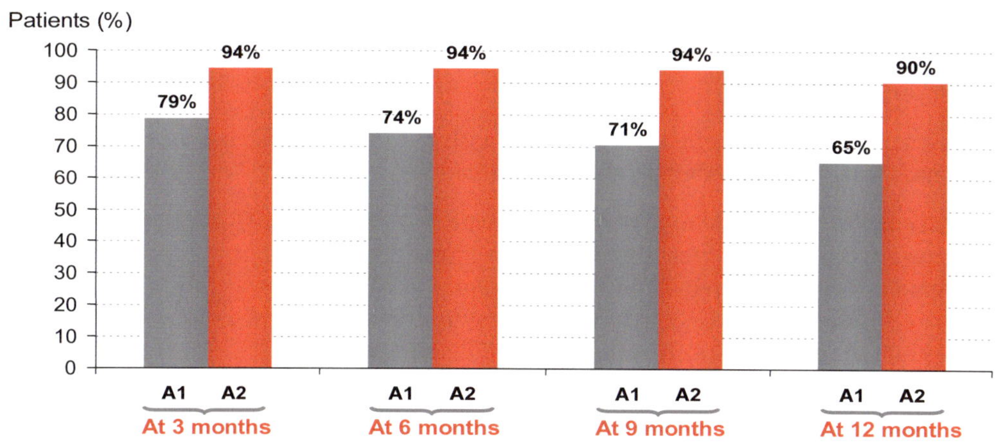

Fig. 4. Cumulative percent of patients with esophagitis grade A in remission in groups A1 (omeprazole 20 mg on demand) and A2 (omeprazole 10 mg QID) at 3, 6, 9, and 12 months of maintenance therapy by number of patients with esophagitis grade A concluding the study in these groups (per-protocol)

2.7 PPI refractory GERD

Patient with GERD are named refractory to PPIs when they do not respond to PPI standard dose BID . Potential etiologies may be gastrointestinal (GI) or non-GI related. The GI etiologies can be esophageal or nonesophageal, and the former may be reflux or nonreflux related.

There are 3 major categories of reflux related causes:

1. First category is reflux with ongoing acid exposure. Etiologies include incorrect medication dose timing, medication noncompliance, residual pathologic acid secretion, rapid PPI metabolism, a hypersecretory state, a significant anatomic abnormality like a large hiatal hernia, excess reflux during tLESRs, or defective esophageal mucosal barrier function.
2. Second category is reflux of nonacid material from either the stomach or the duodenum (e.g., bile).
3. Third category is reflux of normal amounts of weakly acidic or alkaline contents into a hypersensitive esophagus.

The non-reflux–related esophageal causes include dysmotility syndromes such as achalasia, esophageal spasm, or scleroderma; eosinophilic esophagitis; pill esophagitis; and infectious esophagitis.

In the absence of structural, motility, or inflammatory causes, functional heartburn or function chest pain should be considered.

Nonesophageal causes of reflux-type symptoms include gallbladder disease, malignancy in the GI system or surrounding organs, cardiovascular disease, and musculoskeletal disease (Dellon ES & Shaheen NJ, 2010).

After we are sure that patient adheres to the treatment recommendations and PPIs are prescribed BID, further diagnostic procedures are necessary. It is beyond the scope of this Chapter to discuss this procedures in more detail.

2.8 Surgery and GERD

Surgery is a therapeutic option in patients with GERD if GERD has been objectively confirmed. Surgery is an option in individuals who:

1. Have failed medical management (inadequate symptom control, several regurgitation in case of big hiatal hernias, medication side effects.
2. Do not to want to be on life long PPI treatment.
3. Have extraesohageal GERD syndrome (asthma, hoarseness, chronic cough, NCCP, aspiration) and have a positive response to PPI therapy.

Preoperatively workup includes: esophagogastroduodenoscopy, pH-metry, esophageal manometry, barium swallow. Patient should be operated in high volume centers with experiences in GERD laparoscopic surgery. The Nissen fundoplication has, in many series, been found superior to other procedures, with symptomatic improvement occurring in 85 % to 90 % of patients. This procedure originally involved passage of the gastric fundus behind the esophagus to encircle the distal 6 cm of the esophagus. Most surgeons choose to perform a loose ("floppy") Nissen fundic wrap that is about 1 to 2 cm in length including a posterior crural repair. (Ellis FH Jr, 1992). In patients with weak propulsive peristalsis a parcial fundoplication is recommended (anterior fundoplication, Toupet parcial posterior fundoplication).

Up to 20 % of patients will have postoperative dysphagia or gas-bloat syndrome and up to 10 % will need revisional surgery after laparoscopic fundoplication (Lamb PJ,et al. 2009).

Several randomized controlled trials have compared surgical therapy with medical therapy with a follow-up from 1 to 10,6 years. The majority of studies showed that patients need PPIs after operation in up to 21 % of cases, one study showed that this percentage is much higher -62 % (Spechler SJ, et al, 2001; Dassinger MS,et al, 2004; Kamolz T, et al. 2005; Zaninotto G,et al, 2007).

There has been some randomized controlled trials evaluating cost between medical (omeprazole) and surgical therapy (open total and partial fundoplication) over a period up to 10 years. One modeling study found that the cost-equivalency point for medical and surgical therapy was at 10 years (Heudebert GR, et al, 1997) , whereas another still reported lower cost with medical therapy at 10 years (Arguedas MR, e tal, 2004).

Barrett's esophagus is present in 1.65% of the general population, in 8.6% of symptomatic GERD patients presenting to a tertiary care center, and in 10.8% of patients undergoing antireflux surgery . Barrett's esophagus (neoplasia not present) is associated with a significantly increased risk for developing esophageal adenocarcinoma (approximately 100-fold) over that of the general population (Ronkainen J, et al, 2005; Rex DK, et al, 2003, Attwood SE, et al, 2008). Antireflux surgery does not alter the need for continued surveillance endoscopy in patients with Barrett's esophagus. The available evidence is inconclusive about the effect of antireflux surgery on patients with Barrett's esophagus.

3. Side effects of long term PPI therapy

The risk of minor adverse effects from proton pump inhibitors use is 1%-3%, with rates of withdrawal from clinical research studies being 1%-2%, with no significant differences noted between the PPIs (Langtry HD,&Wilde MI, 1997; Laine L, et al 2000).The most common side effects of PPI therapy are: headache, diarrhea and abdominal pain with frequency up to 4 %, what is less than in H 2 blockers (Relly JP, 1999).

Serious adverse effects are rare. Acute interstitial nephritis is a rare complication of PPI treatment (a class effect) which can be potentially reversible if we think on it early enough. Otherways it can lead to acute renal failure. PPIs' metabolites most probably act as a hapten in an autoimmune process in renal interstitium (Geevasinga N, 2006). Hepatitis or disrupted visual disturbances are very rare adverse effect of PPI use (Koury SI, et al ,1998; Garcia Rodriges LA,et al 1996).

PPI are very frequent used as a maintenance therapy in some indications listed above. They are also very frequently used without proper indication, what can be a reason for mayor concern. Up to 60 % of PPI prescriptions, especially in primary care, are without appropriate indications (Nardino RJ, et al, 2000 ;Batuwitage BT, et al, 2007).

Long term PPI use can have influence on human physiology in different ways:

1. long term hypochlorhydria can influence Ca, Fe, Mg, Vit B12 absorbtion, and can increase risk for enteric infections
2. hypergastrinemia can have an effect on parathyroid gland, enterochromaffin cells, or gastric histology
3. interactions with other drugs through cytochrome P450
4. idiosyncratic effects

3.1 Effects of PPIs on absorbtion of minerals and vitamins

Clacium - Calcium solubility is important for its absorbtion . Acid facilitates release of ionized calcium from insoluble calcium salts (Nordin BE, 1997; Sheikh MS, et al 2007). Several studies have tried to evaluate the importance of acid for calcium absorbtion . Four out of five studies found decreased absorbtion of calcium in older patients on PPI therapy (Graziani G, et al, 1995; Graziani G, et al, 2002 ; Hardy P, et al, 1998 O'Connell MB,et al, 2005; Serfaty-Lacrosniere C, et al ,1995).

Iron- Nonheme iron is a mayor source of dietary iron and is predominantly in the form of ferric iron. Iron absorbtion is directly related to the capacity of gastric juice to release iron contained in food (Chorad ME& Shade SG , 1968; Bezwoda W, et al, 1978).

In a group of patients with Zollinger Ellison syndrome on long term PPI therapy for an everage of 6 years, no association was found with decreased stores of body iron or iron deficiency (Stewart CA, et al 1998).

Magnesium - several cases of hypomagnesaemia were associated with long term PPI treatment. Prompt resolution of normal magnesium concentration occurred in two weeks after PPI discontinuation or switch to H2 receptor antagonist . The pathophysiologic mechanism for magnesium deficiency is not understood (Epstein M, et al, 2006; Cuny T & Disdsanayake A, 2008;).

Vitamin B 12- gastric acid and pepsin release vit B12 from protein in food and allows vit B12 to bind to R protein and to intrinsic factor in duodenum (Doscherholmen A& Swaim WR, 1973; Festen HP, 1991). The majority of studies did not find that longterm PPI use reduce the vitamin B12 reabsorbtion. Only in the study which included older patients with Zollinger Ellison syndrome, vitamin B 12 serum concentration was significantly reduced. (Schenk BE ,et al, 1999; Insogna KL ,2009; McColl KE , 2009;).

3.2 Effect on bone metabolism

Long term PPI therapy can affect bone metabolism and cause osteoporosis through three potential mechanisms:

- calcium absorbtion,
- hypergastrinemia
- vitamin B12 deficiency.

The effect of PPI therapy on calcium metabolism has been already described. Hypergastrinemia can led to parathyroid hyperplasia which can increase bone resorbtion and reduce cortical bone mineral density, but clinical data are limited. (*Mizunashi* K,,et al ,

1993). Vitamin B12 is involved in osteoblast activity and bone formation. Patients with marginally low levels of vitamine B12 were 4,5 fold more likely to have osteoporosis than dose with normal levels (*Stone KL* , et al, 2004; *Tucker KL; Dhonukshe-Rutten RA* , et al, 2003). Vitamin B12 deficiency can lead to neurologic complications that can also increase the risk of falls (Sato Y, et al, 2005).

Several epidemiologic studies on the use of PPIs and risk for osteoporotic hip fractures have been published. A population based study using UK general practice research database (UK GPRD) observed a 44 % increased risk for hip fractures among patients older than 50 years on PPIs , with significant dose- and duration- response effects (Yang YX, et al, 2006). A population based study from Canada (Targownik LE, et al, 2008) associated long-term PPI exposure with a significant increase in risk of osteoporotic fractures (> 7 years of PPI exposure: OR, 1.92; 95% CI,1.16 -3.18; hip fractures > 7 years of PPI exposure: OR, 4.55; 95% CI, 1.68 -12.29).The problem of retrospective studies is bias due to confounding. In the nested case control studies using UK GPRD , Kaye et al did not find increased risk of fractures in patients on PPI therapy. Factors such as osteoporosis, vitamin B12 deficiency and prior fractures were among the leading reasons for exclusion , what makes it difficult to generalize the findings (Kaye JA & Jick H. 2008). Targownik et al conducted a cross-sectional and longitudinal analysis of patients referred for dual-energy X-ray absorptiometry scan . They did not associate PPI therapy with prevalent osteoporosis or with significant decreases in BMD over time (Targownik LE, et al, 2010).

3.3 PPIs and infection

Gastric acid acts as a barrier that keeps bacteria from colonizing the upper gastrointestinal tract. The increased bacterial colonization of the stomach observed in PPI users might be associated with pulmonary micro aspiration (Laheij RJ , et al, 2004; Theisen J, et al, 2000). Two retrospective studies found an increased risk for community- acquired pneumonia with current use of PPI (Laheij RJ , et al, 2004; Gulmez SE , et al, 2007). Both studies observed an inverse relationship between the magnitude of the association and the duration of PPI exposure. The weakest association was observed among current users who used the drug for the shortest duration. A third study conducted using the UK GPRD did not find an association between current use of PPIs and a significant increase in risk of community-acquired pneumonia. (*Sarkar M* , et al, 2007) This study accounted for several highly influential confounders that were not considered in the previous studies. It also showed the inverse relationship between duration of current PPI therapy and risk of pneumonia by demonstrating the greatest increase in risk of community-acquired pneumonia in individuals who were issued a new PPI prescription in the past 48 hours. A similar pattern of risk increase was observed with H2RAs. These observations are inconsistent with a causal association mediated by acid suppression or immunosuppression. In fact, they indicate a protopathic bias (ie, drugs given to relieve early symptoms might be temporally associated with the subsequent illness).

Several studies and a meta analysis by Leonard have observed a 2 to 3 fold increase in the risk of nosocomial or community associated Clostridium difficile or other enteric infections in patients on PPI therapy (Leonard J , et al, 2007; Wilcox MH , et al, 2008; Elphick DA, et al, 2005). All the studies are retrospective and some have small number of patients included.

At the moment no PPIs given as once-daily dose truly increase gastric pH >4 for more than 15 hours per day. A large randomized control trials are needed before PPIs can be blamed for increased infection risk.

3.4 PPIs and gastric mucosa

Fundic gland polys can appear after long term PPI therapy. Patients on PPIs have fourfold increased incidence of fundic glands polyps, which have no malignant potential (El-Zimaity HM , et al 1997; Raghunath AS , et al, 2005;).

If a patients on PPI therapy have Helicobacter pylori (H pylori) infection, antrum predominant inflammatory phenotype can change to corpus predominant, what can accelerate atrophy and intestinal metaplasia. (Uemura N , et al, 2000). The first Maastricht Consensus recommended H pylori eradication in all GERD patients before they are enmbarked to PPI maintenance therapy (EHPSG, 1997).

H pylori eradication may cause regression of gastric atrophy or intestinal metaplasia (Tepeš B , et al 1999; Sung JJ , et al 2000; Rocco A , et al , 2002; Ito M & Haruma K, 2002).

Mild / modest hypergastrinemia is a physiologic response to reduction in acid secretion due to PPI therapy. Diffuse linear or micronodular hyperplasia of enterochromaffin like cells is observed in 10 % to 30 % of patients on chronic PPI therapy, mainly in H pylori positive patients. Dysplasia or carcinoid have never been described in long term PPI users (Solcia E , et al, 1992; Genta RM, et al, 2003).

Gastrin has trophic effect on tissues through the gastrointestinal tract (Wang TC , et al, 1996). In several studies no increase in colorectal polyps or cancer have been noticed in patients on maitennance PPI therapy (Robertson DJ, et al, 2007; Singh M,,et al, 2007; Van Soest EM, et al, 2008).

3.5 PPIs and clopidogrel

PPIs are metabolized by hepatic cytochrome P 450 system, predominantly by CYP2C19, and to lesser extent by CYP3A4 (Ishiazaki T& Horai Y, 1999). Clopidogrel is a pro-drug converted to an active metabolite by cytochrome P450 CYP2C19. Clopidogrel active metabolite irreversibly binds to the platel adenosine diphosphate P2Y receptor and inhibits platelet aggregation (Gurbel PA,et al, 2009). The common metabolic pathway can theoretically be a reason for drug-drug interaction that can have an impact on clopidogrel activity.

The OCLA study first showed that omeprazole significantly decreased clopidogrel inhibitory effect on platel P2Y12 as assessed by VASP phosphorilation test (Gilard M , et al, 2008). In in vitro study Di Angiolillo found that metabolic drug-drug interaction exists between clopidogrel and omeprazole but not between clopidogrel and pantoprazole (Angiolillo DJ,et al, 2011).

Several retrospective studies pointed out that concomitant use of PPI and clopidogrel may be associated with adverse cerebrovascular events and myocardial infarction (Gupta E, et al, 2009; Ho PM, et al, 2009; Juurlink DN, et al, 2009; Pezalla E, et al, 2008; Rassen JA, et al, 2009). Meta analysis of 13 studies by Kwork showed no significant association between PPI use and clopidogrel and overall cerebrovascular or cardiovascular mortality (Kwork CS, et al, 2010).

The only two randomized prospective clinical trials, Triton TIMI 38 and Cogent (O'Donoghue ML, et al, 2009; Bhatt DL, et al, 2010) did not find any association between PPI use and risk of cerebrovascular or cardiovascular morbidity or mortality. Cogent data indicated that use of omeprazole with clopidogrel reduced the risk of gastrointestinal events compared with clopidogrel plus placebo, without increasing the risk of cardiovascular events.

4. Conclusions

PPIs are the therapy of choice for GERD patients. Ussually PPIs are prescribed QID for two to three months. One third of patients will need PPI BID. All GERD patients with Extraesophageal syndromes will need PPI BID for three to six months. Patients should be informed about lifestyle modifications and use of antacids for acid breakthrough.Those patients with ERD, Extraesophageal syndromes and Barrett esophagus need maintenance treatment with the lowest dose of PPI that keep them in remission.

Surgery is a therapeutic option for patients who do not have complete therapeutic response with PPI therapy, who do not want to take PPIs lifelong or for those with proven GERD and Extraesophageal syndromes. Long term therapy can have some side effects especially on bone metabolism and can increase risk of enteric infections. The majority of long term side effects data are from epidemiologic or retrospective studies. To be able to clearly answer those questions we need prospective randomized controlled studies.

5. References

Angiolillo DJ, Badimon JJ, Saucedo JF, Frelinger AL, Michelson AD, Jakubowski JA, LaCreta FP, Hurbin F, Dubar M. Differential effects of omeprazole and pantoprazole on clopidogrel incl healthy subjects: randomized, placebo-controlled, crossover comparison studies. Clinical Pharmacology& Therapeutics. 2011;89:65-74.

Arguedas MR, Heudebert GR, Klapow JC, Centor RM, Eloubeidi MA, Wilcox CM, Spechler SJ Re-examination of the cost-effectiveness of surgical versus medical therapy inpatients with gastroesophageal reflux disease: the value of longterm data collection. American Journal of Gastroenterology 2004; 99:1023–1028.

Attwood SE, Lundell L, Hatlebakk JG, Eklund S, Junghard O, Galmiche JP, Ell C, Fiocca R, Lind T Medical or surgical management of GERD patients with Barrett's esophagus: the LOTUS trial 3-year experience. Journal of Gastrointestinal Surgery 2008; 12: 1646–1654 (discussion 1654–1645)

Barham CP, , Gotley DC, Mills A, Alderson D. Precipitating causes of acid reflux episodes in ambulant patients with gastro-oesophageal reflux disease. Gut 1995; 36:505-510.

Batuwitage BT, Kingham JG, Morgan NE, Bartlett RL. Inappropriate prescribing of proton pump inhibitors in primary care. Postgraduate Medical Journal 2007; 83: 66-68.

Bell NJV, Burget D, Howden CW ,Wilkinson J, Hunt RH. Appropriate acidsuppression for the management of gastro-oesophageal reflux disease. Digestion 1992;51(suppl 1):59–67.

Bezwoda W, Charlton R, Bothwell T, Torrance J, Mayet F. The importance of gastric hydrochloric acid in the absorption of nonheme food iron. Journal of Laboratory and Clinical Medicine 1978; 92:108–116.

Bhatt DL, Cryer BL, Contant CF,Cohen M, Lanas A, Schnitzer TJ, Shook TL, Lapuerta P, Goldsmith, MA, Laine, L, Scirica BM, Murphy SA, Cannon CP, for the COGENT Investigators. Clopidogrel with or without Omeprazole in Coronary Artery Disease. The New England Journal of Medicine 2010; 363:1909-1917.

Chorad ME, Shade SG. Ascorbic acid chelates in iron absorbtion: a role for hydrochloric acid and bile . Gastroenterology 1968; 55: 35- 45.

Charbel S, Khandwala F, Vaezzi MF. The role of esophageal pH monitoring in symptomatic patients on PPI therapy. American Journal of Gastroenterology 2005; 100: 283-289.

Crawley JA, Schmitt CM. How satisfied are chronic heartburn sufferd with their prescription medications ? results of the patient unmet needs survey. Journal of Current Medical Research and Opinion 2000;7: 29-34.

Cuny T, Disdsanayake A. Severe hypomagnesaemia in long-term users of proton-pump inhibitors. Clinical Endocrinology 2008; 69:338–341.

Dassinger MS, Torquati A, Houston HL, Holzman MD, Sharp KW, Richards WO Laparoscopic fundoplication: 5-year follow-up. American Surgery 2004; 70:691–694 (discussion 694–695)

Dean BB, Gano AD Jr, Knight K, Ofman JJ, Fass R. Effectiveness of proton pump inhibitors in nonerosive reflux disease. Clinical Gastroenterology and Hepatology 2004;2:656-664.

Dellon ES, Shaheen NJ. Persistent reflux symptoms in the proton pump inhibition era: the changing face of gastroeoesophageal reflux disease. Gastroenterology 2010; 139: 7-13.

Dent J, El Serag HB, Wallander MA,Johansson. Epidemiology of gastroesophageal reflux disease:a systematicreview. Gut 2005; 54: 710-717.

DeVault KR, Castell DO, American College of Gastroenterology. Updated guidelines for the diagnosis and treatment of gastroesophageal reflux disease. American Journal of Gastroenterology. 2005;100: 190–200.

Dhonukshe-Rutten RA, Lips M, de Jong N, Chin A, Paw MJ, Hiddink GJ, van Dusseldorp M. Vitamin B-12 status is associated with bone mineral content and bone mineral density in frail elderly women but not in men. Journal of Nutrition 2003;133:801–807.

Donnellan C, Sharma N, Preston C, Moayyedi P. Medical treatments for the maintenance therapy of reflux oesophagitis and endoscopic negative reflux disease. Cochrane Database Syst Rev 2005;2:CD003245. Doscherholmen A, Swaim WR. Impaired assimilation of egg Co 57 vitamin B 12 in patients with hypochlorhydria and achlorhydria and after gastric resection. Gastroenterology 1973; 64: 913–919.

Drossman D. Rome II: The functional gastrointestinal disorders.3rd ed. McLean,VA: Degnon Associates,Inc., 2006:369-418.

Ellis FH Jr. The Nissen fundoplication. Ann Thorac Surg 1992; 54:1231-1235.

Elphick DA, Chew TS, Higham SE, Bird N, Ahmad A,Sanders DS. Small bowel bacterial overgrowth in symptomatic older people: can it be diagnosed earlier? Gerontology 2005; 51: 396-401

El Serag HB, Aguirre TV, Davis S, Kuebeler M, Bhattacharyya A, Sampliner RE Proton pump inhibitors are associated with reduced incidence of dysplasia in Barrett's esophagus. American Journal of Gastroenterology 2004; 99:1877-1883.
El-Zimaity HM, Jackson FW, Graham DY. Fundic gland polyps developing during omeprazole therapy. Am J Gastroenterol 1997; 92: 1858-1860.
Epstein M, McGrath S, Law F. Proton-pump inhibitors and hypomagnesemic hypoparathyroidism. New England Journal of Medicine 2006; 355: 1834–1836.
Eslick GD, Jones MP, Talley NJ. Non-cardiac chest pain: prevalence,risk factors, impact and consulting–a population-based study. Alimentary Pharmacology and Therapy 2003;17:1115–1124.
European Helicobacter Pylori Study Group. Current European concepts in the management of Helicobacter pylori infection. The Maastricht Consensus Report. Gut 1997; 41: 8-13.
Festen HP. Intrinsic factor secretion and cobalamin absorption. Physiology and pathophysiology in the gastrointestinal tract. Scandinavian Journal of Gastroenterology, Supplement 1991;188:1–7.
Garcia Rodriges LA, Mannino S,Wallander MA, Lindblom B.A cohort study of the ocular safety of anti-ulcer drugs. British Journal of Clinical Pharmacology 1996; 42: 213-216.
Geevasinga N, Coleman PL, Webster AC, Roger S. Proton pump inhibitors and acute intestinal nephritis. Clinical Gastroenterology and Hepatology 2006; 4: 597-604.
Genta RM, Rindi G, Fiocca R, Magner DJ, D'Amico D, Levine DS. Effects of 6-12 months of esomeprazole treatment on the gastric mucosa. American Journal of Gastroenterollogy 2003; 98: 1257- 1265.
Gilard M, Arnaud B, Cornily JC, Le Gal G, Lacut K, Le Calvez G, Mansourati J, Mottier D, Abgrall JF, Boschat J.Influence of omeprazole on the antiplatelet action of clopidogrel associated with aspirin. Journal of the American College of Cardiology 2008; 51: 256- 260
Gill SK, O'Brien L, Einarson TR, Koren G. The safety of proton pump inhibitors (PPIs) in pregnancy: a meta-analysis. American Journal of Gastroenterology 2009; 104:1541.
Graziani G, Badalamenti S, Como G, Gallieni M, Finazzi S, Angelini CC. Effect of gastric acid secretion on intestinal phosphate and calcium absorption in normal subjects. Nephrology Dialialysis Transplantation. 1995;10:1376–1380.
Graziani G, Badalamenti S, Como G, Gallieni M, Finazzi S, Angelini C. Calcium and phosphate plasma levels in dialysis patients after dietary Ca-P overload. Role of gastric acid secretion. Nephron 2002;91:474– 479.
Gupta E, Bansal D, Sotos J, Olden K. Risk of adverse clinical outcomes with concomitant use of clopidogrel and proton pump inhibitors following percutaneous coronary intervention. Digestive Disease and Science 2009; 55:1964-1968.
Gurbel PA, Antonio Mj, Tantry US. Recent developments in clopidogrel pharmacology and their relation to clinical out come. Expert Opinion on Drug Metabolism& Toxicology 2009; 5: 989- 1004.
Gulmez SE, Holm A, Frederiksen H, Jensen TG, Pedersen C,. Hallas J. Use of proton pump inhibitors and the risk of community-acquired pneumonia: a population-based case-control study. Archives of Internal Medicine 2007;167:950-5.
Hatlebakk JG, Katz PO, Castell DO. Proton pump inhibitors: better acid suppression when taken before a meal than without a meal. Alimentary Pharmacology et Therapeutics 2000;14(10):1267–1272.

Hampel H, Abraham NS, El-Serag HB. Meta-analysis: obesity and the risk for gastroesophageal reflux disease and its complications. Annual Internal Medicine 2005; 143:199.

Hardy P, Sechet A, Hottelart C, Oprisiu R, Abighanem, O, Said S. Inhibition of gastric secretion by omeprazole and efficiency of calcium carbonate on the control of hyperphosphatemia in patients on chronic hemodialysis. Artificial Organs 1998;22:569–573.

Hatlebakk JG, Katz PO, Kuo B, Castell DO. Nocturnal gastric acidity and acid breakthrough on different regimens of omeprazole 40mg daily. Alimentary Pharmacology and Therapeutics. 1998;12:1235–1240.

Heudebert GR, Marks R, Wilcox CM, Centor RM . Choice of long-term strategy for the management of patients with severe esophagitis: a cost-utility analysis. Gastroenterology 1997; 112: 1078–1086

Hirshovici T, Fass R. Nonerosive reflux disease (NERD) –an update. Journal of Neurogastroenterology and Motility 2010; 16:8-21.

Ho PM, Maddox TM, Wing L, Fihn SD, Jesse RL, Peterson ED, Rumsfeld JS. Risk of adverse outcomes associated with concomitant use of clopidogrel and proton pump inhibitors following acute coronary syndrome. The Journal of the American Medical Association 2009; 301: 937–944.

Insogna KL. The effect of proton pump-inhibiting drugs on mineral metabolism. American Journal of Gastroenterol ogy2009; 104 Suppl 2: S2-S4.

Ishiazaki T, Horai Y. Review article: cytochrome P450 and the metabolism of proton pump inhibitors- emphasis on rabeprazole. Alimentary Pharmacology and Therapeutics 1999; 3: 27-36.

Ito M, Haruma K. Helicobacter pylori eradication therapy improves atrophic gastritis and intestinal metaplasia: a 5-year prospective study of patients with atrophic gastritis. Alimentary Pharmacology and Therapetics 2002; 16: 1449-56.

Johansson KE, Ask P, Boeryl B, Fransson SG, Tibbling L. Oesophagitis, signs of reflux,and gastric acid secretion in patients with symptoms of gastro-oesophageal reflux disease. Scandinavian Journal of Gastroenterology1986; 21: 837-847.

Johnson DA, Benjamin SB, Vakil NB, Goldstein JL, Lamet M Esomeprazole once daily for 6 months is effective therapy for maintaining healed erosive esophagitis and for controlling gastroesophageal reflux disease symptoms: a randomized, double-blind, placebo-controlled study of efficacy and safety. American Journal of Gastroenterology 2001;96:27–34.

Jones RH, Hungin AP, Philips J,Mills JG. Gastro-esophageal reflux disease in primary care in Europe: clinical presentation and endoscopic findings. European Journal of General Practice 1995; 1: 149-154. Juurlink DN, Gomes T, Ko DT, Szmitko PE, Austin PC, Tu JV, Henry DA, Kopp A, Mamdani MM: A population-based study of the drug interaction between proton pump inhibitors and clopidogrel. Canadian Medical association Journal 2009 180:713-718

Kahrilas PJ; Shaheen NJ,Vaezi M. AGA technical review: management of gastrooesophageal reflux disease. Gastroenterology 2008; 135: 1392-1413.

Katz PO, Castell DO. Gastroesophageal reflux disease during pregnancy.Gastroenterology Clinics of North America. 1998 Mar;27(1):153-67.

Kaltenbach T, Crockett S, Gerson LB. Are lifestyle measures effective in patients with gastroesophageal reflux disease? An evidence-based approach. Archive Internal Medicine 2006; 166:965.

Kamolz T, Granderath FA, Schweiger UM, Pointner R . Laparoscopic Nissen fundoplication in patients with nonerosivereflux disease. Long-term quality-of-life assessment and surgical outcome. Surgical Endoscopy 2005; 19:494–500.

Kaye JA, Jick H. Proton pump inhibitor use and risk of hip fractures in patients without major risk factors. Pharmacotherapy 2008; 28:951–959.

Khan M, Santana J, Donnellan C, Preston C, Moayyedi P. Medical treatment in the short term management of reflux esophagitis. Cochrane Database Systematic Review 2007;2: CD003244.

Koury SI, Stone CK, La Charité DD. Omeprazole and the development of acute hepatitis. European Journal of Emergency Medicine 1998; 5: 467-469.

Kwork CS, Loke YK. Meta-analysis: the effects of proton pump inhibitors on cardiovascular events and mortality in patients receiving clopidogrel. Alimentary Pharmacology and Ther apeutics 2010; 31: 810-823.

Laheij RJ, Sturkenboom MC, Hassing RJ, Dieleman J, Stricker BH, Jansen JB. Risk of community-acquired pneumonia and use of gastric acid-suppressive drugs.The Journal of the Americam Medical association 2004; 292:1955-1960.

Laine L, Ahnen D, McClain C, Solcia E, Walsh JH. Review article: potential gastrointestinal effects of long-term acid suppression with proton pump inhibitors. Alimentary Pharmacology and Therapeutics 2000; 14: 651-668.

Lamb PJ, Myers JC, Jamieson GG, Thompson SK, Devitt PG. Long-term outcomes of revisional surgery following laparoscopic fundoplication. British Journal of Surgery 2009; 96:391- 397.

Langtry HD, Wilde MI. Lansoprazole. An update of its pharmacological properties and clinical efficacy in the management of acid-related disorders. Drugs 1997; 54: 473-500.

Larson JD, Patatanian E, Miner PB Jr, Rayburn WF, Robinson MG. Reflux symptoms during pregnancy. Obstetrics and Gynecology 1997;90:83 –87.

Leonard J, Marshall JK, Moayyedi P. Systematic review of the risk of enteric infection in patients taking acid suppression. American Journal of Gastroenterology 2007; 102:2047–2056.

Lind T, Havelund T, Carlsson R, Anker-Hansen 0, Glise H, Hernqvist H, Junghard 0 , Lauritsen K,. Heartburn without oesophagitis: efficacy of omeprazole therapy and features determining therapeutic response. Scandinavian Journal of Gastroenterology 1997;32:974-979.

Locke GR, III, Talley NJ, Fett SL, Zinsmeister AR, Melton LJ, III. Prevalence and clinical spectrum of gastroesophageal reflux: a population-based study in Olmsted County, Minnesota. Gastroenterology 1997; 112(5):1448-1456.

McColl KE. Effect of proton pump inhibitors on vitamins and iron. American Journal of Gastroenterol 2009; 104 Suppl 2: S5-S9.

Mizunashi K, Furukawa Y, Katano K, Abe K. Effect of omeprazole, an inhibitor of. H+,K(+)-ATPase, on bone resorption in humans. Calcified Tissue International. 1993;53:21–25.

Moayyedi P, Talley Nj. Gastro-oesophageal reflux disease. Lancet 2006; 367: 2086-2100.

Nardino RJ, Vender RJ, Herbert PN. Overuse of acid-suppresive therapy in hospitalized patients. American Journal of Gastroenterology 2000; 95: 3118-3122.

Nordin BE. Calcium and osteoporosis.Nutrition 1997;13: 664-686.

O'Connell MB, Madden DM, Murray AM, Heaney RP, Kerzner LJ. Effects of proto pump inhibitors on calcium carbonate absorption in women: a randomized crossover trial. American Journal of Medicine 2005;118:778–781.

O'Donoghue ML, Braunwald E, Antman EM, Murphy SA, Bates ER, Rozenman Y,. Pharmacodynamic effect and clinical efficacy of clopidogrel and prasugrel with or without a proton-pump inhibitor: an analysis of two randomised trials. Lancet 2009;374:989–997.

Pace F, Tonini M, Pallotta S, Molteni P, Porro GB. Systematic review: maintenance treatment of gastro-oesophageal reflux disease with proton pump inhibitors taken 'on-demand'. Alimentary Pharmacology and Therapeuticsd. 2007;26:195–204.

Peghini PL, Katz PO, Bracy NA, Castell DO . Nocturnal recovery of gastric acid secretion with twice-daily dosing of proton pump inhibitors. American Journal of Gastroenterology. 1998;93:763–767.

Pezalla E, Day D, Pulliadath I. Initial assessment of clinical impact of a drug interaction between clopidogrel and proton pump inhibitors. Journal of the American College of Cardiology 2008; 52: 1038–1039.

Raghunath AS, O'Morain C, McLoughlin RC. Review article:the long-term use of proton-pump inhibitors. Alimentary Pharmacology and Therapeutics 2005; 22 Suppl 1: 55-63.

Rassen JA, Choudhry NK, Avorn J, Schneeweiss S. Cardiovascular outcomes and mortality in patients using clopidogrel with proton pump inhibitors after percutaneous coronary intervention or acute coronary syndrome. Circulation 2009; 120: 2322–2329.

Relly JP. Safety profile of the proton-pump inhibitors. Am J Health Syst Pharm 1999 ;56 (Suppl 4):S 11-17.

Rex DK, Cummings OW, Shaw M, Cumings MD, Wong RK,Vasudeva RS, Dunne D, Rahmani EY, Helper DJ Screening for Barrett's esophagus in colonoscopy patients with and without heartburn. Gastroenterology 2003; 125:1670–1677

Richter JE, Campbell DR, Kahrilas PJ, Huang B, Fludas C. Lansoprazole compared with ranitidine for the treatment of nonerosive gastroesophageal reflux disease. Archives of Internal Medicine 2000;160:1803-1809.

Robertson DJ, Larsson H, Friis S, Pedersen L, Baron JA, Proton pump inhibitor use and risk of colorectal cancer: a population-based, case-control study. Gastroenterology 2007; 133:755-760.

Rocco A, Suriani R, Cardesi E, Venturini I, Mazzucco D, Nardone G. Gastric atrophy and intestinal metaplasia changes 8 years after Helicobacter pylori eradication. A blind, randomized study. Minerva Gastroenterology and Dietology. 2002; 48: 175-8.

Ronkainen J, Aro P, Storskrubb T, Johansson SE, Lind T, Bolling-Sternevald E, Vieth M, Stolte M, Talley NJ, Agreus L.Prevalence of Barrett's esophagus in the general population:an endoscopic study. Gastroenterology 2005; 129:1825–1831

Sachs G, Shin JM, Briving C, Wallmark B. and Hersey S. The pharmacology of the gastric acid pump: the H+,K+ ATPase. Annual Revue Pharmacology and Toxicology 1995;35:277–305.

Sachs G, Shin JM, Howden CW. Review article: the clinical pharmacology of proton pump inhibitors. Alimentary Pharmacology and Therapeutics 2006;23(Suppl 2):2– 8.

Sarkar M, Hennessy S, Yang YX. Proton-pump inhibitor use and the risk for community-acquired pneumonia. Annals of Internal Medicine. 2008;149:391-398.

Sato Y, Honda Y, Iwamoto J, KanokoT, Satoh K. Effect of folate and mecobalamin on hip fractures in patients with stroke: a randomized controlled trial.The Journal of the American Medical association. 2005 ; 293:1082–1088.

Serfaty-Lacrosniere C, Wood RJ, Voytko D, Saltzman JR, Pedrosa M, Sepe TE, Russell RR. Hypochlorhydria from short-term omeprazole treatment does not inhibit intestinal absorption of calcium, phosphorus, magnesium or zinc from food in humans. Journal of the American College of Nutrition 1995;14:364–368.

Sheikh MS, Santa Ana CA, Nicar MJ, Schiller L R, Fordtran JS. Gastrointestinal absorbtion of calcium from milk and calcium salts. New England Journal of Medicine 1987; 317: 532-536.

Shabajee N, Lamb EJ, Sturgess I, Sumathipala RW. Omeprazole and refractory hypomagnesaemia. British Medical Journal 2008; 337: a425.

Schenk BE, Kuipers EJ, Klinkenberg-Knol EC, Bloemena EC, Sandell M, Nelis GF, Snel P, Festen HP Atrophic gastritis during long-term omeprazole therapy affects serum vitamin B12 levels. Alimentary Pharmacology and Therapeutics 1999; 13: 1343-1346.

Shi S, Klotz U. Proton pump inhibitors: an update of their clinical use and pharmacokinetics. European Journal of Clinical Pharmacology 2008;64:935–951.

Shin JM, Sachs G. Pharmacology of proton pump inhibitors. Current Gastroenterology Reports 2008;10:528–534.

Singh M, Dhindsa G, Friedland S, Triadafilopoulos G. Long-term use of proton pump inhibitors does not affect the frequency, growth, or histologic characteristics of colon adenomas. Alimentary Pharmacology and Therapeutics. 2007; 26:1051-1061.

Sjostedt S, Befrits R, Sylvan A, Harthon C, Jorgensen L, Carling L, Modin S,. Stubberod A, Toth E, Lind T. Daily treatment with esomeprazole is superior to that taken on-demand for maintenance of healed erosive oesophagitis. Alimentary. Pharmacology and Therapeutics. 2005;22:183-191.

Smout AJPM. Endoscopy negative acid reflux disease. Alimentary Pharmacology and Therapeutics1997; 11:81-85.

Solcia E, Fiocca R, Havu N, Dalväg A, Carlsson R. Gastric endocrine cells and gastritis in patients receiving long-term omeprazole treatment. Digestion 1992; 51 Suppl 1: 82-92.

Spechler SJ, Lee E, Ahnen D, Goyal RK, Hirano I, Ramirez F, Raufman JP, Sampliner R, Schnell T, Sontag S, Vlahcevic ZR,Young R, Williford W .Long-term outcome of medical and surgical therapies for gastroesophageal reflux disease: follow-up of a randomized controlled trial. The Journal of the American Medical association 2001; 285:2331–2338.

Stewart CA, Termanini B, Sutliff VE, Serrano J, Yu F, Gibril F, Jensen RT. Iron absorption in patients with Zollinger-Ellison syndrome treated with long-term gastric acid antisecretory therapy. Alimentary Pharmacol ogy and Therapetics 1998;12:83-98.

Stone KL, Bauer DC, Sellmeyer D, Cummings SR. Low serum vitamin. B12 levels are associated with increased hip bone loss in older women: a prospective study. Journal of Clinical Endocrinology & Metabolism 2004;89:1217–21.

Sung JJ, Lin SR, Ching JY. Atrophy and intestinal metaplasia one year after cure of H. pylori infection: a prospective randomized study. Gastroenterology 2000; 119:7-14.

Targownik LE, Lix LM, Metge CJ, Prior HJ, Leung S, Leslie WD. Use of proton pump inhibitors and risk of osteoporosis-related fractures. Canadian Medical association Journal. 2008;179:319-326.

Targownik LE, Lix LM, Metge CJ, Prior HJ, Leung S, Leslie WD. Proton-pump inhibitor use is not associated with osteoporosis or accelerated bone mineral density loss. Gastroenterology 2010;138:896-904.

Tepeš B, Kavčič B, Zaletel-Kragelj L, Gubina M,. Ihan A, Poljak M, Križman I. Two to four year histological follow up of gastric mucosa after H. pylori eradication Journal of Pathology 1999; 188:24-29

Tepeš B. Extraesophageal symptoms and signs of gastroesophageal reflux disease. Zdravniski vestnik 2006; 75: 247- 251.

Tepeš B, Štabuc B, Kocijančič B, Ivanuša M. Maintenance Therapy of Gastroesophageal Reflux Disease Patients with Omeprazole. Hepato-Gastroenterology 2009; 56: 67-74.

Theisen J. Nehru D. Citron D. Johansson J. Hagen JA, Crookes PF, DeMeester SR. Suppression of gastric acid secretion in patients with gastroesophageal reflux disease results in gastric bacterial overgrowth and deconjugation of bile acids. Journal of Gastrointestinal Surggery 2000; 4: 50-54.

Tucker KL, Hannan MT, Qiao N, Jacques PF, Selhub J, Cupples LA. Low plasma vitamin B12 is associated with lower BMD: the Framingham Osteoporosis Study. J ournal of Bone and Mineral Research. 2005;20:152-158.

Uemura N, Okamoto S, Yamamoto S, Matsumura N, Yamaguchi S, Mashiba H, Sasaki N. Changes in Helicobacter pylori-induced gastritis in the antrum and corpus during long-term acid-suppressive treatment in Japan. Alimentary Pharmacology and Therapetics 2000; 14: 1345-1352.

Vakil N, van Zanten SV, Kahrilas P, Dent J, Jones R, Global Consensus GroupThe Montreal definition and classification of gastroesophageal reflux disease: a global evidence-based consensus. American Journal of Gastroenterology. 2006a;101(8):1900-1920.

Vakil N, Guda N, Partington S. The effect of over the counter ranitidine 75 mg on night time heartburn in patients with erosive oesophagitis on daily proton pump inhibitor maintenance therapy. Alimentary Pharmacology and Therapeutics 2006b; 23: 649-653.

Vakil NB, Shaker R, Johnson DA, Kovacs T, Baerg RD, Hwang C, D'Amico D. The new proton pumpinhibitor esomeprazole is effective as a maintenance therapy in GERD patients with healed erosive oesophagitis: a 6-month,randomized, double-blind, placebo-controlled study of efficacy and safety. Alimentary Pharmacology and Therapeutics 2001;15:927–935.

Van Soest EM, van Rossum LG, Dieleman JP. Proton pump inhibitors and the risk of colorectal cancer. American Journal of Gastroenterology. 2008; 103:966-973.

Wang TC, Koh TJ, Varro A, Cahill RJ, Dangler CA, Fox JG, Dockray GJ. Processing and proliferative effects of human progastrin in transgenic mice. Journal of Clinical Investigation. 1996 ;98:1918–1929. .

Wilcox MH, Mooney L, Bendall R, Settle CD, Fawley WN. A case-control study of community-associated Clostridium difficile infection. Journal of Antimicrobial Chemotherapy 2008;62:388–396.

Yang YX, Lewis JD, Epstein S, Metz DC. Long-term proton pump inhibitor therapy and risk of hip fracture. The Journal of the American Medical Association 2006;296:2947–2953.

Zaninotto G, Portale G, Costantini M, Rizzetto C, Guirroli E, Ceolin M, Salvador R, Rampado S, Prandin O, Ruol A, Ancona E Long-term results (6–10 years) of laparoscopic fundoplication. Journal of Gastrointestinal Surgery 2007; 11:1138–1145

7

E3710, Long-Acting PPI as New Approach for the Treatment of Unmet Medical Needs for GERD

Kotaro Kodama[1], Hideaki Fujisaki[1], Hideo Tonomura[1], Miwa Jindo[1], Misako Watanabe[1], Junichi Nagakawa[1] and Noriaki Takeguchi[2]
[1]*Eisai Co., Ltd.,*
[2]*Toyama Medical and Pharmaceutical University*
Japan

1. Introduction

Gastroesophageal reflux disease (GERD) is a spectrum of multifunctional disorder caused by the failure of the normal antireflux mechanism with frequent acid reflux. Patients with GERD experience primary symptoms of heartburn and/or acid regurgitation. The patients with GERD have erosive esophagitis, peptic strictures, Barrett esophagus or evidence of extraesophageal diseases such as chest pain, pulmonary symptoms or symptoms in ear, nose and throat symptoms, while others have no apparent mucosal injury by endoscopic diagnosis (non-erosive GERD) [Armstrong, 2005]. GERD is a chronic, relapsing disorder requiring long term management. The pathophysiological mechanism of GERD is complicated. The decreased lower esophageal sphincter pressure, night time reflux, impaired mucosal defense factors, bile reflex, delayed gastric emptying, visceral hypersensitivity, hiatal hernia, insufficient esophageal clearance, physiological comorbidity and concomitant functional bowl diseases are implicated in the refractory mechanism of GERD [Castell et al., 2004; Fass and Sifrim, 2009].

GERD impairs both the quality of life (QOL) and work productivity of patients, so that they need to receive adequate remedy [Wahlqvist et al., 2008]. The goals of treatment for GERD are three folds; control of symptoms, healing of erosion and the maintenance of remission of esophagitis for prevention from complications such as stricture, Barrett esophagus and esophageal malignancy. Although presently available proton pump inhibitors (PPIs) made a large contribution to the treatment for GERD, their clinical efficacy still has some limitations. Further, the degree of acid control is inadequate for some patients as follows. First, about 30 % of patients still remain unhealed or unsatisfied symptom relief, even when the dose or dosing frequency of current PPIs is increased [Fass et al., 2005]. Second, healing rates with current PPIs at 8 weeks are relatively sufficient, whereas those at 4 weeks are not satisfactory and still need to be improved [Castell et al., 2002]. Third, there are still GERD patients whose esophagitis remain unhealed even after 8 weeks treatment with currently available PPIs, especially among patients in Los Angeles grades C and D, having high-grade esophagitis with transverse mucosal breaks, and with inadequate symptom resolutions [Castell et al., 2002]. Fourth, the long-term maintenance study showed that 10-20% of GERD patients administered once-daily PPI relapsed within 6 months [Katz et al., 2006]. Fifth, symptom relief with once-daily PPIs administration was achieved in only 60-70% of GERD patients at 8 weeks [Katz et al., 2006].

GERD is evoked by the reflux of gastric contents including acid and pepsin; therefore, intragastric pH have extremely impact on GERD severities. The healing rate of GERD at 8 weeks is closely correlated with the maintenance of the intragastric pH over 4-holding time [Armstrong, 2004]. The comparison study in respect of intragastric pH with current PPIs in GERD patient was performed. As the result, esomeprazole given once daily was superior to other PPIs regarding intragastric pH over 4-holding time at day 5 [Minder et al., 2003]. However, since its effect lasted only 14 h per day, the intragastric pH fell below 4 in the remaining of the day. In achieving appropriate intragastric pH control, neither double-dose nor twice a day administration with current PPIs were fully effective for the patients with refractory GERD [Fass and Shfirm, 2009; Saches et al., 2010; Hershcovici and Fass, 2011]. An extended release formulation or a pro-drug approach has been recently addressed, while unstable pharmacokinetics and pharmacodynamics would be induced due to different individual absorption and metabolic capacities.

We expected that long-acting PPI, even given once daily, may control appropriate intragastric pH and that it would be promising for the treatment of these unmet medical needs of GERD. We evaluated about 500 compounds newly synthetized, finding one promising compound, a mixture of two optical isomers. Thus, we confirmed that R-isomer was a feasible candidate with the results of the comparative studies of both isomers on pharmacology, pharmacokinetics, CYP inhibition and metabolism by dog and human liver microsomes.

We finally determined that E3710, sodium(*R*)-2-[4-(2,2-dimethyl-1,3-dioxan-5-yl) methoxy-3, 5- dimethylpyridin-2-yl] methylsulfinyl-1 *H*-benzimidazole (Fig. 1), would be useful with once-daily administration for the treatment of GERD as new PPI with potent and long-acting acid neutralization [Kodama et al., 2010]. We compared the effects of E3710 on 24-h intragastric pH with that of esomeprazole to predict clinical superiority and usefulness by using newly established measurement system in gastric fistula dogs. In a clinical study, a cross-over design including placebo is performed to assess the efficacy of PPIs with accuracy. We investigated a cross over study design in gastric fistula dogs to confirm the long-acting effect of E3710 in comparison with esomeprazole.

2. Methods

2.1 Materials

E3710 was synthesized at Eisai (Ibaraki, Japan). Esomeprazole magnesium trihydrate was purchased from Kemprotec Ltd. (Middlesbrough, UK). Male 11-week old New Zealand White rabbits (Kitayama Labes, Nagano, Japan) and male 1-3 year old mongrel dogs (Kitayama Labes, Gifu, Japan) were maintained at a temperature of 23°C (20-26°C) and a humidity of 55% (40-70%) and on a 12-h light/dark cycle. All experiments were approved by the Animal Care and Use Committee at the Eisai Tsukuba Research Laboratories.

Chemical structure

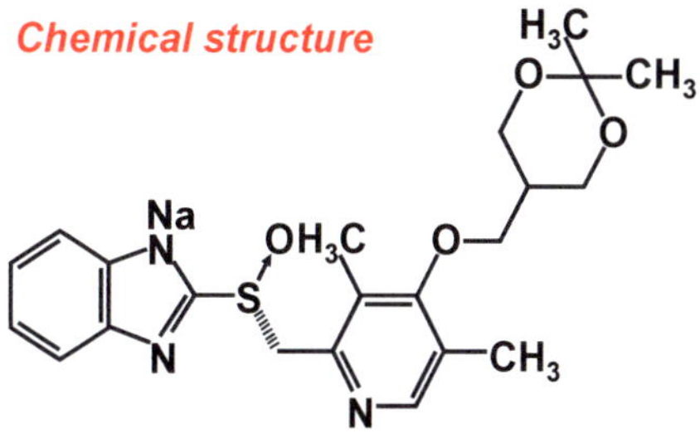

Sodium(*R*)-2-[4-(2,2-dimethyl-1,3-dioxan-5-yl) methoxy-3, 5-dimethylpyridin-2-yl] methylsulfinyl-1 *H*-benzimidazole

Mechanism of action

Irreversible inhibition on H^+,K^+-ATPase

Potential Indications

Acid related diseases:

- **Peptic ulcer**
- **Duodenal ulcer**
- **GERD (erosive and symptomatic)**
- **Prophylaxis of nonsteroidal anti-inflammatory drugs-induced ulcer**
- ***Helicobacter pylori* infection**
- **Upper gastrointestinal bleeding**
- **Zollinger-Ellison syndrome**

Fig. 1. Features of E3710

2.2 *In vitro* experiments

Inhibitory effects of E3710 on H^+,K^+-ATPase activity under several pH conditions were estimated and compared with the effects on Na^+,K^+-ATPase activities. The inhibitory mechanism of E3710 on H^+,K^+-ATPase is compared with that of esomeprazole (PPI), SCH28080 (P-CAB: potassium-competitive acid blocker) and famotidine (Histamine H_2 receptor antagonist). E3710, esomeprazole, SCH28080 and famotidine were dissolved in methanol and ouabain was dissolved in distilled water. The concentration of reagent is expressed as a final concentration.

2.2.1 Measurement of H^+,K^+-ATPase and Na^+,K^+-ATPase activities

H^+,K^+-ATPase prepared from pig gastric mucosa was incubated with E3710 (0.3-30 μmol/L at pH 6.1 or 1-30 μmol/L at pH 7.4), esomeprazole (0.3-30 μmol/L at pH 6.1 or 1-30 μmol/L at pH 7.4) or vehicle for 30 min at 37°C. KCl (or distilled water) and gramicidin were added, followed by incubation for 10 min. Then, Mg–ATP (pH 7.4) was added, followed by incubation for 10 min. After stopping the enzyme reaction, the amount of inorganic phosphorus released from ATP was determined.

To measure the inhibitory effects under acidic conditions, gastric microsomal membranes enriched in H^+,K^+-ATPase were isolated in a vesicular form, and accumulation of H^+ in the presence of ATP, Mg^{2+}, K^+ and valinomycin (K^+ ionophore) was established. The inhibitory effects of PPIs under this acidic condition can mimic the inhibition in the luminal canalicular acidic space. H^+,K^+-ATPase was mixed with E3710 (0.01-3 μmol/L), esomeprazole (0.01-3 μmol/L) or vehicle in a solution containing KCl (or NaCl) and valinomycin. The reaction was started by adding of Mg–ATP, and H^+,K^+-ATPase activity was measured for 30 min. H^+,K^+-ATPase activity was assayed by the coupled-enzyme method for last 10 min.

Na^+,K^+-ATPase prepared from porcine cerebral cortex was mixed with E3710 (0.3-100 μmol/L), esomeprazole (0.3-100 μmol/L), ouabain (0.01-10 μmol/L) or vehicle in a solution containing KCl, NaCl and 1 mmol/L ouabain (or distilled water). The reaction was started by the addition of Mg–ATP, and Na^+,K^+-ATPase activity was measured for 30 min. Na^+,K^+-ATPase activity was assayed by the coupled-enzyme method for last 10 min.

2.2.2 Investigation of the inhibitory mechanism on H^+,K^+-ATPase

The irreversibility of the inhibitory effects on H^+,K^+-ATPase activity was studied using the inhibitor dilution method. H^+,K^+-ATPase was preincubated with 100 μmol/L E3710, 100 μmol/L esomeprazole, 10 μmol/L SCH28080 or vehicle for 30 min at 37°C in buffer (pH 6.1). Then, H^+,K^+-ATPase activity was measured under two conditions: with or without dilution of the preincubated reaction mixture. KCl (or distilled water), gramicidin and Mg-ATP (pH 7.4) were added, followed by incubation for 10 min under the undiluted condition or 20 min under the diluted condition. After stopping the enzyme reaction, the amount of inorganic phosphorus released from ATP was determined.

The interaction of PPI with cysteine groups of H^+,K^+-ATPase was investigated using DTT (a sulfhydryl reducing agent). H^+,K^+-ATPase was incubated with 30 μmol/L E3710, 10 μmol/L esomeprazole, 10 μmol/L SCH28080 or vehicle, in coexistence with DTT (0.1-3 μmol/L) or distilled water, for 30 min at 37°C in buffer (pH 6.1). KCl (or distilled water) and gramicidin were added, followed by incubation for 10 min at 37°C. Then, Mg–ATP (pH 7.4) was added, followed by incubation for 10 min at 37°C. After stopping the enzyme reaction, the amount of inorganic phosphorus released from ATP was determined.

The inhibitory effects on acid secretion were investigated in isolated rabbit gastric glands. The gastric glands were incubated with E3710 (0.03-10 μmol/L), esomeprazole (0.03-10 μmol/L) or famotidine (0.3-100 μmol/L for db-cAMP stimulation and 0.03-10 μmol/L for histamine stimulation) in a solution containing [^{14}C]aminopyrine (0.1 μCi/mL) at 37°C for 30 min. Then, secretagogue (1 mmol/L db-cAMP or 0.1 mmol/L histamine) was added, followed by incubation for 30 min. Then the levels of radioactive [^{14}C]aminopyrine present in the supernatant and the pellet were measured using a liquid-scintillation counter. The ratio of the weak base [^{14}C]aminopyrine in the supernatant and pellet was used as a measure of the acid-secretory activity in the gastric glands.

2.3 *In vivo* experiments

Effects of E3710 on histamine-induced gastric acid secretion and 24-h intragastric pH in gastric fistula dogs underwent surgery to create gastric fistulae were studied to confirm its long-acting inhibitory effects. E3710 and esomeprazole were suspended in 0.5% methyl cellulose (MC) and intraduodenally administered.

2.3.1 Measurement of histamine-stimulated gastric acid secretion

Twelve dogs under surgery to create gastric fistula and divided into two groups: one received 0.1, 0.2, 0.4 or 0.8 mg/kg E3710 or the 0.5% MC vehicle alone (n=6) and the other received 0.2, 0.4, 0.8 or 1.6 mg/kg esomeprazole or the 0.5% MC vehicle alone (n=6). Each experiment used a 6 x 5 cross-over study design for both drugs including the vehicle and each experiment was carried out over two consecutive days. On day 1, gastric acid secretion was stimulated by intravenously infusing 50 or 75 μg/kg/min histamine over 180 min and gastric juice were collected every 20 min. Sixty minutes after the start of histamine infusion, 0.5% MC, E3710 or esomeprazole was administered intraduodenally. On day 2, 24 h after 0.5% MC, E3710 or esomeprazole administration, histamine was infused intravenously over 120 min and gastric juice were collected every 20 min (Fig. 2).

The volume of gastric juice was determined, and then the concentration of acid was measured by titrating 0.5 mL of gastric juice with 0.04 mol/L NaOH solution to pH 7.0 using a Titration Workstation. The gastric acid output was calculated using the following formula: gastric acid secretion (mEq/20 min) = volume of gastric juice (ml/20 min) × acid concentration (mEq/ml). The inhibitory effects of the drugs were measured for the 0-2 h time period after administration on day 1 and the 24-26 h time period after administration on day 2. In another study, blood sampling was made 0.25, 0.5, 1, 2 and 6 h after intraduodenal administration of E3710 or esomeprazole under the same condition in Fig. 2 for pharmacokinetic (PK) data.

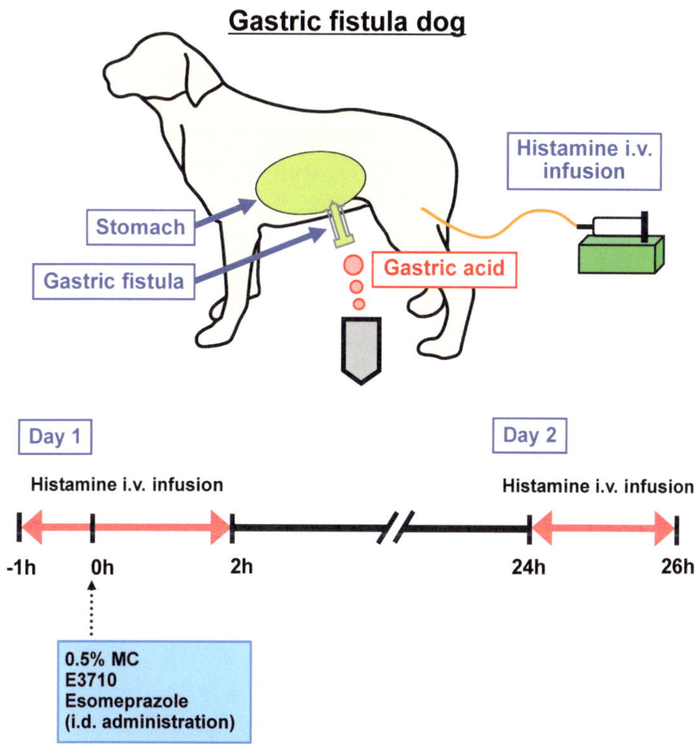

Fig. 2. The measurement system and experimental protocol for histamine-stimulated gastric acid secretion in gastric fistula dogs. i.d.: intraduodenal

2.3.2 Measurement of intragastric pH over 24 h

Glass pH electrode was inserted through gastric fistula to be immobilized in position to measure the intragastric pH changes. Intragastric pH was recorded by pH data recorder under the condition where dogs can move around and drink water freely during the experiment (Fig. 3).

We basically carried out three separate intragastric stimulations according to 3-times food intake schedule in the standard clinical trial for the evaluation of efficacy of PPI. We thus used histamine stimulation at a time appropriate for "breakfast" followed by two feeds at times appropriate for "lunch" and "dinner".

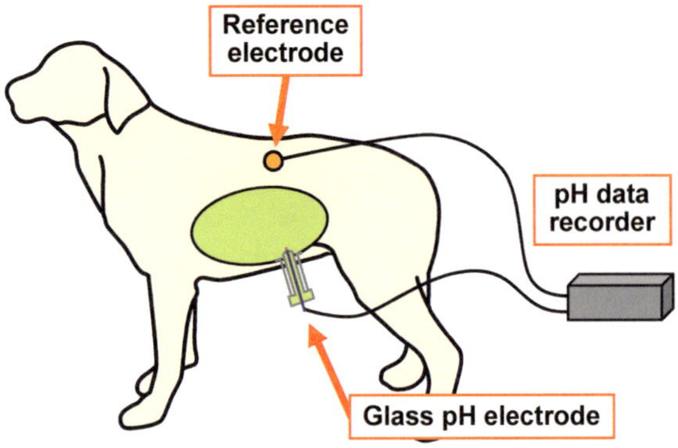

Fig. 3. The measurement system of 24-h intragastric pH in gastric fistula dogs

First, we evaluated the effect of histamine stimulation (as breakfast) on 24-h intragastric pH intraduodenally administered by E3710 to confirm the effect of breakfast intake. Experimental protocol was summarized in Fig. 4. After with or without intravenous histamine infusion for 40 min, E3710 both at 0.4 and at 0.8 mg/kg were intraduodenally administered. The measurement of intragastric pH over 24 h commenced at around 10:00 AM, and values were recorded every 10 s using ambulatory pH monitoring system (PH-101ZG; Chemical Instruments Co., Ltd, Tokyo, Japan) carried in a canine jacket, and the data were downloaded to a computer and analyzed using the W-IPC pH analysis program (Chemical Instruments Co. Ltd.). Two meals, each of ~225 g DS-A pellet diet (Oriental Yeast Co., Ltd., Tokyo), were offered to each animal separately at about 13:00 (as lunch) and 18:00 (as dinner).

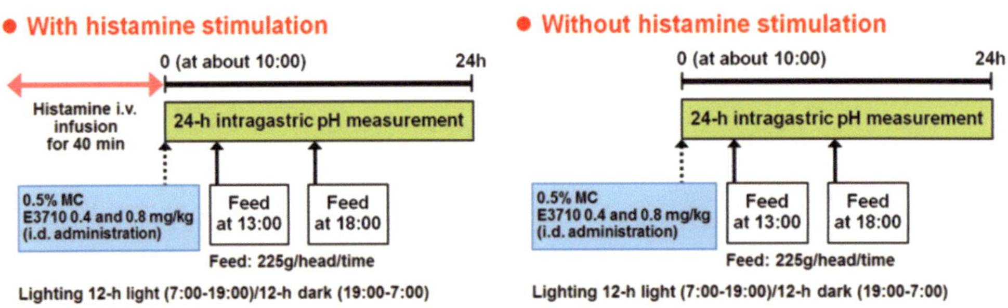

Fig. 4. Experimental protocol for measurement of effect of breakfast on 24-h intragastric pH by E3710 in gastric fistula dogs

Second, we obtained the dose dependent effects of E3710 and esomeprazole. Experimental protocol of comparative studies of E3710 with esomeprazole on 24-h intragastric pH was presented in Fig. 5. After infusion of histamine intravenously for 40 min (as breakfast) 0.5% MC, E3710 (0.2, 0.4 and 0.8 mg/kg) or esomeprazole (0.8 and 1.6 mg/kg) was administered intraduodenally. Third, in a clinical study a cross-over design including placebo is performed to assess the efficacies of PPIs with accuracy. A 6 x 3 cross-over design studies, using 0.5% MC, 0.4 mg/kg E3710 and 1.6 mg/kg esomeprazole (n=6), were carried out to confirm the long-acting inhibitory effects of E3710 compared to esomeprazole.

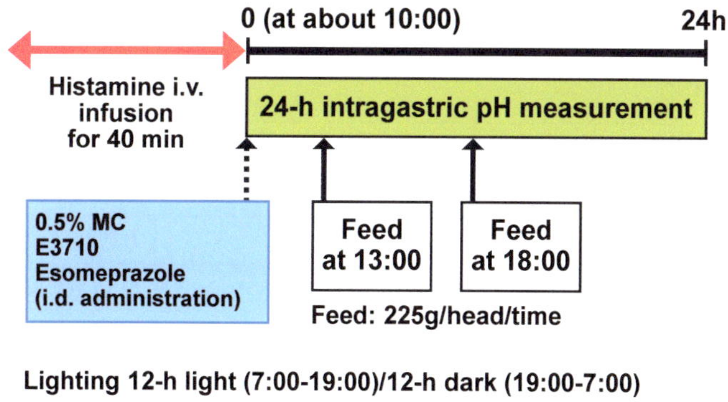

Fig. 5. Experimental protocol of comparative studies of E3710 with esomeprazole on 24-h intragastric pH in gastric fistula dogs

2.4 Statistical analysis

All data were expressed as means ± SEM. In *in vitro* experiments, the mean IC_{50} and 95% confidence intervals (CI) were calculated based on the IC_{50} values generated from separated sigmoid curves. In *in vivo* experiments, ED_{50} values were calculated by linear regression and the potency ratio with 95% CIs were calculated using two-by-three assay. Difference in the intragastric pH between with histamine stimulation and without histamine stimulation was analyzed using t-test. Differences in the intragastric pH between E3710 and 0.5% MC or esomeprazole and 0.5% MC were analyzed using Dunnett's multiple range test in a dose escalation study. Intragastric pH was evaluated using one-way analysis of variance followed by Tukey's multiple comparison test in a cross over study. Two-sided probability (p) values < 0.05 were considered statistically significant. Statistical analyses were performed using the SAS software package version 8.1 (SAS Institute Japan Ltd., Tokyo, Japan).

3. Results

3.1 Summary of *in vitro* studies

The inhibitory effects of E3710 and esomeprazole on H^+,K^+-ATPase activity were dependent on pH condition (Table 1). Ouabain inhibited Na^+,K^+-ATPase activity with an IC_{50} value of 0.43 μmol/L (95% CI 0.41–0.45). In contrast, both E3710 and esomeprazole were very poor inhibitors of Na^+,K^+-ATPase with IC_{50} values greater than 100 μmol/L.

	IC_{50} (μM)		
	Acidic condition	pH 6.1	pH 7.4
E3710	0.28 (0.17-0.44)	4.2 (3.8-4.7)	>30
Esomeprazole	0.53 (0.47-0.59)	2.3 (2.1-2.5)	>30

Table 1. Inhibitory effects of E3710 and esomeprazole on pig gastric H^+,K^+-ATPase activity. Each data represents mean from 3 independent experiments in performed in duplicate. Vesicles accumulated H^+ under the acidic condition, and did not accumulate H^+ under the conditions of medium pH 6.1 and 7.4. The 95% CIs are expressed in the parenthesis.

E3710 and esomeprazole inhibited acid secretion of isolated rabbit gastric glands stimulated by db-cAMP or histamine. By contrast, famotidine inhibited only acid secretion stimulated by histamine (Table 2).

	IC_{50} (μM)	
	db-cAMP	Histamine
E3710	0.40 (0.28-0.59)	0.27 (0.12-0.58)
Esomeprazole	0.53 (0.29-0.99)	0.41 (0.22-0.74)
Famotidine	>100	0.35 (0.25-0.48)

Table 2. Inhibitory effects of E3710 and esomeprazole on acid secretion of isolated gastric glands. Each data represents mean from 4 independent experiments in performed in duplicate. The 95% CIs are expressed in the parenthesis.

In dilution studies, 100 μmol/L E3710 inhibited H^+,K^+-ATPase activity by 55.4% and by 58.5% when the reaction mixture was diluted. Similarly, 100 μmol/L esomeprazole inhibited H^+,K^+-ATPase activity by 91.1% when undiluted and by 93.0% after dilution. In contrast, 10 μmol/L SCH28080 inhibited H^+,K^+-ATPase activity by 80.5% but by 7.0% after dilution. Accordingly, the inhibitory effects of E3710 and esomeprazole on H^+,K^+-ATPase activity were not reversed by diluting the drug concentration in the medium, whereas that of SCH28080 was reversed. DTT antagonized the inhibitory effects of E3710 and esomeprazole on H^+,K^+-ATPase, however not that of SCH28080 (Fig. 6).

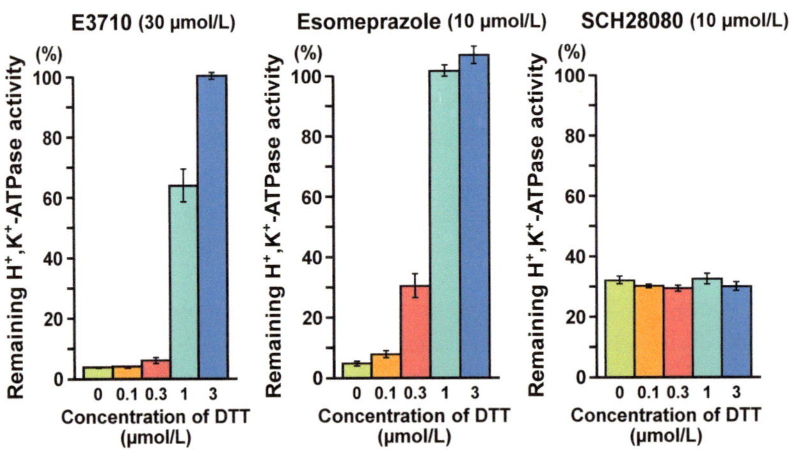

Fig. 6. Effects of the concomitant presence of DTT on the inhibition of H^+,K^+-ATPase activity with E3710, esomeprazole or SCH28080 at indicated concentrations. Each data point represents the mean ± SEM from three independent experiments performed in duplicate.

3.2 Summary of *in vivo* studies

3.2.1 Inhibitory effect of E3710 on histamine-stimulated gastric acid secretion

E3710 inhibited gastric acid secretion in a dose-dependent manner and at 0.4 and 0.8 mg/kg fully inhibited gastric acid secretion within 1 h of administration. Even 24 h after administration, these sustained inhibitory effect was still observed after histamine stimulation (Fig. 7).

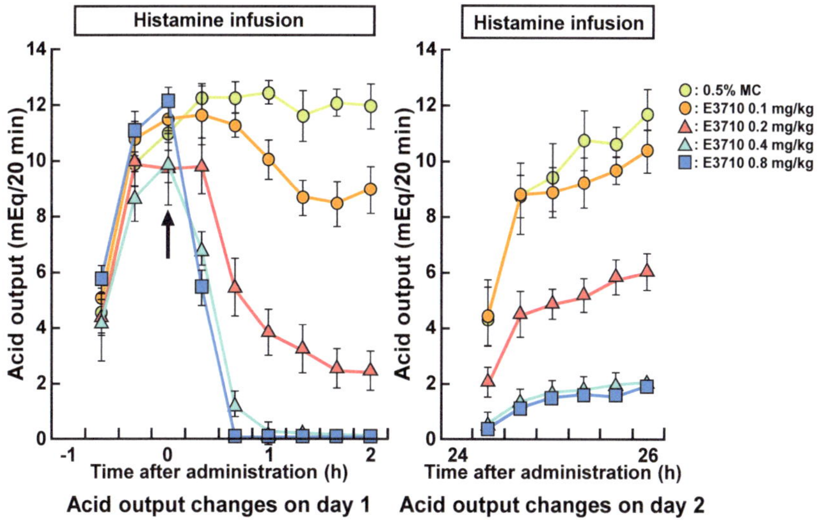

Fig. 7. Effect of E3710 on histamine-stimulated gastric acid secretion in gastric fistula dogs. E3710 was administrated at the arrow (time zero). Results are expressed as the mean ± SEM of 6 dogs (6 x 5 cross-over study).

Esomeprazole also inhibited histamine-stimulated gastric acid secretion 1 h after administration. However 24-26 h after administration these inhibitory effect was not sustained in the way seen with E3710 (Fig. 8).

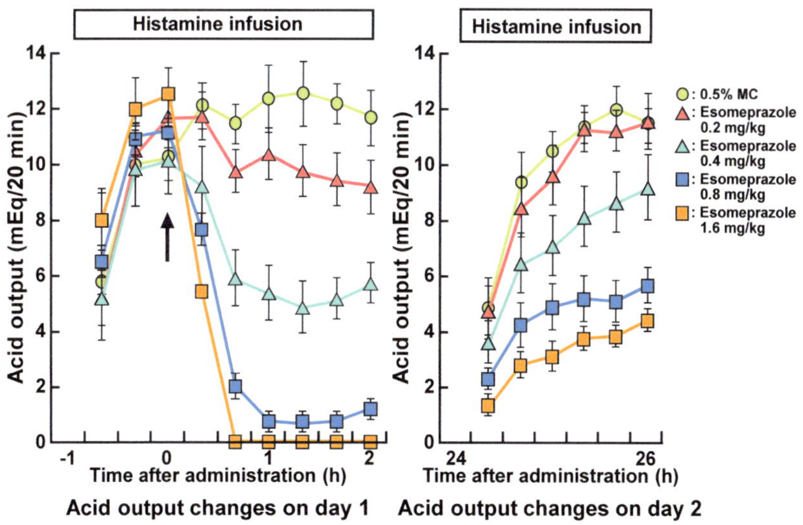

Fig. 8. Effect of esomeprazole on histamine-stimulated gastric acid secretion in gastric fistula dogs. Esomeprazole was administered at the arrow (time zero). Data are expressed as the mean ± SEM of 6 dogs (6 x 5 cross-over study).

The ED_{50} values for E3710 (liner regression range: 0.1, 0.2 and 0.4 mg/kg) and esomeprazole (liner regression range: 0.2, 0.4 and 0.8 mg/kg) during 0-2 h and 24-26 h after administration are shown in Table 3. The potency ratio for E3710 to esomeprazole during 0-2 h and 24-26 h after administration was 2.3 (95% CI: 1.9 - 2.6) and 2.8 (95% CI: 2.2 - 3.6), respectively.

	ED_{50} (mg/kg)	
	0-2 h	24-26 h
E3710	0.18 (0.15-0.20)	0.22 (0.19-0.27)
Esomeprazole	0.40 (0.37-0.43)	0.71 (0.58-0.99)

Table 3. The ED_{50} values of E3710 to esomeprazole on histamine-induced gastric acid secretion in gastric fistula dogs

E3710 (mg/kg)	N	T max (h)	Cmax (µg/mL)	AUC (µg•h/mL)	$T_{1/2}$ (h)
0.1	4	0.25	0.16	0.22	0.77
0.2	4	0.31	0.30	0.49	1.01
0.4	4	0.25	0.54	0.65	0.76
0.8	4	0.25	1.74	2.56	0.70

Table 4. PK data of E3710 in gastric fistula dogs.

Esomeprazole (mg/kg)	N	T max (h)	Cmax (µg/mL)	AUC (µg•h/mL)	$T_{1/2}$ (h)
0.2	4	0.25	0.27	0.24	0.59
0.4	4	0.25	0.40	0.36	0.47
0.8	4	0.25	0.81	0.72	0.52
1.6	4	0.25	1.73	1.64	0.58

Table 5. PK data of esomeprazole in gastric fistula dogs.

3.2.2 Effect of E3710 on 24-h intragastric pH with or without histamine stimulation

Effect of E3710 on intragastric 24-h pH profile was reduced in without histamine stimulation in comparison of that with histamine stimulation (Fig. 9, 10).

Mean pH at 0.4 mg/kg of E3710 and the % of time with pH≥4/24 h at 0.4 and 0.8 mg/kg of E3710 were significantly reduced without histamine stimulation (Fig. 10).

Time course changes of intragastric pH with E3710 (Fig. 11) and esomeprazole (Fig. 12) was summarized. E3710 and esomeprazole elevated the mean intragastric pH in a dose-dependent manner and increased %of time with pH≥4/24 h, compared to the 0.5% MC (Table 6).

In a cross over study, E3710 even at one fourth of esomeprazole dose rapidly elevated intragastric pH, and E3710 kept higher intragastric pH in comparison with esomeprazole almost during 24 h (Fig. 13). Thus mean intragastric pH of E3710 group was relatively higher, compared with that of esomeprazole. These potencies of E3710 were the same results observed in dose-dependent study (Fig. 11 and 12). In both E3710- and esomeprazole-treated groups the intragastric pH gradually dropped after the maximum pH-elevating effects had been reached. The intragastric pH in the esomeprazole-treated group dropped below 4 just after midnight (between 1:00 to 3:00), while that in the E3710-treated group was substantially above pH4 during the same time period. In terms of intragastric pH profile during night-time (0:00-04:00), E3710 is superior to that of esomeprazole.

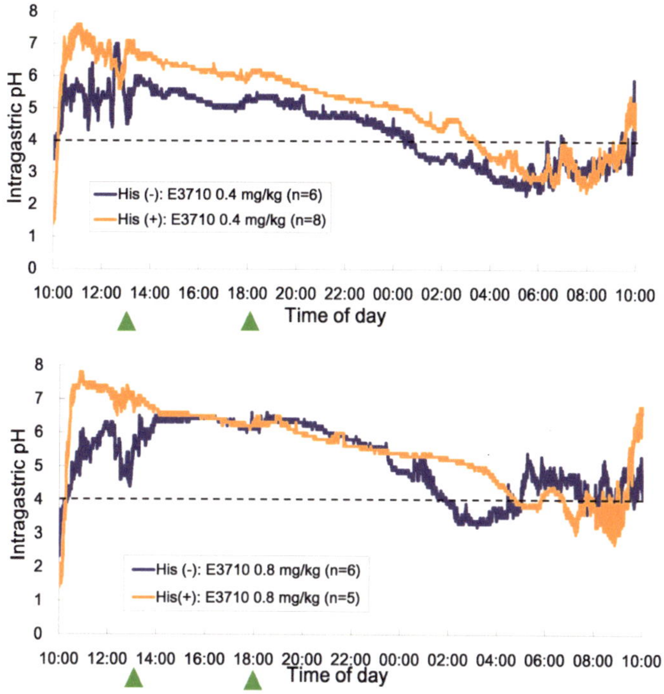

Fig. 9. Profiles of E3710-administered intragastric pH under with or without histamine stimulation in gastirc fistula dogs. His (+): Histamine infusion was performed approximately from 9:10 to 9:50. His (-): No treatement was performed approximately from 9:10 to 9:50. E3710 was intraduodenally administrated at about 10:00. Arrows indicate feeding time.

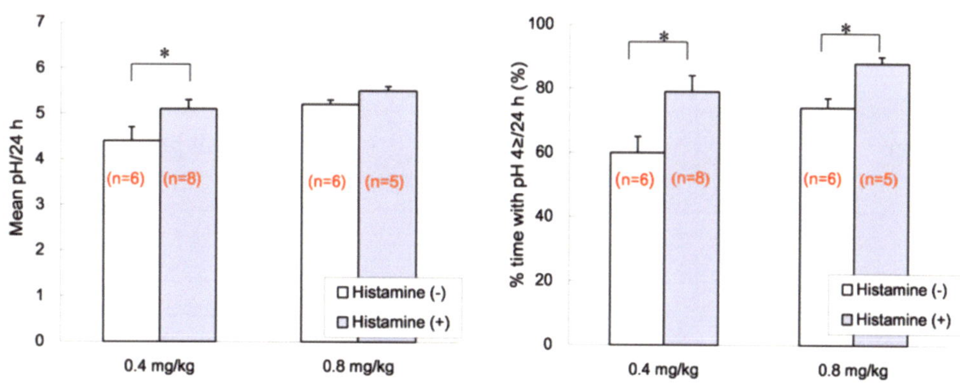

Fig. 10. Effect of histamine stimulation on E3710-administered intragastric pH profile in gastric fistula dogs. Data are expressed as the mean ± SEM. *p<0.01 versus Histamine (-).

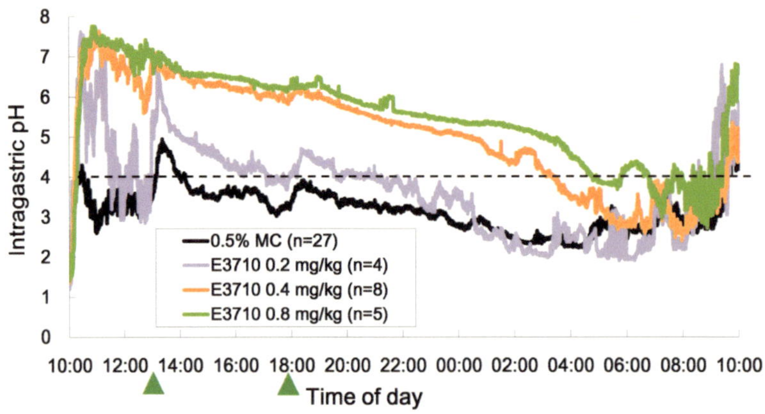

Fig. 11. Profiles of E3710 on intragastric pH in gastric fistula dogs. Histamine infusion was performed approximately from 9:10 to 9:50. E3710 was intraduodenally administrated at about 10:00. Arrows indicate feeding time.

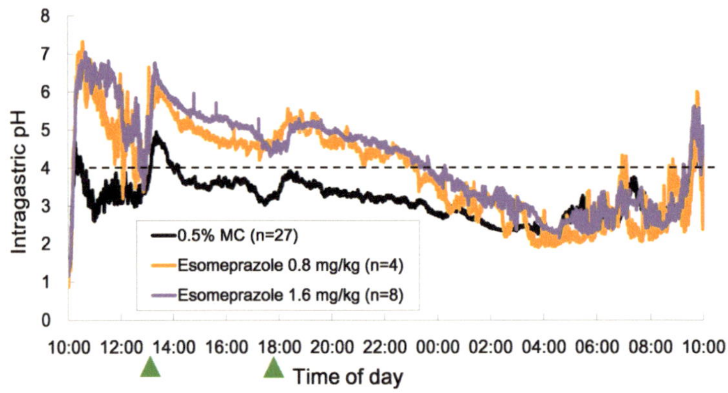

Fig. 12. Profiles of esomeprazole on intragastric pH in gastric fistula dogs. Histamine infusion was performed approximately from 9:10 to 9:50. Esomeprazole was intraduodenally administrated at about 10:00. Arrows indicate feeding time.

Treatment	Dose (mg/kg)	N	Mean pH/24 h	% Time with pH≥4/24 h
0.5% MC		27	3.2 ± 0.1	17 ± 3
E3710	0.2	4	3.7 ± 0.2	40 ± 6*
	0.4	8	5.1 ± 0.1**	79 ± 3**
	0.8	5	5.5 ± 0.1**	88 ± 2**
Esomeprazole	0.8	4	4.0 ± 0.2*	55 ± 3**
	1.6	8	4.3 ± 0.1**	59 ± 4**

Table 6. Effects of E3710 and esomeprazole on 24-h intragastric pH in gastric fistula dogs. Data is expressed as the mean ± SEM. *p<0.01, **p<0.001 versus the 0.5% MC

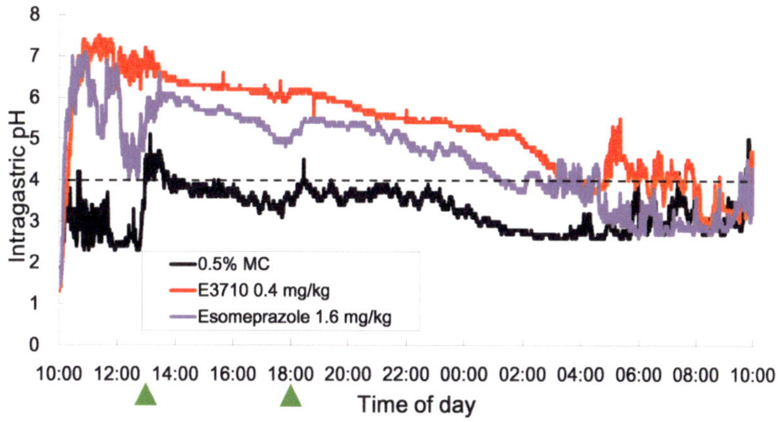

Fig. 13. Profiles of intragastric pH in gastric fistula dogs in cross over study. Histamine infusion was performed approximately from 9:10 to 9:50. E3710 or esomeprazole was intraduodenally administrated at about 10:00. Arrows indicate feeding time. (6 x 3 cross-over study).

The mean intragastric pH in the E3710 group was higher than that in the esomeprazole group, although the difference was not statistically significant. The %of time with pH≥4/24 h was significantly longer in the E3710-treated group than in the esomeprazole-treated group (Table 7).

Treatment	Mean pH/24 h	% of time with pH≥4/24 h
0.5% MC	3.3 ± 0.2	20 ± 5
E3710 0.4 mg/kg	5.3 ± 0.3**	82 ± 5 **, #
Esomeprazole 1.6 mg/kg	4.6 ± 0.3*	61 ± 7**

Table 7. Effects of E3710 and esomeprazole on 24-h intragastric pH in gastric fistula dogs in a cross over study. Data are expressed as the mean ± SEM. *$p<0.01$, **$p<0.001$ versus the 0.5% MC; #$p<0.05$ versus the esomeprazole.

4. Discussion

4.1 Summary of preclinical experiments

E3710 irreversibly inhibited H^+,K^+-ATPase which is responsible for the final common pathway of hydrochloric acid secretion in gastric parietal cells *in vitro*, especially under acidic condition. The inhibitory effect of E3710 on H^+,K^+-ATPase activity was antagonized by DTT and not reversed by diluting the drug concentration in the medium, suggesting that the pharmacological active form (sulfenamide) inhibited the H^+,K^+-ATPase activity via formation of covalent disulfide bridges with cysteine groups on this enzyme [Sachs et al., 2006]. E3710 inhibited the acid secretion similar to the mode of action of esomeprazole, but unlike histamine H_2 receptor antagonist. In gastric fistula dogs, E3710 potently inhibited the histamine-stimulated gastric-acid secretion with potency 2.3 and 2.8 times higher than that of esomeprazole at 0-1 h and 24-26 h posttreatment, respectively. Moreover, E3710 immediately elevated intragastric pH above 4 and provided prolonged and better intragastric pH control compared with esomeprazole over a 24 h period.

4.2 Effects of E3710 on 24-h intragastric pH

It is well known that PPIs inhibit the activated proton pumps induced by food intake. Breakfast is commonly given after the oral PPIs administrations in many clinical trials. The study showed that better acid suppressions were observed when PPIs were taken before breakfast than without breakfast. When taking the PPIs, the median % of time with pH ≥ 4/8 h (from 8:00 until 16:00 with lunch at 12:00) was 83% with breakfast in comparison with that of 58% without breakfast (P=0.01) [Hatlebakk et. al., 2000]. In our experiment each dog did not necessary simultaneously finish breakfast when we fed in the morning, therefore we used intravenous histamine infusion instead of breakfast to evoke an assured H^+,K^+-ATPase activation. We also confirmed that the effects of E3710 on mean pH and % of time with pH ≥4/24 h were significantly reduced without histamine stimulation.

Although GERD affects patients during the day as well as the night, the symptoms of heartburn and regurgitation during the night time have a greater negative impact on QOL in such a way as to interrupt sleep patterns and to increase the risk of esophageal and respiratory complications [Shaker et al., 2004]. The pattern of reflux during the day is usually postprandial and promptly cleared. The occurrence of reflux during sleep is relatively less frequent but events are significantly longer and are associated with delayed acid clearance. This is partly caused by such factors as 1) reduced saliva production, which would otherwise protect the esophageal tissue and neutralize acidic reflux events, 2) decline in the frequency of swallowing, which contributes to the volume gastric acid cleared, 3) prone position during the night, which delays the clearance of acid compared with an upright position during the day. Furthermore, nocturnal acid breakthrough (NAB), defined as a period of intragastric pH below 4 for more than 1 h at night during PPI therapy [Peghini et al., 1998], has been suggested as a possible refractory causes for GERD. Even though currently available PPIs are administered twice a day before breakfast and before dinner, NAB cannot be sufficiently controlled [Hatlebakk et al., 1998]. Clinical significance of NAB for GERD has been uncertain, while it has been suggested as a possible refractory causes for GERD. The night-time esophageal acid exposures, including the mean number of acid reflux episodes, mean % time esophageal pH<4 in were significantly higher in the PPI failing group compared with PPI success group [Hershcovici et al., 2011].

In a cross-over study E3710 at 0.4 mg/kg didn't completely hold intragastric pH≥4 during night, although the intragastric pH remained substantially above pH4 during midnight (between 1:00 to 3:00). On the contrary, that of the esomeprazole-treated group dropped below 4 during the same period. Considering that NAB in midnight in comparison with that in early morning may be a high risk factor to cause heartburn which leads sleeping disturbance and reduction of QOL, E3710 would show better symptom relief during night than esomeprazole does. The doubling dose has been used to deal with heartburn not responding to current PPIs, while this approach hasn't fully succeeded [Fass and Shfirm, 2009; Saches et al., 2010]. Regarding the dose-dependent efficacy of the % of time with pH ≥4/24 h of esomeprazole in GERD patients, the slight elevation was observed from 61.4% at 40 mg (clinical standard dose) to 65.8% at 80 mg (clinical double dose) [Armstrong, 2004] with the similar elevation from 55% at 0.8 mg/kg to 59% at 1.6 mg/kg in gastric fistula dogs

(Table. 6). It seems the clinical efficacy of esomeprazole may reach its maximum even at double dose. On the contrary, the % of time with pH≥4/24 h with E3710 was increased from 79% at 0.4 mg/kg to 88% at 0.8 mg/kg in gastric fistula dogs (Fig. 12). These results revealed that a dose escalation of E3710 would be a promising way to control 24-h intragastric pH in an appropriate manner. Accordingly, E3710 would be more useful for the treatment of NAB in comparison with esomeprazole.

4.3 A hypothesis for the long-acting effect of E3710 based on the acid-induced split mechanism

The plasma half-life of E3710 (0.70-1.01 h: mean 0.81 h: Table 4) was relatively longer than that of esomeprazole (0.47-0.59 h: mean 0.54 h: Table 5) in gastric fistula dogs. Moreover, the AUC levels of E3710 were higher than those of esomeprazole under the same dose comparison. We assumed that these different PK parameters may account for a long-acting of E3710.

Besides plasma half-life, we speculated another long-acting mechanism of E3710 with respect of chemical features. We calculated the distribution coefficient (oil/water) of E3710 and esomeprazole at pH 7.4 (blood) and pH 1.0 (stomach) by PhysChem ver 12.01 (Advanced Chemistry Development, Canada) as an index of lipophilicity (Fig. 14). PPIs including E3710 are absorbed from intestine into blood and reach in the canalicular space of gastric parietal cells finally crossing the basolateral and apical membranes of the parietal cell owing to the highly lipophilic characteristics of PPIs. The distribution coefficient (oil/water) of E3710 is calculated to be 3.3-fold greater than that of omeprazole at neutral pH, indicating that E3710 more quickly reach in the canalicular space than omeprazole. PPIs are pro-drugs and their acid activated compound bind with Cys residues in H^+,K^+-ATPase from the canalicular side (not from the intracellular side). A recent study indicates that the transformation of PPI into its activated states requires very low pH (less than 1) [Shin et al., 2004]. This indicates that the activation of PPIs occurs only near the proton exit site of H^+, K^+-ATPase that is actively secreting acid. One particular feature of E3710 is the following. E3710 has 2, 2-dimethyl-1, 3-dioxane moiety. This dimethyl group is unstable in the strong acidic space and the isopropyl group including the dimethyl group is splitted leaving two OH groups in the remaining main body, which gives a higher hydrophilicity. The distribution ratio of the acid activated form of E3710 at pH 1 is calculated to be 1/6-fold that of omeprazole; that is, the acid activated form of E3710 is more hydrophilic than that of acid-activated omeprazole. A higher hydrophilic property of the acid-activated E3710 gives a higher accumulation power in the strongly acidic canalicular space because of its less membrane-permeability, which may contribute to the long-acting acid-inhibitory effect.

4.4 Summary of pharmacokinetics, toxicology and clinical study of E3710

4.4.1 Pharmacokinetic features

E3710 shows weak or no inhibitory effects on CYPs in human liver microsomes and revealed weak or no induction of CYPs in primary culture of human hepatocytes, indicating that E3710 would show low potential of drug-drug interaction. Regarding CYP3A4, E3710 was also found to be a weak mechanism-based inhibitor of this isozyme. E3710 was shown to be a substrate and a weak inhibitor of multidrug resistance 1 glycoprotein.

E3710

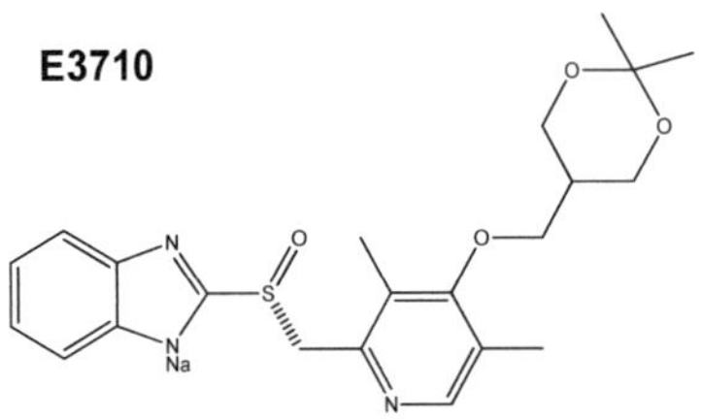

Log D=2.87 (pH=7.4)

E3710 active form

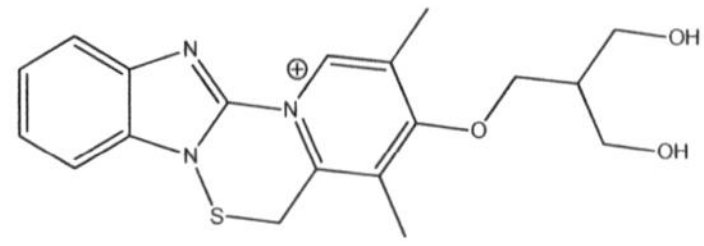

Log D=1.47 (pH=1.0)

Esomeprazole

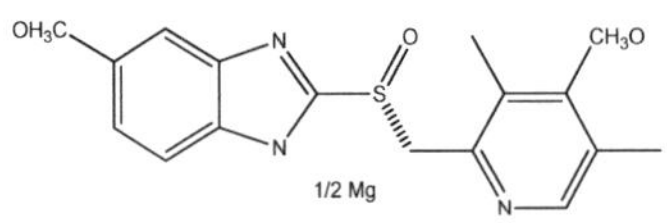

Log D=2.35 (pH=7.4)

Esomeprazole active form

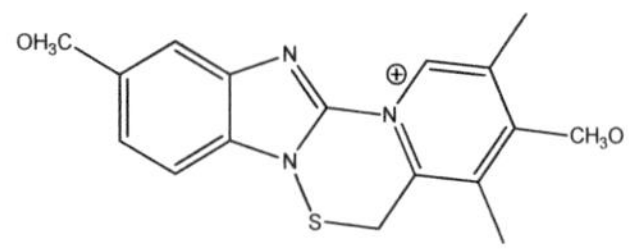

Log D=2.26 (pH=1.0)

Fig. 14. Anticipated log D values of E3710, esomeprazole and their active forms.

The primary metabolic enzyme for E3710 in human microsomes was CYP3A4 and contributions of another CYP were negligible. The metabolism of E3710 and its efficacy may be less affected by CYP2C19 polymorphism, unlike other PPIs such as omeprazole, lansoprazole where CYP2CY19 pathway is a significant metabolic pathway. Besides for GERD, PPIs are widely used with clopidogrel, an antiplatelet drug, to reduce the risk of gastrointestinal bleeding. Clopidogrel is converted to its active form mainly through CYP2C19 and this active metabolite reduces the cardiovascular event based on its platelet inhibitory effect [Disney et al., 2011]. Antiplatelet efficacy of clopidogrel therefore may be reduced in patients with receiving medicine which is metabolized by CYP2C19. In these days, there is growing concern about concomitant use of omeprazole with clopidogrel may be associated with the risk to reduce platelet inhibition and to increase cardiovascular events. Although clinical relevant interactions of PPIs with clopidogrel was not clearly clarified so far [Disney et al., 2011], European Medical Agency released a statement and FDA issued the warning letter on the concomitant use of these drugs [Laine and Hennekens, 2010]. As the metabolism of E3710 was less involved with CYP2C19, we expect that possibility of E3710 to interfere with clopidogrel may be low.

4.4.2 Toxicological features

E3710 inhibited human ether-a-go-go related gene (hERG) tail current with the IC_{50} value of 88.2 μmol/L, but it showed no effect on action potential at concentrations of 5 and 50 μmol/L. Similarly, cardiovascular safety study *in vivo* using the telemetry in conscious dogs indicated that E3710 had no effects on heart rate, blood pressure or electrocardiogram parameters, including QT intervals up to 30 mg/kg. E3710 up to 1000 mg/kg did not induce any effects on the respiratory function parameters and it up to 100 mg/kg had no effects on any observation/measurement in the central nervous system toxicity study in rats. These results suggested that E3710 is a low risk for adverse effects on the cardiovascular, respiratory and central nervous system.

The level for no observed adverse effect in 4-week repeated oral dose toxicity study was 10 mg/kg in rats and 3 mg/kg in dogs. The toxicological profile of E3710 is similar to those of other compounds in the same class. E3710 has been shown to have a tendency to exert its effect in more acidic state in comparison with esomeprazole (acidic condition in Table 1). Based on the results of several genotoxicity studies such as Ames test, mouse lymphoma thymidine kinase assay *in vitro*, rat micronucleus assay and rat liver unscheduled DNA synthesis *in vivo*, the genotoxic risk of E3710 is low. E3710 for 26 weeks administration showed no evidence of a carcinogenic potential in the strain of mice including $p53^{+/-}$ heterozygous knockout mice.

4.4.3 Study on the safety and tolerability in humans

The clinical ascending single and multiple dose studies of E3710 were carried out to examine its safety, tolerability and PKs in non-erosive GERD patients. For 14 days of continuous oral administration, the C_{max} and AUC increased in approximately proportion to doses and no accumulation upon multiple dosing. E3710 is well tolerated up to 180 mg designed as the maximum dose and no serious safety issues were observed at any doses. In summary, there were no clinically significant safety issues and the overall safety profile was similar to other PPIs in the clinical studies so far.

4.5 Competitive landscape with new concept in future acid related diseases

Besides of PPIs as gastric acid inhibitors, many pharmacological approaches such as P-CAB, transient lower esophageal sphincter relaxation (TLESR) inhibitors, transient receptor potential vanilloid (TRPV) 1 antagonist have been developing for the treatment of GERD (Fig. 15).

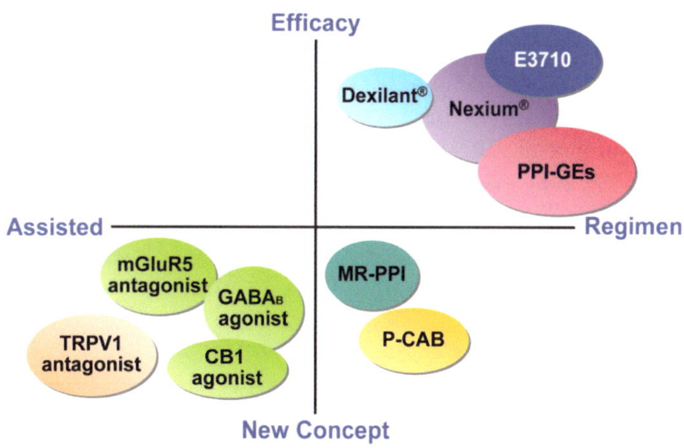

Fig. 15. Competitive landscape with new concept in future acid related diseases. Nexium®: esomeprazole, Dexilant®: dexlansoprazole modified-release, PPI-GEs: proton pump inhibitor generics, MR-PPI: modified-release proton pump inhibitor, P-CAP: potassium-competitive acid blocker, mGluR5: metabotropic glutamate receptor 5, GABAB: gamma-aminobutyric acid B, CB1: cannabinoid receptor 1, TRPV1: transient receptor potential vanilloid 1.

4.5.1 P-CAB

P-CAB inhibits H^+,K^+-ATPase based on different mechanism from PPIs. In contrast to the covalent biding and irreversible mechanism of action of PPIs, P-CAB binds to the potassium binding site of H^+,K^+-ATPase and result in its enzyme inhibition in a potassium-competitive manner with reversible inhibition. P-CAB doesn't need to be transferred its active form unlike to PPI; therefore, P-CAB would rapidly inhibit gastric acid secretion. The onset of relief of GERD symptoms may be related to the rapidity to the intragastric pH elevation. P-CAB has been expected to show the fast onset of heartburn relief, whereas this favorable clinical benefit has not been delivered so far. Full effect of gastric acid inhibition was actually observed on the first day of AZD0865 administration in Ph I study [Sachs et al., 2010]; however no dose response was observed regarding the time to sustained absence of heart burn among AZD0865-treated groups (25, 50 and 75 mg) in both GERD and non-erosive GERD patients [Kaharilas et al., 2007; Dent et al., 2008]. Moreover, AZD0865-treated groups didn't achieve faster sustained heartburn relief in comparison with esomeprazole (40 mg). Despite the long research history similar to PPI, no P-CAB has been launched up to now. A new type P-CAB, TAK-438, is only under Ph II trials in Japan [Sachs et al., 2010].

4.5.2 TLESR inhibitor

The lower esophageal sphincter plays a critical role in regulating flow across the gastro-esophageal junction by generating a tonic pressure to prevent reflux of gastric contents into the esophagus. TLESR is an episode of lower esophageal relaxation that occurs unrelated to swallowing [Kessing et al., 2011], and it is considered to be the underlying refractory factors for GERD treatment with PPIs. Many receptors in central nervous system is involved in TLESR, hence several approaches for TLESR inhibitors mediated through $GABA_B$, metabolic glutamine (mGlu) and cannabinoid (CB) receptors have been developed to enhance the lower esophageal sphincter constriction for blocking the gastric acid and non-acid reflux. Although $GABA_B$ receptor agonist (baclofen, R-baclofen, AZD9343, lesogaberan: AZD3355), mGlu receptor 5 antagonist (ADX10059, AZD2066, AZD2516) and CB1 agonist (D9-THC) reduced the TLESR, central nerve side effects such as headache and drowsiness, and low compliance (need to be taken twice or three times a day) were observed in clinical studies [Blondeau, 2010; Kessing et al., 2011]. Lesogaberan which was administered twice daily as add-on treatment to PPI ameliorated heartburn and regurgitation symptoms in persistent GERD symptoms even daily PPI therapy [Boeckxstaens et al., 2011]; however these effects were not adequate. Potent TLSER inhibitor without side effects is likely to be favorable as an add-on treatment for patients of GERD with PPIs in the future.

4.5.3 TRPV1 antagonist

Many patients show hypersensitivities to heat and acid; therefore, transient receptor TRPV1 might be a potential target for the remedy of refractory GERD. In the clinical study of TRPV1 antagonist, AZD1386, healthy volunteers were subjected to painful heat, mechanical, electrical stimulation similar to acid-induced hyperalgesia in esophagus. The skin and deep pressure pain was used as somatic controls. AZD1386 elevated the heat pain threshold in the esophagus and skin. Favorable safety profile was observed, dose dependent increases in body temperature were observed [Krarup et al., 2011]. This pursuit is still in smoke.

4.6 E3710 in the future

In the light of these disappointing situations for approaches associated with other mechanism, PPIs provide the most effective pharmacotherapy for treating acid related diseases (ARDs) with respect of efficacy and safety at present. We expect that E3710 with long-acting suppressive effects on gastric acid secretion would keep longer intragastric pH over-4 holding time in comparison with current PPIs for the treatment of the unmet medical needs of GERD. GERD is known as a common gastroesophageal disorder with a high prevalence rate at 10-20% in the USA [Dent et al., 2005]. The prevalence of GERD in Asia was reported to be relatively lower, while the recent research presented that the prevalence of symptom-based GERD and endoscopic reflux esophagitis has increased [Jung, 2011]. The adoption of a Western lifestyle accompanied by diet with high fat and energy, smoking and alcohol consumption, and increases in body mass index, obesity and metabolic syndrome may account for the increased prevalence rate of GERD in these areas [Goh, 2011]. According to better diagnosis system such as endoscope and questionnaire, GERD would be perceived as major gastroesophageal diseases all over the world.

In addition to GERD, there are still unmet medical needs in the treatment of patients with ARDs including NSAID (nonsteroid anti-inflammatory drug) -related ulcers, gastrointestinal bleeding, and *Helicobacter pylori* eradication. The widespread use of NSAID and aspirin would involve the risk of drug-related ulcers especially for the patients including personal history of complicated ulcer diseases, concurrent use of NSAID or aspirin, use of high doses, concurrent use of anticoagulant, personal history of uncomplicated peptic ulcer disease, age>70 and concurrent use of steroid. For these patients, concomitant use of promising PPIs with NSAID and/or aspirin would be useful to protect ulcers [Katz et al., 2006; Scarpignato and Pelosini, 2006]. E3710 possesses the appropriate stability in the point view of physical and chemical characteristics, combinational formulation of E3710 with NSAID and/or aspirin therefore may be expected. The co-therapy of PPIs with aspirin reduced not only upper gastrointestinal bleeding, but also cardiovascular events due to the increased aspirin adherence. This concomitant use is likely to be cost-effective [Saini et al., 2005]. In order to induce platelet aggregation, clot formulation and stability, a sustained intragastric pH>6 is necessary. The current PPIs are not able to maintain intragastric pH>6 for prolonged periods. The potent and long-acting PPI would be feasible for the treatment of gastrointestinal bleeding [Katz et al., 2006; Scarpignato and Pelosini, 2006]. The success rate of *Helicobacter pylori* eradication therapy depends on intragastric pH, so a long-acting PPI would be acceptable [Katz et al., 2006; Scarpignato and Pelosini, 2006]. Optimizing the control of intragastric pH would also be beneficial in these ARDs, so that a potent and long-acting PPI such as E3710 would be expected to offer improved clinical outcomes for patients with these ARDs as well as GERD.

Concerns have been expressed about the increased risk with long-term PPIs administration such as bone fracture, community-acquired pneumonia and in hospital-acquired *Clostridium difficile* diarrhea and malabsorption of nutrients etc. [Kushner and Peura, 2011]. Given that the potent and long-acting intragastric acid neutralization would lead to faster resolution of symptoms, faster healing of lesions, better responses in severe lesions and less frequent relapses for GERD, patients administered with E3710 would lead to sufficiently healed for only 4- or 6-weeks treatment instead of a standard 8-weeks treatment and less incidence of recurrence. These shorted remedy periods with E3710 may result in the reduced these warnings. As a consequence, E3710 would provide a cost-effective and a valid therapy, improving patients' QOL for GERD in clinic, especially for intractable with current PPIs.

In conclusion, E3710, a newly synthesized long-acting PPI, could achieve potent and a long-acting suppression of gastric acid production. E3710 provides cost-effective and improved therapy for the treatment of unmet medical needs of GERD as well as other ARDs.

5. References

Armstrong, D. (2004). Review article: gastric pH - the most relevant predictor of benefit in reflux disease? *Aliment Pharmacol Ther,* Vol.20, Suppl.5, (October), pp. 19-26, ISSN 1365-2036.

Armstrong, D. (2005). Gastroesophageal reflux disease. *Curr Opin Pharmacol,* Vol.5, No.6, (December), pp. 589-595, ISSN 1471-4892.

Blondeau, K. (2010). Treatment of gastro-esophageal reflux disease: the new kids to block. *Neurogastroenterol Motil,* Vol.22, No.22, (August), pp.836-840. ISSN 1350-1925.

Boeckxstaens, GE.; Beaumont, H.; Hatlebakk, JG.; Silberg, DG.; Björck, K.; Karlsson, M. & Denison, H. (2011). A novel reflux inhibitor lesogaberan (AZD3355) as add-on treatment in patients with GORD with persistent reflux symptoms despite proton pump inhibitor therapy: a randomised placebo-controlled trial. *Gut,* Vol. 60, No.9 (September), pp. 1182-1188, ISSN 0017-5749.

Castell, DO.; Kahrilas, PJ.; Richter, JE.; Vakil, NB.; Johnson, DA.; Zuckerman, S.; Skammer, W. & Levine, JG. (2002). Esomeprazole (40 mg) compared with lansoprazole (30 mg) in the treatment of erosive esophagitis. *Am J Gastroenterol,* Vol.97, No.3, (March), pp.575-583, ISSN 0002-9270.

Castell DO.; Murray JA.; Tutuian R.; Orlando RC. & Arnold R. (2004). Review article: the pathophysiology of gastro-oesophageal reflux diseases-oesophageal manifestations. *Aliment Pharmacol Ther,* Vol.20, Suppl.9, (December), pp. 14-25, ISSN 1365-2036.

Dent, J.; El-Serag, HB.; Wallander, MA. & Johansson, S. (2005). Epidemiology of gastro-oesophageal reflux disease: a systematic review. *Gut,* Vol.54, No.5, (May), pp. 710-717, ISSN 0017-5749.

Dent, J.; Kahrilas, PJ.; Hatlebakk, J.; Vakil, N.; Denison, H.; Franzén, S. & Lundborg, P. (2008). A randomized, comparative trial of a potassium-competitive acid blocker (AZD0865) and esomeprazole for the treatment of patients with nonerosive reflux disease. *Am J Gastroenterol,* Vol.103, No.1, (January), pp. 20-26, ISSN 0002-9270.

Disney, BR.; Watson, RD.; Blann, AD.; Lip, GY. & Anderson, MR. (2011). Review article: proton pump inhibitors with clopidogrel--evidence for and against a clinically-important interaction. *Aliment Pharmacol Ther,* Vol.33, No.7, (April), pp. 758-767, ISSN 1365-2036.

Fass, R.; Shapiro, M.; Dekel, R. & Sewell, J. (2005). Systematic review: proton-pump inhibitor failure in gastro-oesophageal reflux disease--where next? *Aliment Pharmacol Ther,* Vol.22, No.2, (July), pp. 79-94, ISSN 1365-2036.

Fass, R. & Sifrim, D. (2009). Management of heartburn not responding to proton pump inhibitors. *Gut,* Vol. 58, No. 2, (February), pp. 295-309, ISSN 0017-5749.

Goh, K-L. (2011). Gastroesophageal reflux disease in Asia: A historical perspective and present challenges. *J Gastroenterol Hepatol,* Vol.26, Suppl.1, (January), pp. 2-10. ISSN 0017-5749.

Hatlebakk, JG.; Katz, PO.; Kuo, B. & Castell, DO. (1998). Nocturnal gastric acidity and acid breakthrough on different regimens of omeprazole 40 mg daily. *Aliment Pharmacol Ther,* Vol.12, No.12, (December), pp.1235-1240, ISSN 1365-2036.

Hatlebakk JG.; Katz, PO.; Camacho-Lobato, L. & Castell, DO. (2000). Proton pump inhibitors: better acid suppression when taken before a meal than without a meal. *Aliment Pharmacol Ther,* Vol.14, No.10, (October), pp. 1267-1272, ISSN 1365-2036.

Hershcovici, T. & Fass, R. (2011). Pharmacological management of GERD: where does it stand now? *Trends Pharmacol Sci,* Vol.32, No.4, (April), pp. 258-264, ISSN 0165-6147.

Hershcovici, T.; Jha, LK.; Cui H.; Powers, J. & Fass, R. (2011). Night-time intra-oesophageal bile and acid: a comparison between gastro-oesophageal reflux disease patients who failed and those who were treated successfully with a proton pump inhibitor. *Aliment Pharmacol Ther,* Vol.33, No.7, (April), pp. 837-844, ISSN 1365-2036.

Jung, HK. (2011). Epidemiology of gastroesophageal reflux disease in Asia: a systematic review. *J Neurogastroenterol Motil,* Vol.17, No.1, (January), pp. 14-27, ISSN 2093-0879.

Kahrilas, PJ.; Dent, J.; Lauritsen, K.; Malfertheiner, P.; Denison, H.; Franzén, S. & Hasselgren, G. (2007). A randomized, comparative study of three doses of AZD0865 and esomeprazole for healing of reflux esophagitis. *Clin Gastroenterol Hepatol,* Vol.5, No.12, (December), pp. 1385-1391, ISSN 1542-3565.

Katz, PO.; Scheiman, JM. & Barkun, AN. (2006). Review article: acid-related disease--what are the unmet clinical needs? *Aliment Pharmacol Ther,* Vol.23, Suppl. 2, (June), pp. 9-22, ISSN 1365-2036.

Kodama, K.; Fujisaki, H.; Kubota, A.; Kato, H.; Hirota, K.; Kuramochi, H.; Murota, M.; Tabata, Y.; Ueda, M.; Harada, H.; Kawahara, T.; Shinoda, M.; Watanabe, N.; Iida, D.; Terauchi, H.; Yasui, S.; Miyazawa, S. & Nagakawa, J. (2010). E3710, a new proton pump inhibitor, with a long-lasting inhibitory effect on gastric acid secretion. *J Pharmacol Exp Ther,* Vol.334, No.2, (August), pp. 395-401, ISSN 1521-0103.

Krarup, AL.; Ny, L.; Astrand, M.; Bajor, A.; Hvid-Jensen, F.; Hansen, MB.; Simrén, M.; Funch-Jensen, P. & Drewes, AM. (2011). Randomised clinical trial: the efficacy of a transient receptor potential vanilloid 1 antagonist AZD1386 in human oesophageal pain. *Aliment Pharmacol Ther,* Vol.33, No.10, (May), pp. 1113-1122, ISSN 1365-2036.

Kessing, BF.; Conchillo, JM.; Bredenoord, AJ.; Smout, A. & Masclee, AA. (2011). Review article: the clinical relevance of transient lower oesophageal sphincter relaxations in gastro-oesophageal reflux disease. *Aliment Pharmacol Ther,* Vol.33, No.6, (March), pp. 650-661, ISSN 1365-2036.

Kushner, PR. & Peura, DA. (2011). Review of proton pump inhibitors for the initial treatment of heartburn: Is there a dose ceiling effect? *Adv Ther,* Vol.28, No.5, (May), pp. 367-88, ISSN 0741-238X.

Laine, L. & Hennekens, C. (2010). Proton pump inhibitor and clopidogrel interaction: fact or fiction? *Am J Gastroenterol,* Vol.105, No.1, (January), pp. 34-41, ISSN 0002-9270.

Miner, P Jr.; Katz, PO.; Chen, Y. & Sostek, M. (2003). Gastric acid control with esomeprazole, lansoprazole, omeprazole, pantoprazole, and rabeprazole: a five-way crossover study. *Am J Gastroenterol,* Vol.98, No.12, (December), pp. 2616-2620, ISSN 0002-9270.

Peghini, PL.; Katz. PO.; Bracy, NA. & Castell, DO. (1998). Nocturnal recovery of gastric .acid secretion with twice-daily dosing of proton pump inhibitors. *Am J Gastroenterol,* Vol.93, No. 5, (May), pp. 763-767, ISSN 0002-9270.

Sachs, G.; Shin, JM. & Howden, CW. (2006). Review article: the clinical pharmacology of proton pump inhibitors. *Aliment Pharmacol Ther,* Vol.23, Suppl.2, (June), pp. 2-8, ISSN 1365-2036.

Sachs, G.; Shin, JM. & Hunt, R. (2010). Novel approaches to inhibition of gastric acid secretion. *Curr Gastroenterol Rep,* Vol.12, No.6, (December), pp. 437-447, ISSN 1522-8037.

Saini, SD.; Fendrick, AM. & Scheiman, JM. (2011). Cost-effectiveness analysis: cardiovascular benefits of proton pump inhibitor co-therapy in patients using aspirin for secondary prevention. *Aliment Pharmacol Ther,* Vol.34, No.2, (July), pp. 243-51, ISSN 1365-2036.

Scarpignato, C. & Pelosini, I. (2006). Review article: the opportunities and benefits of extended acid suppression. *Aliment Pharmacol Ther,* Vol.23, Suppl.2, (June), pp. 23-34, ISSN 1365-2036.

Shaker, R.; Brunton, S.; Elfant, A.; Golopol, L.; Ruoff, G. & Stanghellini, V. (2004). Review article: impact of night-time reflux on lifestyle - unrecognized issues in reflux disease. *Aliment Pharmacol Ther,* Vol.20, Suppl.9, (December), pp. 3-13, ISSN 1365-2036.

Shin, JM.; Cho, YM. & Sachs, G. (2004). Chemistry of covalent inhibition of the gastric (H^+, K^+)-ATPase by proton pump inhibitors. *J Am Chem Soc,* Vol.126, No.25, (June), pp. 7800–7811, ISSN 0002-7863.

Wahlqvist, P.; Karlsson, M.; Johnson, D.; Carlsson, J.; Bolge, SC. & Wallander, MA. (2008). Relationship between symptom load of gastro-oesophageal reflux disease and health-related quality of life, work productivity, resource utilization and concomitant diseases: survey of a US cohort. *Aliment Pharmacol Ther,* Vol.27, No.10, (May), pp. 960-970, ISSN 1365-2036.

8

Laparoscopic Total Fundoplication for Refractory GERD: How to Achieve Optimal Long-Term Outcomes by Preoperative Instrumental Assessment and a Standardized Technique

Paolo Limongelli et al.[*],[**]
Department of General and Hepato-Pancreato-Biliary Surgery S.M., Loreto Nuovo Hospital, Naples
Italy

1. Introduction

Gastroesophageal reflux disease (GERD) is one of the most common gastrointestinal disease among adults in Europe and USA. A recent consensus conference (the Montreal Consensus) defined GERD as "a condition which develops when the reflux of stomach contents causes troublesome symptoms and/or complications". Symptoms were considered to be " troublesome" if they adversely affected an individual's well-being. GERD can lead to both esophageal and non-esophageal symptoms. The most common typical symptoms of GERD are heartburn and regurgitation. Non-esophageal GERD symptoms include chronic aspiration with cough and laryngitis (Shaheen & Ransohoff, 2002). At its core, GERD is the failure of the antireflux barrier, allowing abnormal amounts of reflux of gastric contents into the esophagus (Dodds et al., 1982). The primary treatment modality for GERD is acid suppression therapy, in particular by use of PPI (Castell et al., 2002). However, consideration should be given for surgery if the following indications exist: complications of GERD (such as peptic stricture or Barrett's esophagus), extraesophageal manifestations (chest pain, pulmonary symptoms), failed medical management, or desire to discontinue medical treatment despite adequate symptomatic control. Minimal invasive anti-reflux surgery can be considered an effective GERD therapy, with its mechanical function both in the short and long term period. Several different ways of fashioning a total fundoplication lead to different outcomes. This chapter addresses the technical details of the antireflux technique we adopted without modifications for all patients with GERD. In particular it

---

[*] Salvatore Tolone, Gianmattia del Genio, Antonio d'Alessandro, Gianluca Rossetti, Luigi Brusciano, Giovanni Docimo, Roberto Ruggiero, Simona Gili, Assia Topatino, Vincenzo Amoroso, Giuseppina Casalino, Alfonso Bosco, Ludovico Docimo and Alberto del Genio
Second University of Naples, Division of General and Bariatric Surgery, Naples, Italy
[**]Paolo Limongelli and Salvatore Tolone gave the same contribution to the chapter

aims to discuss the appropriate selection of patients undergoing laparoscopic fundoplication and the relation between wrap and the physiology of the esophagus. In fact, selecting gastroesophageal reflux disease (GERD) patients for surgery on the basis of traditional pH-monitoring or endoscopy, may be challenging, particularly if endoscopy is negative (i.e. NERD patient), or presenting "uncommon" GERD with clinical symptoms (Charbel et al., 2005). Combined multichannel intraluminal impedance pH monitoring (MII-pH) is able to physically detect each episode of intraesophageal bolus movements, enabling identification of either acid or non-acid reflux episodes and thus establish the association of the reflux with symptoms. Since the mechanism of fundoplication is to physically block gastric refluxate to enter into the esophageal lumen by restoring the competence of the lower esophageal sphincter (LES), the routine use of MII-pH in the preoperative evaluation may offer objective parameters for a more accurate indication to surgery. At the same time, some authors assume that a total fundoplication expose the patient to a delayed transit of the swallowed bolus and thus to an increased risk of dysphagia, especially when a peristaltic dysfunction is present. However, few studies have reported the effects of total fundoplication on peristalsis, bolus transit and increased risk of dysphagia by means of objective data; this was mainly due to the exposure to radiations and a difficulty of completing studies by the use of combined manometry and videofluoroscopy.

Multichannel intraluminal impedance combined with traditional esophageal manometry (MII-EM) provides an objective assessment of the transit and clearance of a standardized bolus, and to study the esophageal motility. Montenovo et al. have recently reported the inefficacy of preoperative use of MII and manometry to predict postoperative dysphagia of patients who underwent Nissen fundoplication, based on a postoperative symptom questionnaire. However, no pre- or postoperative evaluation of the effects of fundoplication on the esophageal function has been reported to date.

We undertook the current study to evaluate by means of MII-EM and combined 24-h pH and multichannel intraluminal impedance (MII-pH) the impact of fundoplication on esophageal physiology. An objective demonstration of the impact of the total wrap on the bolus transit may be helpful in refining the correct indications towards partial or total antireflux wrap.

2. Protocol study

The study involved a consecutive cohort of patients undergoing laparoscopic total fundoplication for refractory GERD, with information recorded in a prospectively maintained database, followed up for at least one year. Surgical treatment was offered to PPI- refractory patients with heartburn and regurgitation as their predominant symptoms. Patients were considered PPI refractory if 40 mg omeprazole was insufficient for lasting suppression of symptoms and if, following an increase in dosage to 40 mg two or three times daily, symptoms recurred after return to 40 mg maintenance treatment daily. Patients were included in the present study if upper endoscopy had been performed before surgery, preoperative 24-h combined MII-pH-monitoring demonstrated pathological reflux condition, and objective and subjective outcome had been registered after surgery.

From October 1st 2005 to October 1st 2010, five hundred and twenty-three consecutive patients (298 women and 225 men; mean age 43.7±14.5 years; range 20-65 years) were referred to Esophageal Pathophysiology Center of the First Division of General and

Gastrointestinal Surgery of the Second University of Naples for the suspicion of esophageal diseases. Before subjects entered the study, a specific informed consent was obtained from each.

Surgery was indicated for (1) patients with GERD who were not responding to medical therapy or affected by "nocturnal acid break through" phenomenon; (2) patients not compliant with long-term medical therapy; (3) patients requiring high dosages of drugs; (4) patients too young for lifetime medical treatment; (5) patients performing a particular type of job that does not allow drugs to be taken constantly; (6) patients with atypical GERD who opted for surgery or bile reflux; and (7) patients who decided, in the first instance, for the surgical treatment of typical GERD.

2.1 Clinical evaluation

After a brief interview and examination to assess for the presence and severity of gastrointestinal symptoms and to make anthropometric measurements, all subjects completed a brief symptom assessment questionnaire. The questionnaire incorporated a visual analog scale (modified DeMeester Score) for heartburn, regurgitation, dysphagia, and respiratory symptoms.

2.2 Instrumental assessment

Preoperatively, all patients underwent upper gastrointestinal endoscopy, Combined Multichannel Intraluminal Impedance and Esophageal Manometry (MII-EM) and 24 hours Combined Multichannel Intraluminal Impedance and pH-monitoring (MII-pH), as our routinary preoperative assessment for patients evaluated for antireflux surgery.

Upper gastrointestinal endoscopy was performed according to the international guidelines and the center's current practice criteria that were adopted for the preoperative study of candidates for antireflux therapy. Reflux esophagitis was graded according to the Los Angeles classification, including nonerosive esophageal reflux disease. Biopsies were performed for the histologic confirmation of the diagnosis of Barrett esophagus or when dysplastic lesions were suspected; Barrett esophagus was categorized according to established criteria.

2.2.1 Combined MII-EM protocol

Each patient underwent esophageal function testing using combined MII-EM with a Koenigsberg 10-channel probe (Sandhill EFT catheter; Sandhill Scientific Inc., Highlands Ranch, CO, USA). The 4.5-mm-diameter catheter design has two circumferential solid-state pressure sensors at 5 and 10 cm from the tip and three unidirectional pressure sensors at 15, 20, and 25 cm. Impedance measuring segments consisting of two rings placed 2 cm apart were centered at 7, 10, 15, 20, 25 from the tip. The EFT catheter was inserted transnasally into the esophagus up to a depth of 60 cm and the collection of impedance and pH data (30 Hz) was initiated. Lower esophageal sphincter (LES) was identified using station pull-through technique and the most distal sensor was placed in the high-pressure zone of the LES. Intraesophageal pressure sensors and impedance measuring segments were thus located at 5, 10, 15, 20 cm above the LES and 2, 5, 10, 15, and 20 cm above the LES, respectively. In the supine position, patients were given 10 swallows of 5 cc normal saline and 10 swallows of 5 cc appleasauce consistency viscous material with standardized ionic concentration (Viscous ®, Sandhill Sci.), each 20–30 s apart. Normal saline was used instead of regular water since it has a standardized ionic concentration and provides better impedance changes. Double-swallowing disqualified swallows and these were repeated.

2.2.2 Manometric parameters assessment

Manometric parameters used to characterize swallows included (1) contraction amplitude at 5 and 10 cm above the LES, (2) distal esophageal amplitude (DEA) as average of contraction amplitude at 5 and 10 cm above the LES, (3) onset velocity of esophageal contractions in the distal part of the esophagus (i.e., contraction velocity between 10 and 5 cm above the LES).

During the pull-trough distance of both distal border and proximal border of LES were recorded, as the distance in cm from nares. The LES length was measured, as the difference of distal border and proximal border in cm.

The LES residual pressure was measured as the lowest pressure (excluding respiratory artefacts) during swallow-induced LES relaxation, and the LES resting pressure was calculated as the average (mid respiratory) LES pressure over 4–5 s at the level just distal to the pressure inversion point.

Swallows were classified using the traditional manometric criteria as (1) normal, if contraction amplitudes at 5 and 10cm above the LES were each greater than or equal to 30 mmHg and distal onset velocity was less than 8 cm/s; (2) ineffective, if either of the contraction amplitudes at 5 and 10 cm above the LES was less than 30 mmHg; (3) simultaneous, if the contraction had a distal onset velocity greater than 8 cm/s or retrograde onset and amplitudes at 5 and 10 cm above the LES were each greater or equal to 30 mmHg.

Diagnoses of manometric motility abnormalities were established using criteria published by Spechler and Castell. DES was defined as 20% or more saline swallows with contraction amplitude greater than or equal to 30 mmHg in both distal sites located at 5 and 10 cm above the LES and contraction onset velocity greater than 8 cm/s.

2.2.3 Impedance parameters assessment

Bolus entry at a specific level was identified by the 50% point between 3-s preswallow impedance baseline and impedance nadir during bolus presence. Bolus exit was determined as return to this 50% point on the impedance recovery curve as discussed in previous studies (Fass et al.,1994).

Swallows were classified by MII as showing (1) complete bolus transit if bolus entry occurred at the most proximal site (20 cm above LES) and bolus exit points were recorded in all three distal impedance-measuring sites (i.e., 15, 10, and 5 cm above the LES) and (2) incomplete bolus transit if bolus exit was not identified at any of the three distal impedance measuring sites.

Total bolus transit time was calculated as the time elapsed from bolus entry in the proximal channel 20 cm above the LES to bolus exit in the distal channel 5 cm above the LES when bolus exit present.

Diagnoses of esophageal transit abnormalities were defined as incomplete liquid transit if at least 30% of liquid swallows had complete bolus transit and incomplete viscous transit if at least 40% of viscous swallows had complete bolus transit. These values are based on data from 43 healthy volunteers (Tutuian et al., 2003a).

2.2.4 Combined 24 hour ph-multichannel intraluminal impedance (MII-pH)

Twenty-four-hour ambulatory combined pH-multichannel intraluminal impadance studies were performed to document the presence of GERD. A dedicated MII-pH catheter (with intraluminal impedance segments positioned at 3, 5, 7, 9, 15, and 17 cm above the LES; Sandhill Scientific Inc., Highlands Ranch, CO, USA) was placed transnasally, with the esophageal pH sensor positioned 5 cm above the manometrical determined LES. Patients were invited to signal three or more predominant symptoms that occurred during the recording time, every meal, and changing position in upright or in recumbent, as on the device and a written diary as well. This information was transmitted by the catheter into software integrated into the device (Sleuth System, Sandhill Scientific Inc.). MII-pH data were acquired and analyzed with the Bioview GERD Analysis Software (Sandhill Scientific Inc.). All tracings were carefully reviewed by a single investigator [S.T.] to check correspondence between the results of the computer evaluation and the morphology of each reflux episode. Meal periods and drop in pH, not related to a retrograde movement at impedance (i.e., swallow of acid drink), were excluded from the analysis to improve accuracy of the pH monitoring (Sifrim et al., 2004; Tutuian et al., 2003b). The following variables were assessed: (1) esophageal acid exposure calculated as percentage (%) of time with pH <4 (total, upright, and recumbent), (2) number and quality (acid and non-acid) of reflux detected at MII, and (3) Symptom Index, described according to reported parameters. An abnormal % of time with pH <4 in distal esophagus, a total number of refluxes detected at MII >73, a Symptom Index at least 50%, or the presence of two or all three were considered as parameters useful to indicate antireflux surgery.

Based on the results of MII-pH, the patients were divided into positive pH monitoring (pH+) and negative pH monitoring groups (pH−). This latter were further divided in two sub-groups if the total number of reflux episodes at MII was pathologic (pH-MII+) or the total number of reflux episodes were negative, though the Symptom Index was positive (pH-MII-SI+).

2.3 Surgical technique

Pneumoperitoneum was induced at 12 mmHg via a Verress needle or open Hasson's technique. Five trocars (one 10 mm and four 5 mm) were inserted (one transumbellical, one on the left and one the right emiclavear line in ipocondrium, one in epigastrium and one between umbellical and the left emiclavear line). A steep reverse-Trendelenburg position was applied. The aspirator was inserted in the epigastric trocar to retract the left liver. The height of the gastroesophageal junction was localized by transillumination provided by the endoscope. The procedure began with the section of the anterior peritoneal reflection of the gastroesophageal junction, the surgeon being aware to start the section of the lesser omentum high enough not to cut the vagal branch to the liver. To achieve this step, the assistant employed a Babcock grasper positioned at the anterior esophageal fat pad, which was retracted downward tward the esophagus. After identification of the anterior vagal nerve, the gastrophrenic ligament was sectioned. The dissection was then continued from right to left behind the esophagus until the crura was exposed and the angle of His was abolished, with particular care taken to avoid injury to the posterior vagus.

At this point, an esophageal retractor replaced the Babcock grasper, and a posterior window was created large enough to accommodate fashioning of the wrap. With the help provided by right and left steering of the aspirator, the esophagus was widely mobilized in its mediastinal portion until non-inflammatory periesophageal tissue was reached and the esophagus lay in the abdomen without tension (floppy esophagus). The cruroplasty was accomplished by one simple extracorporeal non-adsorbable knot; only in cases where there a larger defect (>4 cm) were additional sutures required. The 2-cm-long Nissen-Rossetti wrap was fashioned with the anterior wall of gastric fundus passed, if possible, between the esophagus and the posterior vagus nerve. The short gastric vessels were always preserved. The two gastric hemi-valves were sutured with two stitches that never incorporated the esophageal muscular layer. In all cases, to check the calibration of the wrap, at the end of the procedure we performed intraoperative manometry and an endoscopic control (A. del Genio et al., 1997; G. del Genio et al., 2007); whenever a pressure outside the range (20-40 mmHg) was detected or the endoscopic vision of the wrap was not satisfactory (difficult passage of the endoscope through the fundoplication, superior edge of the gastric fundus not included into the wrap), the fundoplication was refashioned correctly.

2.4 Post-operative assessment and follow-up

The same pre-operative questionnaire (incorporating a visual analog scale (0–10) for heartburn, regurgitation, dysphagia, and chest pain) was re-administered to patients at 6 months, 1 and 5 years after surgery. At the 1-year control patients were asked to re-underwent to MII-EM and MII-pH and upper endoscopy when needed.

3. Outcomes

3.1 Patients candidate for laparoscopic total fundoplication

Among 523 patients investigated at MII-pH, 184 patients (35.1%) had one or more MII-pH parameter positive and, for this reason, were submitted to Laparoscopic Nissen-Rossetti Fundoplication and 339 patients (64.9%) had a negative MII-pH exam. Of these, 47.2% of patients complained of abdominal pain, with gastritis at esophagogastroduodenoscopy and underwent eradication of Helicobacter pylori infection (14/47.2) and/or started PPI therapy. The remaining 52.7% of patients were non-responders to PPI.

In particular, 19.7% of patients with symptoms related to the presence of hiatus hernia underwent laparoscopic hernia repair, hiatoplasty, and fundoplication. Twenty-three percent of patients complaining of extraesophageal symptoms (i.e., hoarseness, laryngitis, chest pain, and globus) not related to GERD were referred to otolaryngologists, pulmonologists, or other specialists.

In last cases, the symptoms were suggestive for functional dyspepsia (i.e., bloating, delayed gastric empting), and the patients underwent further clinical–instrumental investigation (i.e., diisopropyl iminodiacetic acid gastric scintigraphy scanning, 24-h intragastric bile monitoring with the Bilitec), and promotility agents like metocloporamide, domperidone, and erythromycin were started.

Among the 184 patients, 53.3% had abnormal pH monitoring (pH+), 27.4% had a normal pH monitoring and a positive number of MII reflux (>73 episodes; pH-MII+), and 19.3% had a normal pH monitoring and number of MII reflux (<73 episodes) and a positive Symptom Index. Twenty-six percent of patients were positive for all the parameters (e.g., pH-monitoring, number of reflux >73, and Symptom Index). All of them underwent to Laparoscopic Nissen-Rossetti fundoplication.

3.2 Clinical outcomes and follow-up

The evaluations were performed a median of 15 days (range 5-35 days) before the fundoplication then 6, 12 and 60 months afterward.

The pre- and post-operative visual analog scale symptom scoring system is reported in table 1.

Mean symptom score ± S.D.	Pre-operative	Post-operative	p
Hearthburn	2.3±0.8	0.2±0.2	<0.05
Regurgitation	1.8±0.9	0.3±0.2	<0.05
Dysphagia	0.3±0.5	0.4±0.1	N.S.
Chestpain	1.6±0.8	0.3±0.2	<0.05
Respiratory symptoms	1.1±0.9	0.3±0.1	<0.05

Table 1. Mean Pre- and Post-operative DeMeester symptom score (modified).

After surgery the incidence of symptoms related to reflux was statistically decreased; no increase in perception of dysphagia was observed.

At 12 months, 98.3% of patients were satisfied of the procedure and expressed the will to undergo the same operation knowing its effects.

Regarding side effects, among 184 patients, 1.6% of patient complained about bloating and hyperflatulence and 3.8% complained about transient dysphagia, totally resolved in 2 months after surgery. All the patients did not restart taking any anti-acid drugs for symptoms above the wrap.

3.3 Instrumental outcomes

3.3.1 Manometric parameters

At 12 months afterward surgery, mean LES resting pressure raised from the pre-operative value of 16.2±7.5 mmHg to 31.1±6.3 mmHg ($p<0.05$). LES relaxing pressure (%) wasn't affected by the wrap (91.7±3.9% pre-operatively vs. 90.1±6.4% post-operatively).

Mean wave amplitude at 5, 10, 15 and 20 cm above LES wasn't affected by the presence of fundoplication, both for liquid and viscous swallows. Also mean distal esophageal amplitude (DEA), both for liquid and viscous swallows, didn't show any significant variation after surgery (88.8±34.6 mmHg vs. 86.6±39.1 mmHg for liquid swallows and 86.5±38.7 mmHg vs. 90.4±29.0 mmHg for viscous swallows).

The mean percentage of normal, ineffective and simultaneous waves didn't change significantly, both for liquid than viscous swallows.

Detailed manometrical data are shown in table 2.

	Pre-operative	Post-operative	P
LESP (mmHg, mean ± S.D.)	20.0± 7.5	31.1 ± 6.3	<0.05
LES % relax	91.7±3.9	92.1±6.4	N.S.
Liquid Swallow (N=150)			
Normal	110	108	N.S.
Ineffective	40	41	N.S.
Simultaneous	0	1	N.S.
Amplitude (mmHg, mean ± S.D.) at 20 cm above LES	49.1±24.5	63.5±39.8	N.S.
Amplitude (mmHg, mean ± S.D.) at 15 cm above LES	49.1±20.2	44.5±17.2	N.S.
Amplitude (mmHg, mean ± S.D.) at 10 cm above LES	82.6±33.8	75.8±37.1	N.S.
Amplitude (mmHg, mean ± S.D.) at 5 cm above LES	95.5±47.0	97.6±43.3	N.S.
DEA	88.8±34.6	86.6±39.1	N.S.
Viscous Swallow (N=150)			
Normal	103	123	N.S.
Ineffective	47	27	N.S.
Simultaneous	0	0	N.S.
Amplitude (mmHg, mean ± S.D.) at 20 cm above LES	51.5±29.9	59.6±39.9	N.S.
Amplitude (mmHg, mean ± S.D.) at 15 cm above LES	44.5±24.3	45.1±23.3	N.S.
Amplitude (mmHg, mean ± S.D.) at 10 cm above LES	75.7±36.3	79±28.6	N.S.
Amplitude (mmHg, mean ± S.D.) at 5 cm above LES	97.5±48.0	101.8±36.6	N.S.
DEA (mmHg, mean ± S.D.)	86.5±38.7	90.4±29.0	N.S.

Table 2. Pre- and Post-operative Esophageal Manometry findings.

3.3.2 Impedance parameters

After total fundoplication, esophageal bolus transit patterns detected at impedance were the followings:

The mean percentage of complete liquid bolus transit was not influenced by surgery (68.8±23.1% vs 75.5±21.8%, pre- and postoperative respectively).

The mean percentage of complete viscous bolus transit improved, raising from 64.4±25.0% to 86.6±15.8% ($p<0.05$) pre- and postoperative respectively.

Mean total bolus transit time, both for liquid and viscous swallows, didn't show a statistically significant, changing from 8.4±1.6 seconds to 9.0±1.9 seconds for liquid swallows and from 8.6±1.0 seconds to 9.3±1.8 seconds for viscous swallows, pre- and postoperative respectively.

Detailed impedance bolus transit data are shown in table 3.

3.3.3 MII-pH parameters

The Nissen-Rossetti antireflux procedure produced an improvement in all categories of the MII-pH over the patients' preoperative values. Esophageal acid exposure (%) of time with pH <4 showed a drastically reduction post-operatively in total, upright, and recumbent position. The overall number of GER episodes was statistically reduced in both the upright and recumbent positions (p<0.05). This reduction was obtained due to the postoperative control of both the acid (p<0.05) and nonacid (p<0.05) GER episodes (tab 4).

Postoperatively, symptom occurrence fell considerably. None of the patients had a positive symptom index. The proportion of physical reflux characteristics (liquid, mixed, gas) did not change after surgery.

	Pre-operative	Post-operative	P
Liquid Swallows (N=150)			
Complete bolus transit	123	113	N.S.
Incomplete bolus transit	27	37	N.S.
Total bolus transit time (sec, mean ± S.D.)	8.46±1.64	9.0±1.96	N.S.
Viscous Swallows (N=150)			
Complete bolus transit	96	130	<0.05
Incomplete bolus transit	54	20	<0.05
Total bolus transit time (sec, mean ± S.D.)	8.6±1.0	9.3±1.8	N.S.

Table 3. Pre- and Post-operative Bolus transit patterns at impedance

	Pre-operative	Post-operative	p
Total % time at pH <4	5.9±2.9	0.4±0.3	<0.05
Upright % time at pH <4	6.5±3.5	0.7±0.8	<0.05
Recumbent % time at pH <4	3.3±2.5	0.2±0.2	<0.05
DeMeester Score (pH)	17.4±8.5	1.6±1.5	<0.05
Total number of reflux (MII)	65.2±45.4	4.4±0.5	<0.05
Upright Total number of reflux (MII)	53.1±43.0	3.1±0.5	<0.05
Recumbent Total number of reflux (MII)	12.1±5.0	1.3±0.5	<0.05
Total acid reflux (MII)	33.4±21.4	1.6±0.6	<0.05
Upright Total acid reflux (MII)	26.5±21	1.3±0.6	<0.05
Recumbent Total acid reflux (MII)	6.9±6	0.3±0.8	<0.05
Total non acid reflux (MII)	31.8±34.1	2.8±0.3	<0.05
Upright Total non acid reflux (MII)	26.7±34.2	1.9±0.7	<0.05
Recumbent Total non acid reflux (MII)	5.1±3.7	0.9±0.4	<0.05

Table 4. Pre-and post operative MII-pH findings (Mean ± S.D.)

4. Discussion

There are objective data to demonstrate that MII-pH used as a routine diagnostic tool for patient candidates for surgery provided a satisfaction rate comparable to classic pH monitoring. It is noteworthy that these positive results were obtained extending the indication to surgery in an additional 40% of patients, with negative pH monitoring (G. del Genio et al., 2008). In the pre-MII era, to establish the need for surgery in patients with negative pH monitoring was a challenging decision.

Data on non-acid reflux episodes and a more precise symptom index correlation helps the surgeon to decide for an antireflux operation vs. medical treatment. Moreover, the possibility of following up the patients operated on by MII-pH helps the surgeons to distinguish a surgical failure from gastroduodenal-associated symptoms.

From a clinical practice standpoint, we identified three useful parameters to select patients for antireflux surgery. The first parameter is the presence of an abnormal time of esophageal exposure to pH <4. This data indicates the total exposure of the mucosa of the esophagus to acid, and its importance is known from the standard pH monitoring. MII-pH improves the affordability of this parameters, living the opportunity of detecting and excluding the acidification due to the swallow of acid drinks (i.e., coke, lemonade, and orange juice). The second parameter selected is the total number of reflux episodes detected at MII. This parameter indicates how many times the esophageal mucosa is exposed to refluxate from the stomach independently from pH. Because PPI therapy is only able to switch reflux from acid to non-acid without modifying the total number of reflux episodes and because the patients with good esophageal clearance are more likely to have negative pH monitoring being more rapid to clean their esophagus, we believe that to find an abnormal number of reflux episodes in nonresponder patients is an indicator for antireflux surgery (Mainie et al, 2006a). This is consistent with our positive outcomes in the group of patients with negative pH monitoring and a positive total number of reflux episodes at MII (pH-MII+) and the fact that Nissen fundoplication protects against both acid and nonacid reflux (G. del Genio et al., 2008). The last parameter, the Symptom index correlation, helps to identify those patients suffering from a specific symptom. In the case of a repeated disabling symptom correlated to reflux, a patient may be offered the opportunity of surgery knowing the chance of solving it, as demonstrated by our positive clinical outcomes in the pH-MII- SI+ group. short-term follow-up and to the absence of a control group. Furthermore, to avoid interferences in pH monitoring, we prefer to perform all MII-pH exams after suspension of anti-acid therapy; this is a not widely accepted method. Moreover, because we use MII-pH to select patients for surgery, the type of reflux (acid vs. non-acid) is not crucial. It is more important to have real quantification of GERD.

Current gastroenterologic research investigating GERD is focused primarily on finding effective drugs for patients not responding to proton pump inhibitors. It is likely that a large portion of these patients are affected by transient lower esophageal sphincter relaxation, nonacid reflux episodes, or both. Currently, the most effective treatment for these patients is antireflux surgery. However, although the effects of fundoplication in eliminating acid reflux and preventing occurrences of transient lower esophageal sphincter relaxation had been reported, its role on nonacid reflux blocking had not been clarified.

Our postoperative data clearly demonstrate that the antireflux wrap acts as an effective functional barrier capable of protecting the esophageal mucosa from both the acid and nonacid GER events, and that this reduction was obtained in both the upright and recumbent positions. This complete protective effect is not surprising. Indeed, the Nissen procedure increases the distal esophageal sphincter pressure to a height three times the preoperative levels and restores the esophagogastric junction competence (Nissen, 1956; M. Rossetti & Hell, 1977). There is no reason to suspect that after the procedure for these patients the acid GER disappears (at pH monitoring) whereas the nonacid GER remains unchanged. This is consistent with the recent observation of Mainie and Castell on the potential worth of fundoplication for patients not responsive to a proton pump inhibitor with a MII-pH positive for nonacid GER (Mainie et al., 2006b).

Furthermore, the MII-pH was a well-tolerated procedure in both the pre- and postoperative settings but added more information than the traditional pH monitoring (e.g., nonacid reflux). Therefore, we suggest its routine use for selecting and following up the candidates for antireflux surgery.

If confirmed by more extensive evaluations, the data of this study may have important clinical implications. Because fundoplication can control also the nonacid reflux, the diagnostic role of MII-pH to identify the correct candidates for surgery is crucial. Indeed, a patient unresponsive to proton pump inhibitors with a pathologic number of nonacid reflux or a positive correlation of the symptoms with nonacid type GER events can be sent to surgery with an objective indication. For this reason, the mean preoperative DeMeester score may appear surprisingly low. Moreover, the data of this study highlight the fact that patients not responsive to medical treatment and with a diagnosis of nonacid GER at MII-pH need to be addressed with an antireflux procedure until new effective drugs become available.

Laparoscopic total fundoplication is currently accepted as the most effective surgical procedure in controlling gastroesophageal reflux disease. However, in the recent past many authors favored the use of a partial wrap especially for patients with defective peristalsis, as the result of a balanced option between the potential risk of postoperative dysphagia and the benefit of reflux control. Later on, partial antireflux procedures reported less favorable outcomes in assuring a good protection from reflux at long-term follow-up (Patti et al., 2004; Scheffer et al., 2004; Heider et al., 2001; Bessel et al., 2000).

Since early 1970s, our group sustained the idea that a correctly fashioned total fundoplication does not increase the risk of postoperative dysphagia. The technique included an extensive transhiatal esophageal mobilization to restore the LES into the abdomen; the preservation of the lesser omentum and short gastric vessels as important mechanisms of preventing the intratoracic migration, télescopage or rotation of the wrap; the routine use of intraoperative manometry and endoscopy to control of the function (i.e. calibration, length) and anatomy of the wrap (the passage through, height in respect of the cardias, and the correct geometry around the probe in reverse vision).

This feature in controlling reflux without increasing the dysphagia is because of the elastic feature of the anterior gastric wall (Nissen-Rossetti), which is able to dilate when the bolus passes through the wrap or to increase the pressure for Laplace's law when the gastric fundus is distended, preventing reflux after a meal (Code, 1968). A practical confirmation can be found in achalasic patients after extended myotomy, suggesting that the total fundoplication itself creates an adequate barrier without impairing the bolus also when the peristalsis is absent and a myotomy has abolished the lower esophageal sphincter pressure (G. Rossetti et al., 2005).

This assumption recently reported by postoperative clinical trials has been based only on postoperative clinical observation of patients with or without a defective peristalsis. We offer objective data to demonstrate that a total fundoplication acts as an effective functional barrier able to protect the esophageal mucosa from both the acid and non-acid events, without affecting the esophageal transit. This is possible because the postoperative restoration of the LES pressure preserves the mechanisms of LES relaxation, that is consistent with the postoperative data of unchanged peristaltic efficiency and amplitude above the wrap, and a preserved bolus transit time.

When checked by semi-solid deglutition, the percentage of complete bolus transit increased. This is not surprising; as previously described it is most probably the consequence of a reduced esophagitis after the antireflux procedure that facilitates itself a better functioning of the esophageal body.

This study did not investigate the esophageal function after a partial fundoplication and did not compare the impact of a total vs. partial wrap in impairing the transit of the bolus. However, because the total fundoplication is largely recognized to be superior in controlling

GERD, an unchanged transit progression of the bolus after the total fundoplication, associated to previous observations of good outcomes at long follow up in patients normal, defective, or absent peristalsis, support the choice of adopting the total fundoplication as a unique antireflux technique based on intention to treat choice. Appropriate preoperative investigation and a correct surgical technique are important in securing these results.

5. Conclusions

Laparoscopic total fundoplication achieved good outcomes and long-term patient satisfaction with few complications and side-effects.

Fundoplication controls both acid and nonacid GER as measured using MII-pH.

Appropriate preoperative investigation and a correct surgical technique are important in securing these results.

MII-pH provides useful information for an objective selection of patient candidates to antireflux surgery. Nissen fundoplication provides excellent outcomes in patients with positive pH and negative pH and positive MII monitoring or Symptom Index association. More extensive studies are needed to definitively standardize the useful MII-pH parameters to select the patient to antireflux surgery.

Total fundoplication acts as an effective functional barrier able to protect the esophageal mucosa from both the acid and non-acid events, without affecting the esophageal transit

6. References

Bessell JR, Finch R, Gotley DC, Smithers BM, Nathanson L, Menzies B. Chronic dysphagia following laparoscopic fundoplication. *Br J Surg* 2000; 87: 1341-1345.

Castell DO, Kahrilas PJ, Richter JE et al. Esomeprazole (40 mg) compared with lansoprazole (30 mg) in the treatment of erosive esophagitis. *Am J Gastroenterol* 2002; 97: 575-83

Charbel S, Khandawala F, Vaezi MF. The role oh esophageal ph monitoring in symptomatic patients on PPI theraphy. *Am J Gastroenterol* 2005; 100: 283-9

Code CF. Motor activity of the stomach. In Code CF. Handbook of Physiology, Washington 1968.

Del Genio A, Izzo G, Di Martino N, Maffettone V, Landolfi V, Martella A, Barbato D. Intraoperative esophageal manometry: our experience. *Dis Esophagus* 1997; 10: 253-261.

Del Genio G, Rossetti G, Brusciano L, Limongelli P, Pizza F, Tolone S, Fei L, Maffettone V, Napolitano V, del Genio A. Laparoscopic Nissen-Rossetti fundoplication with routine use of intraoperative endoscopy and manometry: technical aspects of a standardized technique. *World J Surg* 2007; 31: 1099-1106.

Del Genio G, Tolone S, del Genio F, Rossetti G, Brusciano L, Pizza F, Fei L, del Genio A. Total fundoplication controls acid and non acid reflux: evaluation by pre- and postoperative 24-hour pH-multichannel intraluminal impedance. *Surg Endosc* 2008; 22: 2518-2523.

Dodds WJ, Dent J, Hogan WJ, Helm JF, Hauser R, Patel GK, Egide MS. Mechanisms of gastroesophageal reflux in patients with reflux esophagitis. *N Engl J Med* 1982; 307: 1547-1552.

Fass J, Silny J, Braun J, et al. Measuring esophageal motilità with a new intraluminal impedance device. First clinical results in reflux patients. *Scand J Gastroenterol* 1994;29: 693–702.

Heider TR, Farrell TM, Kircher AP, Colliver CC, Koruda MJ, Behrns KE. Complete fundoplication is not associated with increased dysphagia in patients with abnormal esophageal motility. *J Gastrointest Surg* 2001; 5: 36-41.

Mainie I, Tutuian R, Agrawal A, Adams D, Castel DO. Combined multichannel intraluminal impedance-pH monitoring identifies patients with persistent reflux symptoms on acid suppressive theraphy who benefit from a lapatoscopic Nissen fundoplication. *Br J Surg* 2006; 93: 1483-87.

Mainie I, Tutuian R, Shay S, Vela M, Zhang X, Sifrim D, Castell DO Acid and non-acid reflux in patient with persistent symptoms despite acid suppressive therapy: a multicentre study using combined ambulatory impedance-pH monitoring. *Gut* 2006; 55: 1398-1402.

Nissen R. Eine einfuche Operation zur Beeinflussung der Refluxoesophagitis. *Schweiz Med Wochenschr* 1956; 86: 590-2.

Patti M, Robinson T, Galvani C, Gorodner MV, Fisichella PM, Way LW. Total fundoplication is superior to partial fundoplication even when esophageal peristalsis is weak. *J Am Coll Surg* 2004; 198: 863-870.

Rossetti G, Brusciano L, Amato G, Maffettone V, Napolitano V, Russo G, Izzo D, Russo F, Pizza F, Del Genio G, Del Genio A. A total fundoplication is not an obstacle to esophageal emptying after Heller myotomy for achalasia. Results at a long term follow-up. *Ann Surg* 2005; 241: 614-621.

Rossetti M, Hell K. Fundoplication for the treatment of gastroesophaeal reflux in hiatal hernia. *World J Surg* 1977; 1: 439-44.

Scheffer RCH, Samsom M, Frakking TG, Smout AJPM, Gooszen HG. Long-term effect of fundoplication on motility of the esophagus and esophagogastric junction. *Br J Surg* 2004; 91: 1466-1472.

Shaheen N, Ransohoff DF. Gastroesophageal reflux, Barrett esophagus and esophageal cancer: scientific review. *JAMA* 2002; 287: 1972-1981.

Sifrim D, Castel D, Dent J, Kahrilas PJ. Gastro-oesophageal reflux monitoring review and consensus report on detection and definitions of acid, non-acid, and gas-reflux. *Gut* 2004;53: 1024-31

Tutuian R, Vela MF, Shay SS, Castell DO. Multichannel intraluminal impedance in esophagel function testing and gastroesophageal reflux monitoring. *J Clin Gastroenterol* 2003; 37: 206-15.

Tutuian R, Vela M, Nagammapudur S, et al. Esophageal function testing with combined multichannel intraluminal impedance and manometry: Multicenter study in healthy volunteers. *Clin Gastroenterol Hepato*l 2003;1:174–82.

9

Quality of Life After Anti-Reflux Surgery in Adults

Mehmet Fatih Can, Aytekin Unlu and Gokhan Yagci
Department of Surgery, Division of Gastrointestinal Surgery, Gulhane School of Medicine, Ankara, Turkey

1. Introduction

Concepts of validity are of vital importance in the contemporary health care environment where outcome and Quality of Life (QoL) constructs are seen as relevant end points for evaluating the success of treatment and justifying continued intervention. QoL assessments, though sometimes subtle, have always played a central role in the therapeutic objectives of medicine. While the evaluation of surgical interventions focus primarily on outcomes, judgment regarding the success of the intervention should also take into account the functional, physiological, and social aspects of the disease and its treatment. Particularly, in chronic disease states, patients' QoL may be the most important parameter in assessing the efficacy of surgical treatment.

As in gastroesophageal reflux disease (GERD), most surgical operations target the correction of physiological or anatomical derangements that lead to a disease process. Hence anti-reflux operations are designed to prevent pathological amounts of gastric reflux that create typical (heartburn, regurgitation, dysphagia) and atypical (cough, hoarseness, chest pain, asthma and aspiration) symptoms and signs of damage (esophagitis and Barrett's epithelium). Reflux-related symptoms contribute substantially to patients' decreased QoL. Successful anti-reflux surgery should ameliorate these symptoms, arrest the progression of esophageal damage, and reinstitute lower esophageal sphincter (LES) function (24-h pH or impedance monitoring).

In the postoperative period, objective tests (esophageal manometry, endoscopy, pathological examination of esophageal mucosa, 24-h pH studies) that evaluate the fulfillment of surgery objectives may be needed. However, from the patients' standpoint, the results of these objective tests have little impact on their QoL, as they seek relief for heartburn or regurgitation. Thus, QoL will be improved to the extent that reflux-related symptoms are relieved and surgery-related new symptoms (bloating, difficulty in vomiting, dysphagia, etc.) are not acquired. In the postoperative period, patients should be able to sleep without head elevation, and be able to return to normal dietary routines with little or no need for acid suppression medications.

In order to assess QoL in upper gastrointestinal disease, questionnaires have been developed. The Gastrointestinal Symptom Rating Scale (GSRS), which concentrates on gastrointestinal symptoms (Länroth, 2000), the Psychological General Wellbeing index (PGWB), which gives a general measure of patients' well-being) (Länroth, 2000), and the Visual Analogue Scale (VAS) (Broeders et al., 2011; deBoer et al., 2004; Länroth, 2000; Nord, 1991) Visick grading system (Rijnhart deJong et al., 2008; Velanovich & Karmy-Jones, 1998; Visick, 1948; Zeman & Rózsa, 2005) GERD-Health Related Quality of Life (GERD-HRQL) (Velanovich, 1998), Short-Form 36 (SF-36), and gastrointestinal quality of life index (GIQLI) (Yano et al., 2009), have all been studied for QoL assessment. Questionnaires like GSRS and PGWB may be hard to validate and to apply to different populations, but they may have a role, particularly in prospective randomized studies. The visual analogue scale ranges from 0 (worst possible health status) to 100 and has been validated for QoL assessment after esophageal surgery (deBoer et al., 2004 & Nord, 1991). The Visick grading system is used to evaluate a patient's appreciation of anti-reflux surgery (Table 1 and Table 2). Visick scores correlate well with heartburn (Rijnhart deJong et al., 2008) and a validated questionnaire for reflux symptoms (Velanovich & Karmy-Jones, 1998 & Zeman & Rózsa, 2005). The SF-36 is one of the most frequently used generic tools, and measures eight domains of QoL; namely, physical functioning, role-emotional, level of perceived pain, vitality, mental health, social functioning, and general health. GERD-HRQL and SF-36 have been reported to be reliable, validated, responsive, and appropriate in the assessment of patients with GERD (Amato et al., 2008; Trus et al., 1999; Velanovich, 1998; Velanovich, 1999; Ware et al., 1993). The GIQLI was developed for measuring QoL, especially in patients with gastrointestinal disorders, and is well established and validated. It includes 36 items (the general response to GIQLI is graded from 0-144 points), and five sub-items: gastrointestinal symptoms, emotional status, physical functions, social functions, and stress by medical treatment. Scores for each sub-item are range between 0 and 4; higher scores reflect better QoL.

Grade I	No symptoms
Grade II	Mild symptoms, relieved by age
Grade IIIa	Symptoms relieved by care but patient satisfied with results
Grade IIIb	Symptoms not relieved by care and patient unhappy
Grade IV	No improvement

Table 1. Visick Classification of peptic ulcer surgical results

Grade I	No symptoms, perfect results
Grade II	Patient states that results are perfect, but symptoms can be elicited
Grade III	Mild to moderate symptoms, patient and surgeon satisfied with results
Grade IV	Mild to moderate symptoms, patient and surgeon dissatisfied

Table 2. Modified Visick Classification

2. Results of open fundoplication and follow up

In the pre-laparoscopy era, a large number of clinical reports were published about consecutive patients who were operated on by open fundoplication techniques.

In one study, the authors (Polk & Zeppa, 1971) reported that 994 patients underwent open fundoplication and were followed-up with for 2.5 years postoperatively. Patients had 96% good results symptomatically.

In another study of open surgery, the authors (Bushkin et al., 1977) treated 165 patients with reflux esophagitis by Nissen fundoplication with an average follow-up period of 4 years, during which time 92% of patients remained free of reflux- related symptoms. The prevalence of gas bloat syndrome, which decreased surgery-related patient satisfaction, was 13% in the early postoperative period. However, this symptom either disappeared or was clinically insignificant in 87% of patients during the follow-up period. The authors concluded that Nissen fundoplication was so initially successful that late occurrence symptoms appeared to be uncommon.

Rossetti and colleagues (Rossetti & Heill, 1977) reported long-term results of fundoplication for the treatment of GERD in hiatal hernia in 590 patients, and showed that 87.5% of patients were symptom-free. In 44 patients with complicated GERD, fundoplication produced clinical healing in 84.1% of patients.

In a study in which 100 consecutive patients were treated with Nissen Fundoplication for GERD (DeMeester et al., 1986), of 89 of patients with complete data, 11 cited heartburn and aspiration as their primary symptoms. Data analysis revealed that fundoplication was successful in 91% of patients in controlling reflux symptoms over a 10-year period. The incidence of postoperative gas bloat and increased flatus was lower in patients with preoperative abnormal distal esophageal manometry. The authors thus concluded that Nissen fundoplication can re-establish a competent cardia and control reflux symptoms with minimal side effects.

3. Laparoscopic anti-reflux operations

The long-term results of conventional anti-reflux surgery have been very successful at attaining the desired goal of diminishing reflux-related symptoms (Bushkin et al., 1977; DeMeester et al., 1986; Polk & Zeppa, 1971; Rossetti & Heill, 1977). This proven success stimulated the application of laparoscopic techniques. In 1991, Dallemagne described and reported the results of laparoscopic Nissen fundoplication (Dallemagne et al., 1991). Since then, several studies have demonstrated the safety and efficacy of laparoscopic fundoplication (Hallerbäck et al., 1994; Hinder et al., 1994; Hunter et al., 1996; Jamieson et al., 1994; Watson et al., 1996) (Table 3).

Authors	No. of patients	Follow up (months)	Improvement in reflux related symptoms (%)
Watson (1996)	320	3-24	91
Hunter (1996)	300	12-36	97
Hallerbäck (1995)	142	12	90
Hinder ((1994)	198	6-32	>90
Jamieson (1994)	137	>3	97

Table 3. Reported results of laparoscopic fundoplication

A prospective randomized controlled study comparing laparoscopic and open fundoplication was published by Laine and colleagues in 1997 (Laine et al., 1997). Of the 110 patients enrolled in the study, 55 were randomized to laparoscopic and 55 to open Nissen fundoplication groups. Postoperative recovery, complications, and outcomes at the 3 and 12 month follow-up were compared in the two groups. In both groups, the most common complaints three months after surgery was dysphagia and gas bloating which disappeared by the 12 month follow-up examination. The authors reported that all patients in the laparoscopy group, and 86% of patients in the open group were satisfied with the results (Table 4).

Symptoms	Open	Laparoscopic
No symptoms	70	83
Bloating	7	17
Heartburn	7	0
Dysphagia	13	0
Upper abdominal pain	3	0

Table 4. Postoperative symptoms at 12 month follow up exam.

Since a symptom is a perception derived from various sources, including psychosomatic factors, objective tests may inadequately assess patients' well-being in the postoperative period (Länroth, 2000). This theory is supported by the findings obtained from a study (Kamolz & Pointner, 2002). The authors evaluated the expectations of 70 patients with GERD awaiting laparoscopic anti-reflux surgery. Only two patients stated that they would expect normalization of pH values and healing of esophagitis. The rest of the patients had expectations related to their QoL. Hence, QoL assessment should essentially be implemented in order to evaluate a patient's postoperative satisfaction level. In 1995, Swedish authors Glise and colleagues presented QoL assessments for the first 40 consecutive patients undergoing laparoscopic Rossetti fundoplication (Glise et al., 1995). They used PGWB and GSRS questionnaires 3 months and 8-12 months after operation, and concluded that patients had good QoL scores postoperatively, thus showing that QoL ratings can be used to assess laparoscopic anti-reflux operations. The results also showed that laparoscopic fundoplication was better than no treatment and as good as optimal medical treatment.

In the last two decades, laparoscopic anti-reflux surgery has been shown to improve the QoL in patients with GERD (Bloomston et al., 2003; Broeders et al., 2010a & 2011; Dallemagne et al., 2006; Draisma et al., 2006a & 2006b; Fein et al., 2008; Fernando et al., 2002 & 2003; Gee et al., 2008; Gilliesa et al., 2008; Kamolz et al., 2003 & 2005; Morino et al., 2006; Papasevas et al., 2003; Pessaux et al., 2005; Ravi et al., 2005; Rosenthal et al., 2006). In addition to general QoL assessments, several authors also used QoL measurements to compare the effectiveness of different anti-reflux procedures. For example, Draisma and colleagues (Draisma et al., 2006a) randomized 177 patients with GERD into groups undergoing either laparoscopic (LNF) or conventional Nissen fundoplication (CNF). The authors found no difference in overall patient satisfaction rates, which were 88% and 90%, respectively, and concluded that both procedures were equally effective in achieving successful objective and subjective results (Table 5).

Although the Nissen procedure produces excellent reflux-related symptom control, it may be associated with a high postoperative dysphagia rate and specific side-effects such as the inability to belch and vomit, and gas bloat syndrome. The Toupet procedure is thought to produce less postoperative side-effects than the Nissen procedure (Broeders et al., 2010b) (Figure 1), but the recurrence rate of reflux symptoms may be higher after this procedure, though not every author agrees with this. In two study (Radajewski et al., 2009 & Sgromo et al., 2008), a comparison of QoL outcomes was made between Nissen and Toupet fundoplication. The authors concluded that QoL scores, overall symptom improvement, and patient satisfaction were equivalent.

		LNF (n = 79)	CNF (n = 69)	Redo Surgery (n = 20)†
	General QoL (Mean VAS score 0-100)	67.1 (2.8)	60.5 (3.2)	63.3 (7.0)
	Increase in general QOL (% of preoperative)	27.3%	28.6%	41.9%
Self rated change in reflux symptoms vs preoperative state	Resolved (n)	39	31	7
	Improved (n)	36	30	11
	Unchanged (n)	3	3	2
	Worsened (n)	1	5	0
	Satisfied with outcome [n(%)]	69 (87.3%)	62 (89.9%)	16 (80%)

Table 5. Subjective outcome after LNF and CNF at 5 years after surgery. (Draisma et al., 2006a). LNF: Laparoscopic Nissen Fundoplication, CNF: Conventional Nissen Fundoplication. † Including 1 patient with cicatricial hernia correction.

A common cause of Nissen procedure failure is thoracic herniation of the fundoplication. This is particularly more common when the esophagus is short, or the esophagus is inadequately mobilized. Esophageal shortening is a complication of advanced GERD, but is also common in patients with esophageal stricture, paraesophageal hernia, dysphagia, and Barrett's esophagus. A short esophagus is usually confirmed intraoperatively, whereas only 20% of preoperative diagnosis of short esophagus is confirmed intraoperatively. Collis gastroplasty combined with fundoplication may be a good alternative in patients with advanced GERD. In a study in which the researchers compared laparoscopic Nissen Fundoplication plus Collis gastroplasty with Nissen fundoplication alone (Youssef et al., 2006), improvement of QoL in the postoperative period was comparable to that observed with Nissen fundoplication alone. The authors concluded that Collis gastroplasty combined with Nissen fundoplication provided excellent relief of reflux-related symptoms.

Several studies have shown the safety and feasibility of robot assisted anti-reflux surgery. Two randomized controlled trials (Draisma et al., 2006b & Morino et al., 2006) compared robot assisted versus laparoscopic Nissen fundoplication, and found comparable outcomes; however, costs were higher due to longer operation times and the use of more expensive instruments.

As older patients have a greater incidence of co-morbid diseases, gastroenterologists are often reluctant to refer these patients to surgery due to concerns about increased operative risks. This is partly due to the fact that medical therapy with proton pump inhibitors (PPIs) seem to provide a 93% symptom remission (Lundell et al., 2008), and studies that show both medical and surgical treatments are highly effective, safe and well tolerated (Mahon et al., 2005; Ortiz et al., 1996; Parrilla et al., 2003; Spechler, 1992; Spechler et al., 2001) and improve

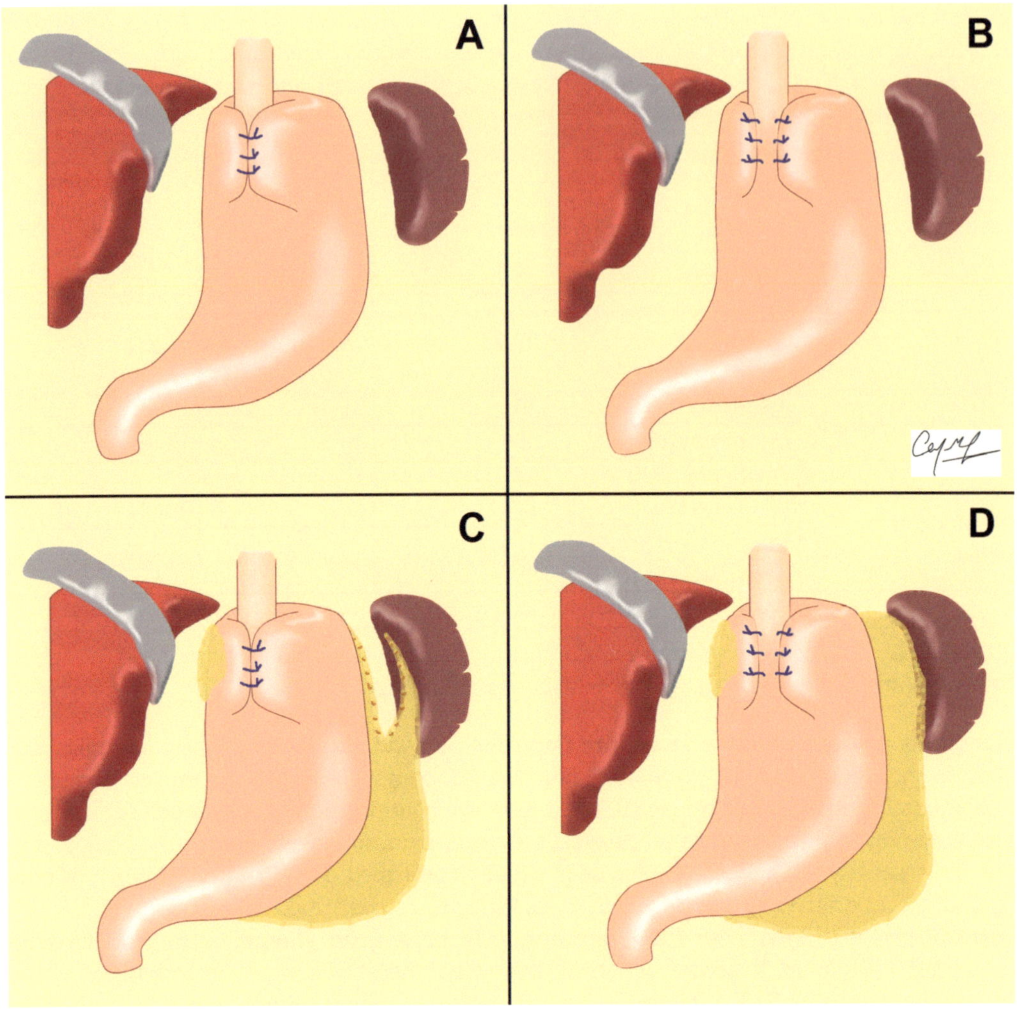

Fig. 1. Illustrated are common kinds of anti-reflux procedures. A: Nissen fundoplication (360 degree fundic wrap), B: Toupet fundoplication (270 degree posterior fundic wrap), C: Nissen fundoplication (short gastric vessels divided), D: Nissen-Rossetti fundoplication (short gastric vessels preserved)

QoL of GERD patients. Gillies and colleagues (Gillies et al., 2008) showed that laparoscopic anti-reflux surgery also improved the QoL of patients whose symptoms were well controlled on medical therapy. In two studies (Fernando et al., 2003 & Wang et al., 2008) in which the investigators compared the outcomes between young and elderly patients who underwent laparoscopic fundoplication, outcomes were similar and QoL scores improved significantly among adult and old patients, despite differences in co-morbid diseases. The authors concluded that laparoscopic fundoplication should be considered as a therapeutic option for older patients with reflux. Paraesophageal hernias are frequently seen in elderly patients, and troublesome heartburn and regurgitation may be present in 23-59% of these patients in addition to obstructive symptoms. Laparoscopic Nissen fundoplication has been found to be equally effective as anti-reflux procedures in both GERD and paraesophageal hernia patients. However, the improvement in QoL is less in these patients due to age-related co-morbidities (Mark et al., 2008).

The choice of surgical procedure (a partial or total-360° fundic wrap) in patients with reflux-related esophageal dismotility is controversial. Theoretically, an 360° wrap may increase the risk of postoperative dysphagia when compared to a partial wrap which decreases the risk of dysphagia, but has a higher likelihood of treatment failure (Baigrie et al., 1997 & Lundell et al., 1996). Reflux-related esophageal disturbances may be improved after successful anti-reflux surgery, possibly due to a compensatory mechanism which overcomes the increased resistance created by fundoplication (Heider et al., 2003 & Scheffer et al., 2004). Ravi and co-workers compared 60 normal esophageal motility patients with 38 esophageal dismotility patients undergoing laparoscopic Nissen fundoplication (Ravi et al., 2005). Esophageal wave amplitude increased in both groups, and 20 patients (53%) in the dismotility group reverted to normal motility after surgery. In the postoperative period, 88% of patients with normal motility, and 89% of patients with dismotility had no symptoms or minor symptoms, with a significant improvement in quality of life six months after surgery. The authors concluded that preoperative dismotility is not a contraindication for total fundoplication. Total fundoplication may cause dysphagia, gas bloat, and inability to belch as a result of increased resistance at the newly created lower esophageal sphincter function. Some measures have been proposed to prevent these surgery-related complications such as mobilization of the gastric fundus by complete division of short gastric vessels to create a floppy wrap. In a randomized study it was found that both dividing and preserving the short gastric vessels provided long term reflux control with no differences in QoL between the two approaches (Mardani et al., 2009).

GERD can be subdivided into erosive (ERD) and non-erosive reflux disease (NERD) depending upon endoscopy findings. Decreased QoL and symptom severity is similar in both ERD and NERD. However, lower response rates to PPI treatment and higher relapse rates have also been reported for patients with NERD. In a study, the authors compared subjective and objective outcomes of Nissen fundoplication in ERD and NERD patients operated on for PPI refractory disease (Broeders et al., 2011). Heartburn, regurgitation, and dysphagia grades were similar postoperatively at the five year follow-up. Moreover, 89% of NERD patients and 96% of ERD patients reported their reflux symptoms as being resolved or improved (Visick score I or II). There was no difference in QoL between the two groups during the follow-up period. Similar results were reported in another study (Kamolz et al., 2005), however QoL improvement was significantly better in the NERD group because the preoperative QoL score (GIQLI) was worse. The authors concluded that laparoscopic surgery is an excellent treatment option for NERD patients. There is not much evidence about the impact of Barrett's esophagus (BE) on the QoL of patients with GERD. BE is frequently associated with severe reflux disease. Kamolz and colleagues (Kamolz et al., 2003) showed that non-BE patients achieved better QoL than those with BE after laparoscopic anti-reflux surgery, and thus concluded that the surgical procedure improved the QoL significantly in all GERD patients with or without BE.

4. Conclusion

Quality of life assessments have a central role in obtaining rapid communication of surgical outcomes. The aforementioned studies and QoL assessments, in addition to ongoing efforts, have provided valuable data for the surgical treatment of GERD. Laparoscopic and open anti-reflux surgery effectively controls disease-related symptoms and significantly improves QoL. However, co-morbid psychiatric disorders, dyspepsia, or aerophagia usually complicate QoL assessments despite appropriate surgical therapies. Furthermore, the presence of numerous QoL tools hinders the easy interpretation and comparison of results. The SF-36 is possibly the most frequently used generic QoL instrument. However, there is still no consensus on clearcut changes on scores representing clinical significance. On the other hand, QoL studies in the postoperative period indicate that anti-reflux surgery, especially laparoscopic Nissen fundoplication, is effective in routine clinical practice.

5. References

Amato G, Limongelli P, Pascariello A & Rossetti G. (2008). Association between persistent symptom and long term quality of life after laparoscopic total fundoplication. *The American Journal of Surgery*, Vol 196, No.4, 582-6.

Baigrie RJ, Watson DI, Myers JC & Jamieson GG. (1997). Outcome of laparoscopic Nissen fundoplication in patients with disordered preoperative peristalsis. *Gut*, Vol.40, No.3, 381-5.

Bloomston M, Nields W & Rosemurg AS. (2003). Symptoms and Antireflu Medication Use Following Laparoscopic Nissen Fundoplication:Outcome at 1 and 4 years. *JSLS* Vol.7, 211-8.

Broeders JA, Draaisma WA, Bredenoord AJ, Smout AJ, Broeders IA & Gooszen HG. (2010). Long-term outcome of Nissen fundoplication in non-erosive and erosive gastro-oesophageal reflux disease. *British Journal of Surgery*; Vol.97, 845–52.

Broeders JA, Mauritz FA, Ahmed Ali U, Draaisma WA, Ruurda JP, Gooszen HG, Smout AJ, Broeders IA & Hazebroek EJ. (2010). Systematic review and meta-analysis of laparoscopic Nissen (posterior total) versus Toupet (posterior partial) fundoplication for gastro-oesophageal reflux disease. *British Journal of Surgery*; Vol.97, No.9, 1318-30.

Broeders JA, Draisma WA, Bredenoord AJ & Smour A.J. (2011). Impact of symptom-reflux association analysis on long term outcome after Nissen fundoplication. *British Journal of Surgery*; Vol.98, 247-54.

Bushkin FL, Neustein CL, Parker TH & Woodward ER. (1977). Nissen fundoplication for reflux peptic esophagitis. *Annals of Surgery*, Vol.185, 672-7.

Dallemagne B, Weerts JM, Jehaes C, Markiewicz S & Lombard R. (1991) Laparoscopic Nissen fundoplication: preliminary report. *Surgical Laparoscopy & Endoscopy*, Vol.1, No.3, 138-43.

Dallemagne B, Weerts J, Markiewicz S, Dewandre JM, Wahlen C, Monami B & Jehaes MC. (2006). Clinical results of laparoscopic fundoplication at ten years after surgery. *Surgical Endoscopy*, Vol.20, 159–65.

deBoer AGEM, vanLanschot JJB, Stalmeier PFM, vonSandick JW & Hulscher BF. (2004). Is a single item visual analogue scale as valid, reliable and responsive as multi-item scales in measuring quality of life? *Quality of Life Research*, Vol.13, 311-20.

DeMeester TR, Bonavina L & Albertucci M. (1986). Nissen fundoplication for gastroesophageal reflux disease: Evaluation of primary repair in 100 consecutive patients. *Annals of Surgery*, Vol.204, 9-20.

Draisma WA, Rijnhart- de Jong HG, Broeders AMJ, Smout A, Furnee E & Gooszen HG. (2006). Five-Year Subjective and Objective Results of Laparoscopic and Conventional Nissen Fundoplication A Randomized Trial. *Annals of Surgery*, Vol.244, 34–41.

Draisma WA, Ruurda JP, Scheffer RCH, Simmermacher RKJ, Gooszen HG, Rijnhart-de Jong, Buskens E, Broeders IA. (2006). Randomized clinical trial of standard laparoscopic versus robot-assisted laparoscopic Nissen fundoplication for gastro-oesophageal reflux disease. *British Journal of Surgery*, Vol.93, No.11, 1351–9.

Fein M, Bueter M, Thalheimer A, Pachmayr V, Heimbucher J, Freys SM & Fuchs KH. (2008). Ten-year Outcome of Laparoscopic Antireflux Surgery. *Journal of Gastrointestinal Surgery*, Vol.12, 1893–9.

Fernando HC, Schauer PR, Rosenblatt M & Wald A. (2002). Quality of Life after Antireflux Surgery compared with Nonoperative management for severe GERD. *Journal of the American College of Surgeons*, Vol.194, No.1, 23-7.

Fernando HC, Schauer PR, Buenaventura PO, Christie NA & Clesa JM. (2003). Outcomes of Minimally Invasive Antireflux Operations in the Elderly: A comparative Review. *JSLS* Vol.7, 311-5.

Gee DW, Andreoli MT & Rattner DW. (2008). Measuring the Effectiveness of Laparoscopic Antireflux Surgery. *Archives of Surgery*, Vol.143, No.5, 482-7.

Gillies RS, Stratford JM., Booth MI & Dehn TC. (2008). Does laparoscopic antireflux surgery improve quality of life in patients whose gastro-oesophageal reflux disease is well controlled with medical therapy? *European Journal of Gastroenterology & Hepatology*, Vol.20, No.5, 430-5.

Glise H, Hallenbäck B & Johansson B. (1995). Quality of life assessments in evaluation of laparoscopic Rossetti fundoplication. *Surgical Endoscopy*, Vol.9, 183-9.

Hallerbäck B, Glise H, Johansson B & Rädmark T. (1994) Laparoscopic Rossetti fundoplication. *Surgical Endoscopy*, Vol.8, 1417-22.

Heider TR, Behrns KE, Koruda MJ, Shaheen NJ, Lucktong TA, Bradshaw B & Farrell TM. (2003). Fundoplication improves disordered Esophageal motility. *Journal of Gastrointestinal Surgery*, Vol.7, 159–63.

Hinder RA, Filipi CJ, Wetscher G, Neary P, DeMeester TR & Perdikis G. (1994). Laparoscopic Nissen fundoplication is an effective treatment for gastroesophageal reflux disease. *Annals of Surgery*, Vol.220, 472-81.

Hunter JG, Trus TL, Branum GD, Waring JP & Wood WC. (1996). A physiologic approach to laparoscopic fundoplication for gastroesophageal reflux disease. *Annals of Surgery*, Vol.223, 673-85.

Jamieson GG, Watson DI, Jones RB & Mitchell PC. Laparoscopic Nissen fundoplication. (1994). *Annals of Surgery*, Vol.220, 137-45.

Kamolz T & Pointner R. (2002). Expectations of patients with GERD for the outcome of laparoscopic antireflux surgery. *Surgical Laparoscopic & Endoscopic Percutaneous Techniques*, Vol.12, No.6, 389-92.

Kamolz T, Granderath F & Pointner R. (2003). Laparoscopic antireflux surgery: Disease-related quality of life assessment before and after surgery in GERD patients with and without Barret's esophagus. *Surgical Endoscopy*, Vol.17, 880-5.

Kamolz T, Granderath FA, Schweiger UM & Pointner R. (2005). Laparoscopic Nissen fundoplication in patients with nonerosive reflux disease: Long-term quality-of-life assessment and surgical outcome. *Surgical Endoscopy*, Vol.19, 494–500.

Laine S, Rantala A, Gullichsen R & Ovaska J. (1997). Laparoscopic versus conventional Nissen fundoplication: A prospective randopmized study. *Surgical Endoscopy*, Vol.11, 440-4.

Länroth H. (2000). Efficiancy of, and quality of life after antireflux surgery. *European Journal of Surgery*, suppl. Vol.585, 34-6.

Mahon D, Rhodes M, Decadt B, Hindmarsh A, Lowndes R, Beckingham I, Koo B & Newcombe RG. (2005). Randomized clinical trial of laparoscopic Nissen fundoplication compared with proton-pump inhibitors for treatment of chronic gastro-oesophageal reflux. *British Journal of Surgery*, Vol.92, 695-9.

Mardani J, Lundell, H. Lőnroth, Dalenback J & Engstrom C. (2009). Ten-year results of a randomized clinical trial of laparoscopic total fundoplication with or without division of the short gastric vessels. *British Journal of Surgery*; Vol.96, 61–5.

Mark LA, Okrainec A, Ferri LE, Feldman LS, Mayrand S & Fried GM. (2008). Comparison of patient-centered outcomes after laparoscopic Nissen fundoplication for gastroesophageal reflux disease or paraesophageal hernia. *Surgical Endoscopy*, Vol.22, 343–7.

Morino M, Pellegrino L, Giaccone C, Garrone C & Rebecchi F. (2006) Randomized clinical trial of robot-assisted versus laparoscopic Nissen fundoplication. *British Journal of Surgery*, Vol.93, 553–8.

Lundell L, Abrahamsson H, Ruth M, Rydberg L, Lönroth H, Olbe L. (1996). Long-term results of a prospective randomised comparison of total fundic wrap (Nissen-Rossetti) or semifundoplication (Toupet) for gastro-oesophageal reflux. *British Journal of Surgery*, Vol.83, 830-5.

Lundell L, Attwood S, Ell C, Fiocca R, Galmiche JP , Hatlebakk J, Lind T & Junghard O. (2008). Comparing laparoscopic antireflux surgery with esomeprazole in the management of patients with chronic gastro-oesophageal reflux disease: a 3-year interim analysis of the LOTUS trial. *Gut*, Vol.57, 1207–13.

Nord E. (1991). The validity of visual analogue scale in determining social utility weights for health states. *International Journal of Health Planning and Management*, Vol.6, 234-42.

Ortiz A, Martinez de Haro LF, Parrilla P, Morales G, Molina J, Bermejo J, Liron R & Aguilar J. (1996). Conservative treatment versus antireflux surgery in Barrett's oesophagus: long-term results of a prospective study. *British Journal of Surgery*, Vol.83, 274-8.

Papasevas PK, Keenan RS, Yeaney WW, Caushay PF, Gagne DS & Landreneau RJ. (2003). Effectiveness of Laparoscopic fundoplication in relieving the symptoms of GERD and eliminating antireflux surgery. *Surgical Endoscopy*, Vol.17, 1200-5.

Parrilla P, Martínez de Haro LF, Ortiz A, Munitiz V, Molina J, Bermejo J & Canteras M. (2003). Long-term results of a randomized prospective study comparing medical and surgical treatment of Barrett's esophagus. *Annals of Surgery*, Vol.237, 291-8.

Pessaux P, Arnaud JP, Delattre JF, Meyer C, Baulieo J & Mosnier H. (2005). Laparoscopic Antireflux Surgery. Five Year Results and Beyond in 1340 Patients. *Archives of Surgery*, Vol.140, 946-51.

Polk HC & Zeppa R. (1971). Hiatal hernia and esophagitis: A survey of indications for operation and technique and results of fundoplication. *Annals of Surgery*, Vol.173, 775-81.

Radajewski R, Hazebroek EJ, Berry H, Leibman S & Smith GS. (2009). Short-term symptom and quality-of-life comparison between laparoscopic Nissen and Toupet fundoplications. *Diseases of the Esophagus*, Vol.22, 84–8.

Ravi N, Al-Sarraf N, Moran T, O'Riordan J, Rowley S, Byrne PJ, Reynolds JV. (2005). Acid normalization and improved esophageal motility after Nissen fundoplication: equivalent outcomes in patients with normal and ineffective esophageal motility. *The American Journal of Surgery*, Vol.190, 445–50.

Rijnhart deJong HG, Draisma WA, Smout AJ, Broeders IA & Gooszen HG. (2008). The Visick Score: a good measure for the overall effect of antireflux surgery? *Scandinavian Journal of Gastroenterology*, Vol.43, 787-93.

Rosenthal R, Peterli R, Guenin MO, von Flüe M & Ackermann C. (2006). Laparoscopic antireflux surgery: Long-term outcomes and quality of life. *Journal of Laparoendoscopic & Advanced Surgical Techniques*, Vol.16, No.6, 557-61.

Rossetti N & Heill K. (1977). Fundoplication for treatment of gastroesophageal reflux in hiatal hernia. *World Journal of Surgery*, Vol.1, 439-43.

Scheffer RC, Samsom M, Frakking TG, Smout AJ & Gooszen HG. (2004). Long-term effect of fundoplication on motility of the oesophagus and oesophagogastric junction. *British Journal of Surgery*, Vol.91, 1466–72.

Sgromo B , Irvine LA, Cuschieri A & Shimi SM. (2008). Long-term comparative outcome between laparoscopic total Nissen and Toupet fundoplication: Symptomatic relief, patient satisfaction and quality of life. *Surgical Endoscopy*, Vol.22, 1048–53.

Spechler SJ. (1992). Comparison of medical and surgical therapy for complicated gastroesophageal reflux disease in veterans. *New England Journal of Medicine*, Vol.326, 786–9.

Spechler SJ, Lee E, Ahnen D, Goyal RK, Hirano I, Ramirez F, Raufman JP, Sampliner R, Schnell T, Sontag S, Vlahcevic ZR, Young R, Williford W. (2001). Long-term outcome of medical and surgical therapies for gastroesophageal reflux disease: follow-up of a randomized controlled trial. *JAMA*, Vol.285, 2331-8.

Trus TL, Laycock WS & Branum GD. (1999). Improvement in quality of life measures after laparoscopic antireflux surgery. *Annals of Surgery*, Vol.229, No.3, 331-6.

Visick AH. (1948). A study of the failures after gastrectomy. *Annals of the Royal College of Surgeons of England*, Vol.3, 266-84.

Velanovich V & Karmy-Jones R. (1998). Measuring gastroesophageal reflux disease: relationships between the Health-Related Quality of Life Score and physiologic parameters. *American Surgeon*, Vol.64, 649-53.

Velanovich V. (1998). Comparison of SF-36 vs a disease specific (GERD-HRQL) quality of life scales for GERD. *Journal of Gastrointestinal Surgery*, Vol.2, 141-5.

Velanovich V. (1999). Comparison of symptomatic and quality of life outcomes of laparoscopic versus open antireflux surgery. *Surgery*, Vol.12 782-8.

Wang W, Huang M, Wei P & Lee W. (2008). Laparoscopic antireflux surgery for the elderly: A surgical and quality-of life study. *Surgery Today*, Vol.38, 305–10.

Watson DI, Jamieson GG, Baigrie RS, Matthew G, Devitt PG & Game PA. (1996). Laparoscopic surgery for gastroesophageal reflux: beyond the learning curve. *British Journal of Surgery*, Vol.83, 1284-7.

Ware JE, Snow KK, Kosinski M & Gandek B. (1993). *SF-36 Health Survey: Manual and Interpretation Guide*. Health Institute, New England Medical Center. ISBN: 1891810065. Boston, USA.

Yano F, Sherif AE, Turaga K, Stadlhuber RJ, Tsuboi K, Ramaswamy S & Mittal SK. (2009). Gastrointestinal quality of life in patients after anti reflux surgery. *Diseases of the Esophagus*, Vol.;22, No.2, 177-84.

Youssef YK, Shekar N, Lutfi R, Richards WO & Torquati A. (2006). Long-term evaluation of patient satisfaction and reflux symptoms after laparoscopic fundoplication with Collis gastroplasty. *Surgical Endoscopy*, Vol.20, 1702–5.

Zeman Z & Rózsa S. (2005). Pschometric documentation of quality of life questionnaire for patients undergoing antireflux surgery (QOLARS). *Surgical Endoscopy*, Vol.19, 257-61.